# Hemodiafiltration – A New Era

# Contributions to Nephrology

## Vol. 168

Series Editor

Claudio Ronco Vicenza

# Hemodiafiltration – A New Era

Volume Editors

Hideki Kawanishi Hiroshima

Akihiro C. Yamashita Fujisawa

59 figures, 7 in color, and 21 tables, 2011

KARGER Basel · Freiburg · Paris · London · New York · Bangalore · Bangkok · Shanghai · Singapore · Tokyo · Sydney

**Contributions to Nephrology**
(Founded 1975 by Geoffrey M. Berlyne)

**Hideki Kawanishi**
Tsuchiya General Hospital
3-30 Nakajima-cho, Naka-ku
Hiroshima 730-8655
Japan

**Akihiro C. Yamashita**
Department of Human and Environmental Science
Shonan Institute of Technology
1-1-25 Tsujido-Nishikaigan
Fujisawa, Kanagawa 251-8511
Japan

Library of Congress Cataloging-in-Publication Data

Hemodiafiltration : a new era / volume editors, Hideki Kawanishi, Akihiro C. Yamashita.
p. ; cm. -- (Contributions to nephrology, ISSN 0302-5144 ; v. 168)
Includes bibliographical references and indexes.
ISBN 978-3-8055-9560-5 (hard cover : alk. paper) -- ISBN 978-3-8055-9561-2 (e-ISBN)
1. Hemodialysis. 2. Blood--Filtration. I. Kawanishi, Hideki. II. Yamashita, Akihiro C. III. Series: Contributions to nephrology ; v. 168. 0302-5144
[DNLM: 1. Hemodiafiltration--methods. 2. Hemodiafiltration--instrumentation. 3. Online Systems. W1 CO778UN v.168 2011 / WJ 378]
RC901.7.H446H46 2011
617.4'61059--dc22

2010033888

Bibliographic Indices. This publication is listed in bibliographic services, including Current Contents® and Index Medicus.


www.karger.com
Printed in Switzerland on acid-free and non-aging paper (ISO 9706) by Reinhardt Druck, Basel
ISSN 0302–5144
ISBN 978–3–8055–9560–5
e-ISBN 978–3–8055–9561–2

# Contents

# Preface

In Japan, the history of online hemodiafiltration (HDF) began in 1982 when it was first performed. However, its use has become widespread since 1990 following the development of an online HDF built-in central dialysis fluid delivery system. The Japanese Society for Hemodiafiltration (JSHDF) was established in 1995. Recently, a JSHDF meeting was held jointly with the Korean Society for Hemodiafiltration, and many clinicians from Asian countries participated.

The 55th Annual Meeting of the Japanese Society for Dialysis Therapy (55th JSDT) was held in Kobe, Japan, June 19–20, 2010, with over 16,000 participants. Both technological and clinical aspects of dialysis therapy for ESRD patients were discussed at the meeting. Two international symposia on HDF of the 55th JSDT were carried out with the titles *'Clinical aspects of HDF – Who to apply HDF?'* and *'Technical aspects of HDF – How to apply HDF?'* following the keynote lecture by Dr. Francesco Locatelli. The authors of this new book are either the speakers of these international symposia or key members of the JSHDF.

Currently the most commonly used dialyzers in Japanese hospitals are so-called 'super' high-flux dialyzers. In Japan, the definition super high-flux membrane dialyzer refers to a clearance of $\beta_2$-microglobulin ≥50 ml/min under a blood flow rate of 200 ml/min and a dialysis fluid flow rate of 500 ml/min. The present share of the market of such dialyzers is over 90%. The main focus of this book is the clinical importance of online HDF that has been re-evaluated on the commonly prescribed conditions with super high-flux membrane dialyzers. Moreover, although HDF has been carried out throughout the world, its clinical benefit has not yet been confirmed sufficiently enough. Therefore, evaluations of the clinical benefits of HDF are another focus as well as new technological developments.

In memory of the late Dr. Kazuo Ota, who served as the first President of the Japanese Society of Hemodiafiltration (1995–2009).

We would like to thank the authors and all the contributors for the enormous effort and the quality of their scientific chapters. We would also like to thank all those who made this publication possible and Karger Publishers for the outstanding editorial assistance.

*Hideki Kawanishi,* Hiroshima, Japan
*Akihiro C. Yamashita,* Fujisawa, Japan

Kawanishi H, Yamashita AC (eds): Hemodiafiltration – A New Era.
Contrib Nephrol. Basel, Karger, 2011, vol 168, pp 1–4

# Dawn of Hemodiafiltration

Kazuo Ota

Tokyo Women's Medical University, Tokyo, Japan

**Abstract**

A brief history of hemodialysis, hemofiltration and hemodiafiltration (HDF) is reviewed with special interest on the development of HDF, including development of dialysis/ultrafiltration membranes, ultrafiltration rate controllers, dialysis fluid delivery systems, and guidelines for water quality required for online HDF treatment.



Needless to say, kidneys purify the blood on the principle of ultrafiltration or hemofiltration (HF). At the beginning of the 20th century, however, there was no such artificial membrane to realize this kind of HF. The history of blood purification therefore started with hemodialysis (HD). The following is a brief history of blood purification, with special interest on the development of hemodiafiltration (HDF) therapy.

## First 60 Years (1914 – Early 1970s)

It is well known that HD was started by Abel et al. [1] who used a collodion tube for their animal experiment in 1913. Later in the 1930s, cellulosic membrane became available and anticoagulant heparin was being refined. In 1945, Kolff [2] succeeded in saving a patient with his rotating-drum artificial kidney.

On the other hand, the history of HF began in the year 1947, the time when Alwall [3] succeeded in removing excess water through cellulosic membrane only applying negative pressure. And the first clinical trial was done by Inoh et al. [4], who developed a DL-II type artificial kidney in 1958. Utilizing 'dog lungs' as membrane, they succeeded in saving patients. The procedure was as follows: first, dog lungs with a bronchial tube were removed and the blood was washed off with dextrin, and so forth. An arterial line was then made between the lung's artery and the patient's artery so that there was a venous line between the lung's vein and patient's vein. Then, through an arterial line, the patient's prediluted blood was sent to the lungs where excess water was removed by negative pressure through the bronchial tube, and the blood was returned to the patient's body through a venous line.

In 1967, Henderson et al. [5, 6] performed an HF experiment with an animal using polysulfone membrane; they undertook the first clinical trial in 1971. In the following year, Kobayashi et al. [7] proposed a new method and termed it the 'extracorporeal ultrafiltration method'. Using a Kiil dialyzer with neither dialysis fluid nor substitution fluid, they removed excess water from a patient's body only by ultrafiltration.

## Middle Molecule Hypothesis and HF

In 1971, when HD and HF were closely related to and competed with each other, Babb and Scribner [8] reported that there should be middle molecules among the waste product in blood that could not be removed by HD. Hearing this theory, which was later known as the 'middle molecule hypothesis', people thought it necessary to develop membranes with large-sized pores and to perform HF using these membranes as hemofilters. In 1974, Rieger et al. [9] and Quellhorst et al. [10] performed HF experiments with collodion membrane, the result of which showed a rise in the removal rate of middle molecules. They also performed clinical trials in 1976 using polyacrylonitrile membrane. Unfortunately however, a problem occurred that when only HF was performed the removal rate of small solutes decreased.

## Development of HDF

With this background, the present author and staff thought it best to combine the method of HD and HF, i.e. HD for removing small solutes and HF for removing middle molecules. In order to control the amount of ultrafiltrate fluid, together with Toray Co., Tokyo, Japan, we developed new equipment which was called an ultrafiltration rate (UFR) controller [11]. The UFR controller had two small fixed-volume chambers, both of which were divided by a piece of silicone rubber membrane. This silicone rubber moved right and left repeatedly to equalize the amount of sending and withdrawing dialysis fluid in a closed circuit. So, if we removed the water from this circuit, the amount was just the amount of ultrafiltration. After completion of the UFR controller, we started clinical HDF in 1977 using a dialyzer with polymethylmethacrylate membrane, and reported our experience in the same year [12].

In 1977 and 1978, great progress was made in studies and clinical applications of HF and HDF. In 1977, Kramer et al. [13] reported continuous arteriovenous hemofiltration and Yamagami et al. [14] reported clinical application of HF. Craddock et al. [15] reported the compliment activation by dialysis membrane, which called our attention to the problem of biocompatibility. In 1978, Leber et al. [16] in Germany reported clinical experiences of HDF, as did we [17].

It was also in 1978 that Henderson and Beans [18] reported the results of clinical online HF. At that time, the substitution fluid required by HF or HDF was put into 1-liter bottles by the pharmaceutical companies. So, not only the cost but also the trouble of connecting tubes or disposing bottles prevented these therapies from becoming popular. In the same year, Bergström [19] devised a new method – sequential HD and HF – the mode of which was shifted from the extracorporeal ultrafiltration method to HD sequentially. Having learned these clinical experiences, Shinzato et al. [20] proposed push-and-pull HDF in 1982. In this epoch-making online system, some amounts of the dialysis fluid flowed into the blood as substitution fluid through the membrane.

## The Current Status of HDF in Japan

At the end of the story, the spread of online HDF in Japan should be discussed. In 1985, the first supplementary machine for HDF (DKR-11) was developed by Nikkiso Co., Tokyo, Japan, and was approved by the Ministry of Health and Welfare of Japan. This machine could perform online HDF including push-and-pull HDF treatment. However, it was used in a limited number of patients in a few hospitals since the quality of water for the online treatment was not an important issue at that time. Later, in 1992, using a conventional UFR controller under a newly devised central dialysis fluid delivery system, online HDF was started in the Kyushu district. Then, in 1994, the Kyushu Society for HDF made a start and in the following year the Japanese Society for HDF was organized.

The first guideline of water quality for online HDF was drafted by the Japanese Society for Dialysis Therapy in 1997, which contributed a great deal to the popularization of HDF. The same issues have also been discussed by the Committee of the International Society for Standardization (ISO) and its final version of the guideline is to be published in the near future. In 2010, three commercial dialysis consoles specifically designed for online HDF will be approved by the Ministry of Health, Labor and Welfare of Japan. From this point of view, we expect the popularization of online HDF treatment.

## References


1 Abel JJ, Rowntree LG, Turner BB: On the removal of diffusible substances from the circulating blood of living animals by dialysis. J Pharmacol Exp Ther 1914;5:275.

2 Kolff WJ: First clinical experience with artificial kidney. Ann Intern Med 1965;62:608–619.

3 Alwall N: On the artificial kidney. I. Apparatus for dialysis of blood in vivo. Acta Med Scand 1944;117:12.

4 Inoh T, Ishi J, Iizuka N, et al: DL-type artificial kidney (in Japanese). Kokyu To Junkann 1958;6:479.

5 Henderson LW, Besarab A, Michaels A, Bluemle LW Jr: Blood purification by ultrafiltration and fluid replacement (diafiltration). Trans Am Soc Artif Intern Organs 1967;13:216.

6 Hamilton R, Ford C, Colton C, Cross R, Steinmuller S, Henderson LW: Blood cleansing by diafiltration in uremic dog and man. Trans Am Soc Artif Intern Organs 1971;17:259–265.

7 Kobayashi K, Shibata M, Katoh K, et al: Studies on development and application of a new method of control of body fluid volume for patients on hemodialysis: extracorporeal ultrafiltration method (ECUM) (in Japanese). J Jpn Soc Nephrol 1972;14:539.

8 Babb AL, Popovich RP, Christopher TG, Scribner BH: The genesis of the square meter-hour hypothesis. Trans Am Soc Artif Intern Organs 1971;17:81–91.

9 Rieger J, Quellhorst E, Lowitz HD, et al: Ultrafiltration for middle molecules in uraemia. Proc Eur Dial Transpl Assoc 1974;11:158.

10 Quellhorst E, Rieger J, Doht B, et al: Treatment of chronic uraemia by an ultrafiltration kidney – first clinical experience. Proc Eur Dial Transpl Assoc 1976;13:314.

11 Ota K, Suzuki T, Era K, et al: Clinical evaluation of a preset ultrafiltration rate controller available for single-pass and hemofiltration systems. Artif Organs 1978;2:141.

12 Ota K, Suzuki T, Ozaku Y, et al: Experiences and problems of hemofiltration and hemodiafiltration (in Japanese). Jin To Toseki 1977;3:681.

13 Kramer P, Wigger, W, Rieger J, et al: Arteriovenous hemofiltration. A new and simple method for treatment of overhydrated patients resistant to diuretics. Klin Wochenschr 1977;55:1121.

14 Yamagami S, Kishimoto S, Ota M, et al: Clinical application of diafiltration system for patients on dialysis (in Japanese). J Jpn Soc Dial Ther 1977;10:483.

15 Craddock PR, Fehr J, Dalmasso AP, Brighan KL, Jacob HS: Hemodialysis leucopenia: pulmonary vascular leukostasis resulting from complement activation by a dialyzer cellophane membranes. J Clin Invest 1977;59:879–888.

16 Leber HW, Wizemann V, Goubeaud G, Rawer P, Schutterle G: Simultaneous hemofiltration/hemodialysis. An effective alternative to hemofiltration and conventional hemodialysis in the treatment of uremic patients. Clin Nephrol 1978;9:115–121.

17 Ota K, Suzuki T, Ozaku Y, Hosino T, et al: Short-time hemodiafiltration using polymethylmethacrylate hemofilter. Trans Am Soc Artif Intern Organs 1978;24:454.

18 Henderson LW, Beans E: Successful production of sterile pyrogen-free electrolyte solution by ultrafiltration. Kidney Int 1978;14:522–525.

19 Bergström J: Ultrafiltration without simultaneous dialysis for removal of excess fluid. Proc Eur Dial Transplant Assoc 1978;15:260–270.

20 Usuda M, Shinzato T, Sezaki R, et al: New simultaneous HF and HD with no infusion fluid. Trans Am Soc Artif Intern Organs 1982;28:24.



Kazuo Ota, MD, PhD
Department of Human and Environmental Science
Shonan Institute of Technology, 1-1-25 Tsujido-Nishikaigan
Fujisawa, Kanagawa 251-8511 (Japan)
Tel./Fax +81 466 30 0234, E-Mail yama@la.shonan-it.ac.jp

Kawanishi H, Yamashita AC (eds): Hemodiafiltration – A New Era.
Contrib Nephrol. Basel, Karger, 2011, vol 168, pp 5–18

# Hemodiafiltration – State of the Art

Francesco Locatelli · Celestina Manzoni · Sara Viganò · Andrea Cavalli · Salvatore Di Filippo

Department of Nephrology, Dialysis and Renal Transplant, Alessandro Manzoni Hospital, Lecco, Italy

**Abstract**

Many observational studies have consistently shown that high-flux hemodialysis (hf-HD) has positive effects on the survival and morbidity of chronic kidney disease stage 5 dialysis (CKD5D) patients when compared with low-flux hemodialysis, but the primary analysis of the prospective randomized Hemodialysis Outcomes (HEMO) study showed that the use of hf-HD was not associated with a significant reduction of the relative risk of mortality. More recently, the Membrane Permeability Outcome (MPO) study found that survival could be significantly improved by use hf-HD compared with low-flux dialysis in high-risk patients as identified by serum albumin ≤4 g/dl and, in a post-hoc analysis, in diabetic patients. Online hemodiafiltration (HDF) is reported as the most efficient technique of using high-flux membranes. Clearances of small solutes like urea are higher than in hemofiltration and of middle solutes like $\beta_2$-microglobulin are higher than in hf-HD. As the number of randomized prospective trials comparing HDF and hf-HD is still very limited, no conclusive data are available concerning the effect of increased convection of online HDF on survival and morbidity in CKD5D patients. A large, randomized controlled study is needed to clinically confirm the theoretical advantages of online HDF.



More than 20 years ago, the hypothesis that the extremely high morbidity and mortality rates of low-flux HD (lf-HD) were associated with inadequate removal of middle molecule solutes (MMs) led to the proposal for an alternative dialysis method: high-flux hemodialysis (hf-HD) [1].

A confirmation of the importance of MMs in uremic toxicity is found in the results of a large retrospective study performed by Leypoldt et al. [2] on a data subset from the USRDS showing a clear correlation between the death rate and the in vitro vitamin $B_{12}$ dialyzer clearance. More recently, experimental data gathered by the EUTox group has revived the interest for middle molecule toxicity [3]. With the advent of hf-HD, many observational studies have consistently shown that high-flux treatments have positive effects on the morbidity and survival of dialyzed patients. However, the 2002 results of the Hemodialysis Outcomes (HEMO) study [4], a prospective, randomized study aimed at verifying the advantages of hf-HD over lf-HD, were very surprising and in some way disappointing insofar as they showed at primary analysis that hf-HD was associated with a non-significant reduction of mortality of 8%, although secondary analyses pointed to an advantage for hf-HD in subgroups of patients [5].

During the course of the HEMO study, the impact of hf-HD on mortality was addressed in another prospective, randomized study: the Membrane Permeability Outcome (MPO) study [6], specifically designed to include a sicker patient population that could take more advantage from hf-HD, in order to provide sufficient statistical power to possibly demonstrate differences in patient survival. Serum albumin ≤4 g/dl was considered an indicator for increased morbidity and mortality risk. Besides, whereas the HEMO study included incident and prevalent patients, who were on dialysis an average of 3.7 years and 60% of them were treated with hf-HD before entry in the study, the MPO study enrolled only incident patients, to avoid early mortality bias (so-called selection of survivors) and a carryover effect of the previous treatment to the actual intervention phase and the reuse of the dialyzer was not allowed. 738 chronic kidney disease stage 5 dialysis (CKD5D) patients were enrolled in 59 European centers (567 of them had serum albumin <4 g/dl and 171 had serum albumin >4 g/dl) and were separately randomized in order to not jeopardize the original study design and have been observed for 3–7.5 years, randomized to two parallel groups, according to high or low flux. 647 patients were eligible to be included in the analysis population. No significant effect of membrane permeability on survival was found in the population as a whole. However, according to the initial study design, hf-HD showed a significant survival benefit in patients at risk for worse outcome, defined by serum albumin <4 g/dl. The relative risk (RR) reduction of mortality in this patient population, after adjustment for confounding factors, was 37%. The total number of deaths observed in the study was 162, 132 of them in the stratum with serum albumin <4 g/dl.

Moreover, a secondary analyses of the HEMO study, namely of patients who were on renal replacement therapy for >3.7 years, showed a significant survival benefit in the high-flux group with a reduction of the relative mortality risk by 32% [5]. In a secondary analysis of the MPO study, a higher survival rate was found in the diabetic population as a whole treated with high-flux compared with low-flux dialysis, with an adjusted RR reduction of 38%. Although this post-hoc analysis was initially not planned in the MPO study, the results are in line with the rationale of the study design and with a post-hoc analysis from the 4D study [7]. This analysis of the 4D study considered only patients who were treated with the same membrane type during the entire follow-up period. Here, the odds ratio for mortality in diabetic patients treated with synthetic low-flux membranes was 59% greater than in those treated with synthetic high-flux membranes. Still, because the patients were not randomly assigned to these membrane types, this post-hoc analysis should be carefully interpreted. In the HEMO study, in contrast to MPO study, no interaction of membrane flux and diabetes status was found. An explanation for this could be a 'selection of survivors' that was unavoidable when enrolling prevalent patients as in the HEMO study, in contrast to the MPO study, in which only incident patients were recruited.

The general applicability of the MPO study results found in patients with relatively low albumin plasma levels and diabetic patients should be seen against the background of an increasing proportion of dialysis patients with inflammation and/or malnutrition and of diabetic nephropathy as primary renal disease or diabetes as comorbidity. Serum albumin is a strong predictor of mortality [8] and related to nutritional and inflammatory status. Epidemiologic studies have confirmed that low serum albumin levels are frequent in HD patients. Owen et al. [9] reported 60% of the patients with serum albumin <4.0 g/dl, which is similar to the more recent figures from the DOPPS study, with 57–86% of the patients with serum albumin below this level [10]. Thus the potential general applicability of the MPO results is impressive.

The causal relation between treatment with hf-HD and survival could lie in the eliminative capacity of high-flux membranes. As shown previously and also in the MPO study, high-flux membranes have a significant removal capacity for $\beta_2$-microglobulin ($\beta_2$-MG – an acknowledged surrogate of the middle molecules) and positively affect serum levels in the long term, which in turn are related to mortality [11].

The current European Best Practice Guidelines (EBPG) on dialysis strategies published in 2007 contain the following recommendation: Guideline 2.1: 'The use of synthetic high-flux membranes should be considered to delay long-term complications of hemodialysis therapy'. Specific indications include: to reduce dialysis-related amyloidosis (evidence level III); to improve control of hyperphosphatemia (level II); to reduce the increased cardiovascular risk (level II); to improve control of anemia (level III)' [12]. The European Renal Best Practice (ERBP) Advisory Board, in the light of the MPO results, published a position statement to change existing guideline 2.1. The Board considers that the MPO study provides sufficient evidence to upgrade the strength of the guidance to a level 1A (strong recommendation, based on high-quality evidence) and that hf-HD should be used in the case of high-risk patients (comparable to the low-albumin group of the MPO study). Because the substantial improvement in an intermediate marker ($\beta_2$-MG) in the high-flux group of the MPO study, the ERBP Advisory Board considers that synthetic high-flux membranes should be recommended even in low-risk patients [13].

During the course of the MPO study, the impact of hf-HD on mortality was addressed in a number of epidemiologic studies, besides in the prospective, randomized, controlled HEMO study which stands as a cornerstone (tables 1, 2). In an analysis of a sample of the US Renal Data System registry, including nearly

**Table 1.** Observational studies on the effect of hf-HD on mortality risk

| Reference (first author) | Design | Treatment (patients, n) | Sample size | % RR reduction | p value |
|---|---|---|---|---|---|
| Hornberger 1992 [38] | historical, prospective | hf-HD (107)<br>lf-HD (146) | 253 | 76 | <0.001 |
| Koda 1997 | historical, prospective | hf-HD (248)<br>lf-HD (571) | 819 | 39 | <0.05 |
| Leypoldt 1999 [2] | historical, prospective | hf-HD<br>lf-HD | 1,771 | 5 | <0.0001 |
| Woods 2000 | historical, prospective | hf-HD (463)<br>lf-HD (252) | 715 | 42 | <0.01 |
| Port 2001 [14] | historical, prospective | hf-HD (3,751)<br>lf-HD (9,040) | 12,791 | 19 | 0.04 |
| Chauveau 2005 [15] | historical, prospective | hf-HD (299)<br>lf-HD (351) | 650 | 38 | 0.01 |
| Krane 2007 [7] | post-hoc analysis of prospective randomized study | hf-HD (241)<br>lf-HD (407) | 648 | 59 | 0.0006 |

14,000 HD patients, the effect of reuse practice and type of dialyzer membranes were addressed. A specific analysis, including only synthetic membranes, revealed the RR for mortality to be 24% higher in patients treated with low-flux than in those treated with high-flux membranes [14]. Similarly, a reduction of the RR for mortality by 38% in the patients on hf-HD versus those on low-flux dialysis was found in a European observational cohort of 650 patients [15].

Moreover, a randomized, prospective, multicenter, 3-year follow-up, controlled clinical trial has been performed in 64 patients enrolled in 20 Italian dialysis centers designed to evaluate the comparative long-term effects of pure convective therapy, online predilution hemofiltration versus ultrapure lf-HD assessing mortality and morbidity outcomes in patients with ESRD [16]. Of 64 patients, 32 were randomly assigned to HD and 32 were randomly assigned to HF. 22 patients completed the follow-up, 11 in each group. The odds ratio of all-cause death was 0.45 for HF compared with HD (p = 0.05). The number of hospitalization events per patient was not significantly different across the two trial arms. Because of the small sample size of this trial, larger randomized controlled trials are needed to get clearer confirmation about the improved survival observed with HF in this study.

In a prospective randomized multicentric trial, Locatelli et al. [17] compared biocompatible and traditional membranes, convective and diffusive treatment

**Table 2.** Randomized studies on the effect of high-flux hemodialysis on mortality risk

| | Design | Treatments (patients) | Sample size | Relative risk reduction | p value |
|---|---|---|---|---|---|
| Locatelli et al. 1996 [17] | randomized, prospective | Cuprophan-HD (132)<br>lf-Ps HD (147)<br>hf-Ps HD (51)<br>HDF Ps (50) | 380 | | NS |
| Eknoyan et al. 2002 [4] | randomized, prospective | hf-HD (921)<br>lf-HD (925) | 1,846 | 8% | NS |
| Locatelli et al. 2009 [6] | randomized, prospective | Albumin ≤ 4 g/dl<br>hf-HD (279)<br>lf-HD (283) | 562 | 37% | 0.032 |
| | randomized, prospective | Albumin > 4 g/dl<br>hf-HD (84)<br>lf-HD (92) | 176 | | NS |
| | randomized, prospective, post-hoc analysis | Diabetics<br>hf-HD (83)<br>lf-HD (74) | 157 | 38% | 0.039 |

hf-HD = High flux hemodialysis; HDF = hemodiafiltration; lf-HD = low flux hemodialysis; Ps = polysulphone.

modalities (cuprophane HD, low-flux polysulphone HD, high-flux polysulphone HD, high-flux polysulphone hemodiafiltration) in 380 patients followed for 24 months. No significant difference in treatment tolerance and cardiovascular stability was demonstrated between the four treatment groups. As stressed in the paper, it is likely that significant differences in cardiovascular stability were not demonstrated because the incidence of intradialytic hypotension in the population as a whole was much lower than expected. Moreover, no difference of mortality between low- and high-flux groups was found, but the study was not designed for this endpoint.

### Online Hemodiafiltration

Hemodiafiltration (HDF), a strategy based on simultaneous diffusive and convective transport, was the first step in the attempt to overcome the major drawback of hemofiltration, that is its low efficiency in small solutes removal.

Clearances of small solutes, like urea, are higher than in hemofiltration and of middle solutes, like $\beta_2$-MG, are higher than in hf-HD. To try to better define the clinical advantages of HDF, we will review some data from clinical studies on the efficacy of this technique, considering several factors possibly related to the high mortality rate of HD patients. It is well known that cardiovascular disease is the major cause of death in these patients and we will analyze the impact of HDF on some of the main cardiovascular risk factors.

Hyperphosphatemia has been associated with increased risk of all-cause mortality, including cardiovascular mortality [18]. By promoting passive and active vascular calcification, hyperphosphatemia is a well-recognized factor implicated in the cardiovascular risk of CKD patients. Adequate control of hyperphosphatemia, a primary target of dialysis adequacy, is rarely achieved. In the DOPPS study, 52% of CKD5D patients are above K-DOQI phosphate recommendation despite the extensive use of phosphate binders [19]. Enhancing phosphate removal by dialysis requires to increase instantaneous phosphate clearance and to enhance duration (or frequency) of treatment. In a study in 16 patients, Zehnder et al. [20] compared the clearance of phosphate during hf-HD and online HDF during two 1-week periods. The results provide evidence that HDF increases the clearance of phosphate. It should be underlined that because of its short length, this study cannot give any information about the possible difference of predialysis phosphatemia levels in the long term in the two treatments.

Recently a 6% decrease in predialysis phosphate levels after 6 months of online HDF has been reported by Penne et al. [21]. However in this study the mean dialyzer surface as well as the mean blood flow were higher in the HDF group as reflected by the spKt/V values equal to 1.6 in HDF and 1.4 in the HD.

Anemia is well recognized, together with hypertension, as the main cause of ventricular hypertrophy in dialysis patients. The difference between conventional HDF (mean replacement fluid 4 l/session), roughly comparable in convection entity to hf-HD, and online HDF (mean replacement fluid 22.5 l/session) was evaluated by Maduell et al. [22] in 37 patients over a period of 1 year. The most interesting result of this study was that online HDF provided a better correction of anemia with lower dosages of erythropoietin. The suggested explanations for these results could be a greater elimination of middle sized molecules reducing erythropoietin response and (or) a better biocompatibility of the system, secondary to a better quality of dialysate due to online treatment. This last possibility is supported by a paper by Schiffl et al. [23] pointing out that the use of ultrapure (filtered, pyrogen-free and sterile) dialysate, reduces the rHu-EPO doses required to maintain hemoglobin levels via a reduction in systemic inflammatory processes.

Several lines of evidence have accumulated showing that microbiological purity of dialysate is a critical component of the complex hemocompatibility network. Transmembrane passage of bacterial-derived products from the dialysate to blood, known as back-transport, has been documented in several studies, occurring either from backfiltration and/or backdiffusion of dialysate contaminants [24]. The problem influences all hemodialysis modalities, since it has been shown that low levels of endotoxin in the dialysate are able to induce the production of cytokines, despite the use of low permeability cellulosic membranes [25]. Chronic inflammation and oxidative stress are highly prevalent in patients with CKD and ESRD, and may contribute to high mortality rates associated with cardiovascular disease. Moreover, advanced glycation end products (AGEs) may represent a novel class of uremic toxins with significant implications for long-term dialysis-related pathological states. Recent studies have indicated that HDF is the most effective method of removing AGEs (mol. wt. 15 kDa). A study by Lin et al. [26] analyzed long-term changes in serum levels among different dialysis modalities (lf-HD, hf-HD and online HDF). In a 6-month study period, predialysis serum AGE levels were significantly lower in patients treated with online HDF. Gerdemann et al. [27], in agreement with Lin's data, found that the predialysis AGE levels of patients on HDF were significantly lower that those of patients on high-flux HD using standard dialysis fluid. However, the difference between the levels of patients on HDF was not significant in comparison with the levels of patients on high-flux HD using ultrapure dialysis fluid.

Cardiovascular instability is the most frequent clinical problem on dialysis. The importance of preventing intradialytic hypotension is mainly related to the need of achieving the patient's dry body weight, thus better controlling hypertension that in CKD5D patients is mainly dependent on fluid overload. A better cardiovascular stability on HDF in comparison to hemodialysis has been reported. A retrospective study by Pizzarelli et al. [28] compared the results during online HDF with those during standard bicarbonate hemodialysis. Online HDF was associated with better cardiovascular tolerance to fluid removal, with a significantly lower incidence of episodes of symptomatic hypotension. The better hemodynamic stability of online HDF was also reported in a prospective, randomized trial by Lin et al. [29]. 111 patients were randomly divided into four groups receiving different frequencies of online HDF and high-flux HD (group 1: HDF three times a week; group 2: HDF twice and high-flux HD once a week; group 3: HDF once and high-flux HD twice a week; group 4: high-flux HD three times a week). Episodes of symptomatic hypotension and mean saline infusion volumes during treatments were significantly reduced when frequencies of online HDF were increased. Of interest, the authors reported a higher predialysis plasma sodium concentration (2.3 mEq/l) in patients with a higher frequency of online HDF, thus suggesting reduced sodium removal, possibly at least partially responsible for the better cardiovascular stability. The same holds true for the results of Maduell et al. [22].

According to the original observation by Maggiore et al. [30] that dialysate temperature set at about 35°C affords a better hemodynamic stability than the standard dialysate temperature of 37–38°C, an alternative hypothesis to explain the reduction of hypotension episodes during online HDF is suggested by Donauer et al. [31] who identify blood cooling as the main blood pressure stabilizing factor in online HDF. During online HDF, an enhanced energy loss within the extracorporeal system occurred, despite identical temperature settings for dialysate and substitution fluids. As a result, the blood returning to the patient was cooler during online HDF than during HD. Moreover, the mean blood temperature was lower in online HDF, even in the patient's circulation, and blood volume was significantly more reduced. The incidence of symptomatic hypotension was similar to that of online HDF by using cooler temperature-controlled HD.

*$\beta_2$-MG.* Until recently, $\beta_2$-MG toxicity was mainly associated with the risk of developing $\beta_2$-MG amyloidosis in long-term dialysis patients. Serum $\beta_2$-MG concentration is now strongly associated with mortality risk in dialysis patients. Post-hoc analysis of the HEMO study has shown that increased $\beta_2$-MG concentrations above a threshold value of 27 mg/l are predictive of an increased risk of death in HD patient. For this reason the $\beta_2$-MG concentrations should be considered as a quite interesting marker of dialysis efficacy. In a study of 58 patients who converted from hf-HD to HDF for 8 months, pre- and posttreatment serum $\beta_2$-MG levels markedly declined compared to hf-HD [32]. On the other hand, Ward et al. [33] performed a prospective clinical trial in 44 patients randomized to online postdilution HDF or high-flux HD for a 12-month study period. There was a similar decrease of pretreatment plasma $\beta_2$-MG concentrations, despite an apparent difference in removal of $\beta_2$-MG as indicated by a significantly higher pre- to posttreatment reduction in plasma $\beta_2$-MG concentration in HDF. With regard to this last point, it should be remembered that a change in plasma concentration of a solute is a good indicator of removal only for solutes distributed in a single pool including plasma. A substantial rebound in posttreatment plasma $\beta_2$-MG concentrations has been reported, suggesting that a single-pool model is not adequate to describe $\beta_2$-MG kinetics.

Paracresol and indoxyl sulfate are the two leading compounds that are implicated in the endothelial dysfunction. Thus increasing removal of these compounds appears highly desirable. Recent studies on highly efficient convective modalities (HDF) have confirmed that low paracresol concentrations were associated with a significant reduction of dialysis patient mortality [34].

A randomized crossover study on 14 patients compared the influence of hf-HD, predilution low-volume (20 l) HDF, and postdilution low-volume (20 l) as well as high-volume (60 l) HDF on removal of the protein-bound solute paracresol [35]. Elimination of paracresol was best during HDF and increased with greater filtration volumes.

Although HDF offers the advantage of increased convective clearance for middle molecules, there is still controversy as to whether reinfusion should occur pre- or postfilter. Predilution limitations include dilution of blood side solute concentration and reduced small solute clearance; postdilution limitations are hemoconcentration, increased fiber clotting, and protein denaturation.

Mid-dilution HDF is a technique that uses a hemodiafilter, OLpUr MD 190 (Nephros, Inc., New York, N.Y., USA), which allows both pre- and post-reinfusion and a reinfusion rates of 10–12 l/h. In a prospective crossover study of 10 patients, mid-dilution HDF was compared to online postdilution HDF [36]. While urea and creatinine clearances were significantly lower, middle molecule removal was higher in mid-dilution HDF over the whole range of investigated solutes including $\beta_2$-MG (mean of 202 vs. 166 ml/min). It is matter of fact that survival, together with quality of life, are the most important outcomes.

In 2006, characteristics and outcomes of patients receiving HDF versus HD in five European countries in the Dialysis Outcomes and Practice Patterns Study [37] were published. The study analyzed 2,165 patients from 1998 to 2001, stratified into four groups: low- and high-flux HD (respectively 63.1 and 25.2% of all patients), and low- and high-efficiency HDF (respectively 7.2 and 4.5% of all patients). High-efficiency HDF patients were associated with a significant 35% lower mortality relative risk (RR = 0.65, p = 0.01) than those receiving lf-HD, while patients receiving low-efficiency HDF were associated with a non-significant 7% lower mortality relative risk (RR = 0.93, p = 0.68) compared to those receiving lf-HD. Strangely enough, these data are not consistent because the effect of flux should be a continuum, while in this study there is no association between hf-HD and survival (even the other side around) and the same holds true for low-volume HFR. Thus, while these results are apparently very impressive, they show only an association and not a demonstration. A selection bias by indication could not be ruled out. As the authors themselves acknowledged, the benefits of HDF must be tested by randomized controlled clinical trials before recommendations can be made for clinical practice. This is particularly true when considering the discrepancies between the results of observational studies and the randomized controlled trials. In 1992, an observational study of Hornberger et al. [38] claimed that patients treated by high-flux HD were associated with a 65% lower relative risk of mortality than those treated with standard HD. On the other hand, in another large observational study comparing convective with diffusive treatments, a 10% non-significant better survival was associated with convective treatments [39]. A recent observational prospective trial [40] evaluated the role of different dialysis modalities on mortality and morbility in 757 hemodialysis patients. After 30 months, HDF was associated with a 22% reduction in relative risk of mortality. A systematic review of randomized controlled trials comparing HD, HF, HDF and acetate-free biofiltration to assess their clinical effectiveness has been performed [41], but because

**Table 3.** Observational and randomized studies on the effect of haemofiltration and/or haemodiafiltration on mortality risk

| | Design | Treatments (patients) | Sample size | Relative risk reduction | p value |
|---|---|---|---|---|---|
| *Observational studies* | | | | | |
| Locatelli et al. 1999 [39] | historical, prospective | HDF or Haemofiltration (188)<br>HD (6,256) | 6,444 | 10% | NS |
| Canaud et al. 2006 [37] | historical, prospective | lf-HD (1,366)<br>hf-HD (546)<br>Low-efficiency HDF (156)<br>High-efficiency HDF (97) | 2,165 | 35%<br>(High-efficiency HDF vs LF-HD) | 0.01 |
| Panichi et al. 2008 | prospective | Bicarbonate-HD* (424)<br>HDF (204)<br>On-line HDF (129) | 757 | 22%<br>(HDF and On-line HDF vs Bicarbonate-HD) | 0.01 |
| *Randomized studies* | | | | | |
| Locatelli et al. 1996 [17] | randomized, prospective | Cuprophan-HD (132)<br>lf-HD (147)<br>hf-HD (51)<br>HDF (50) | 380 | | NS |
| Wizemann et al. 2000 | randomized, prospective | HDF (23)<br>lf-HD (21) | 44 | | NS |
| Santoro et al. 2008 [16] | randomized, prospective | On-line Hemodiafiltration (32)<br>lf-HD (32) | 64 | 55% | 0.05 |

*Including lf-HD (403 patients) and hf-HD (21 patients).

the trials assessed were not adequately powered and had suboptimal method quality, a conclusive definition about the better replacement therapy modality cannot be derived as clearly underlined. However, this systematic review was heavily criticized for its imprecision [42].

As yet, since the number of randomized prospective trials comparing HDF with standard HD is very limited (table 3), no conclusive data is available on the effect of HDF on survival and morbidity in patients with CKD5D. Two further studies are exploring the potential beneficial effect of convection. An Italian prospective multicenter study [43] is comparing online convective treatments (HF and HDF) with standard lf-HD, assuming as primary endpoint cardiovascular stability and blood pressure control and as secondary aims the impact on symptoms, morbidity and mortality. Preliminary data seems to favor online HDF and HF [44]. The Dutch Convective Transport Study (CONTRAST) was initiated in the second quarter of 2004 [45]. The study is conducted in more than 20 centers in The Netherlands and approximately 800 incident and prevalent HD patients will be randomized to either lf-HD or online HDF and followed for 3 years to investigate the effect of increased convective transport by online HDF on all-cause and cardiovascular mortality in chronic HD patients. Unfortunately, this study does not compare hf-HD with online HDF, thus leaving in any case still open the key question of whether online HDF is superior using hard outcomes (like survival) in comparison with hf-HD.

At present, considering the results of the HEMO and MPO studies, there are strong evidence-based data favoring high-flux treatments and suggestions supporting online HDF including the use of ultrapure dialysate. A large randomized controlled study is needed to definitively prove the clinical advantages of online HDF on CKD5D patients.

## References


1 Von Albertini B, Miller JH, Gardner PW, Shinaberger JH: High-flux hemodiafiltration: under six hours/week treatment. Trans Am Soc Artif Intern Organs 1984;30:227–231.

2 Leypoldt JK, Cheung AK, Carroll CE, Stannard C, Pereira BJG, Agodoa LY, Port FK: Effect of dialysis membranes and middle molecule removal on chronic hemodialysis patient survival. Am J Kidney Dis 1999;33:349–355.

3 Vanholder R, Baurmeister U, Brunet P, Cohen G, Glorieux G, Jankowski J, European Uremic Toxin Work Group: A bench to bedside view of uremic toxins. J Am Soc Nephrol 2008;19:863–870.

4 Eknoyan G, Beck GJ, Cheung AK, Daugirdas JT, Greene T, Kusek JW, Allon M, Bailey J, Delmez JA, Depner TA, Dwyer JT, Levey AS, Levin NW, Milford E, Ornt DB, Rocco MV, Schulman G, Schwab SJ, Teehan BP, Toto R, Hemodialysis (HEMO) Study Group: Effect of dialysis dose and membrane flux in maintenance hemodialysis. N Engl J Med 2002;347:2010–2019.

5 Cheung AK, Levin NW, Greene T, Agodoa L, Bailey J, Beck G, Clark W, Levey AS, Leypoldt JK, Ornt DB, Rocco MV, Schulman G, Schwab S, Teehan B, Eknoyan G: Effects of high-flux hemodialysis on clinical outcomes: results of the HEMO study. J Am Soc Nephrol 2003;14:3251–3263.

6 Locatelli F, Martin-Malo A, Hannedouche T, Loureiro A, Papadimitriou M, Wizemann V, Jacobson SH, Czekalski S, Ronco C, Vanholder R, Membrane Permeability Outcome (MPO) Study Group: Effect of membrane permeability on survival of hemodialysis patients. J Am Soc Nephrol 2009;20:645–654.

7 Krane V, Krieter DH, Olschewski M, Marz W, Mann JF, Ritz E, Wanner C: Dialyzer membrane characteristics and outcome of patients with type 2 diabetes on maintenance hemodialysis. Am J Kidney Dis 2007;49:267–275.

8 Goodkin DA, Bragg-Gresham JL, Koenig KG, Wolfe RA, Akiba T, Andreucci VE, Saito A, Rayner HC, Kurokawa K, Port FK, Held PJ, Young EW: Association of comorbid conditions and mortality in hemodialysis patients in Europe, Japan, and the United States: The Dialysis Outcomes and Practice Patterns Study (DOPPS). J Am Soc Nephrol 2003;14:3270–3277.

9 Owen WF, Lew NL, Liu Y, Lowrie EG, Lazarus JM: The urea reduction ratio and serum albumin concentration as predictors of mortality in patients undergoing hemodialysis. N Engl J Med 1993;329:1001–1006.
10 The DOPPS Report, 2004. Available at: http://www.dopps.org/pdf/dopps_report_2004.pdf (accessed June 30, 2007).
11 Cheung AK, Rocco MV, Yan G, Leypoldt JK, Levin NW, Greene T, Agodoa L, Bailey J, Beck GJ, Clark W, Levey AS, Ornt DB, Schulman G, Schwab S, Teehan B, Eknoyan G: Serum $\beta_2$-microglobulin levels predict mortality in dialysis patients: results of the HEMO study. J Am Soc Nephrol 2006;17:546–555.
12 Tattersall J, Martin-Malo A, Pedrini L, Basci A, Canaud B, Fouque D, Haage P, Konner K, Kooman J, Pizzarelli F, Tordoir J, Vennegoor M, Wanner C, ter Wee P, Vanholder R: EBPG guideline on dialysis strategies. Nephrol Dial Transplant 2007;22:ii5–ii21.
13 Tattersall J, Canaud B, Heimburger O, Pedrini L, Schneditz D, Van Biesen W, European Renal Best Practice Advisory Board: High-flux or low-flux dialysis: a position statement following publication of the Membrane Permeability Outcome study. Nephrol Dial Transplant 2010;25:1230–1232.
14 Port FK, Wolfe RA, Hulbert-Shearon TE, Daugirdas JT, Agodoa LY, Jones C, Orzol SM, Held PJ: Mortality risk by hemodialyzer reuse practice and dialyzer membrane characteristics: results from the USRDS dialysis morbidity and mortality study. Am J Kidney Dis 2001;37:276–286.
15 Chauveau P, Nguyen H, Combe C, Chene G, Azar R, Cano N, Canaud B, Fouque D, Laville M, Leverve X, Roth H, Aparicio M, French Study Group for Nutrition in Dialysis: Dialyzer membrane permeability and survival in hemodialysis patients. Am J Kidney Dis 2005;45:565–571.
16 Santoro A, Mancini E, Bolzani R, Boggi R, Cagnoli L, Francioso A, Fusaroli M, Piazza V, Rapanà R, Strippoli GF: The effect of online high-flux hemofiltration versus low-flux hemodialysis on mortality in chronic kidney failure: a small randomized controller trial. Am J Kidney Dis 2008;52:507–518.
17 Locatelli F, Mastrangelo F, Redaelli B, Ronco C, Marcelli D, La Greca G, Orlandini G: Effects of different membranes and dialysis technologies on patient treatment tolerance and nutritional parameters. The Italian Cooperative Dialysis Study Group. Kidney Int 1996;50:1293–1302.
18 Block GA, Klassen PS, Lazarus JM, Ofsthun N, Lowrie EG, Chertow GM: Mineral metabolism, mortality and morbidity in maintenance hemodialysis. J Am Soc Nephrol 2004;15:2208–2218.
19 Young EW, Albert JM, Satayathum S, Goodkin DA, Pisoni RL, Akiba T, Akizawa T, Kurokawa K, Bommer J, Piera L, Port FK: Predictors and consequences of altered mineral metabolism: the Dialysis Outcomes and Practice Patterns Study. Kidney Int 2005;67:1179–1187.
20 Zehnder C, Gutzwiller JP, Renggli K: Hemodiafiltration: a new treatment option for hyperphosphatemia in hemodialysis patients. Clin Nephrol 1999;52:152–159.
21 Penne EL, van der Weerd NC, van der Dorpel MA, Grooteman MP, Lévesque R, Nubé MJ, Bots ML, BlankestijnPJ, ter Wee PM, CONTRAST Investigators: Short-term effects of on-line hemodiafiltration on phosphate control: a result from the randomized controlled Convective Transport Study (CONTRAST). Am J Kidney Dis 2010;55:77–87.
22 Maduell F, del Pozo C, Garcia H, Sanchez L, Hdez-Jaras J, Albero MD, Calvo C, Torregrosa I, Navarro V: Change from conventional haemodiafiltration to on-line haemodiafiltration. Nephrol Dial Transplant 1999;14:1202–1207.
23 Schiffl H, Lang SM, Bergner A: Ultrapure dialysate reduces dose of recombinant human erythropoietin. Nephron 1999;83:278–279.
24 Pereira BJ, Sundaram S, Barrett TW, Butt NK, Porat R, King AJ, Dinarello CA: Transfer of cytokine-inducing bacterial products across hemodialyzer membranes in the presence of plasma or whole blood. Clin Nephrol 1996;46:394–401.

25 Schindler R, Lonnemann G, Shaldon S, Koch KM, Dinarello CA: Induction of interleukin-1 and tumor necrosis factor during in vitro hemodialysis with different membranes. Contrib Nephrol. Basel, Karger, 1989, vol 74, pp 58–65.
26 Lin CL, Huang CC, Yu CC, Yang HY, Chuang FR, Yang CW: Reduction of advanced glycation end product levels by on-line hemodiafiltration in long-term hemodialysis patients. Am J Kidney Dis 2003;42:524–531.
27 Gerdemann A, Wagner Z, Solf A, Bahner U, Heidland A, Vienken J, Schinzel R: Plasma levels of advanced glycation end products during haemodialysis, haemodiafiltration and haemofiltration: potential importance of dialysate quality. Nephrol Dial Transplant 2002;17:1045–1049.
28 Pizzarelli F, Cerrai T, Dattolo P, Tetta C, Maggiore Q: Convective treatments with online production of replacement fluid: a clinical experience lasting 6 years. Nephrol Dial Transplant 1998;13:363–369.
29 Lin CL, Huang CC, Chang CT, Wu MS, Hung CC, Chien CC, Yang CW: Clinical improvement by increased frequency of online hemodiafiltration. Ren Fail 2001;23:193–206.
30 Maggiore Q, Pizzarelli F, Sisca S, Zoccali C, Parlongo S, Nicolò F, Creazzo G: Blood temperature and vascular stability during hemodialysis and hemofiltration. Trans Am Soc Artif Intern Organs 1982;28:523–537.
31 Donauer J, Schweiger C, Rumberger B, Krumme B, Bohler J: Reduction of hypotensive side effects during online haemodiafiltration and low temperature haemodialysis. Nephrol Dial Transplant 2003;18:1616–1622.
32 Lin CL, Yang CW, Chiang CC, Chang CT, Huang CC: Long-term on-line hemodiafiltration reduces predialysis $\beta_2$-microglobulin levels in chronic hemodialysis patients. Blood Purif 2001;19:301–307.
33 Ward RA, Schmidt B, Hullin J, Hillebrand GF, Samtleben W: A comparison of on-line hemodiafiltration and high-flux hemodialysis: a prospective clinical study. J Am Soc Nephrol 2000;11:2344–2350.
34 Bammens B, Evenepoel P, Keuleers H, Verbeke K, Vanrenterghem Y: Free serum concentrations of the protein-bound retention solute *p*-cresol predict mortality in hemodialysis patients. Kidney Int 2006;69:1081–1087.
35 Bammens B, Evenepoel P, Verbeke K, Vanrenterghem Y: Removal of the protein-bound solute *p*-cresol by convective transport: a randomized crossover study. Am J Kidney Dis 2004;44:278–285.
36 Krieter DH, Falkenhain S, Chalabi L, Collins G, Lemke HD, Canaud B: Clinical cross-over comparison of mid-dilution hemodiafiltration using a novel dialyzer concept and post-dilution hemodiafiltration. Kidney Int 2005;67:349–356.
37 Canaud B, Bragg-Gresham JL, Marshall MR, Desmeules S, Gillespie BW, Depner T, Klassen P, Port FK: Mortality risk for patients receiving hemodiafiltration versus hemodialysis: European results from the DOPPS. Kidney Int 2006;69:2087–2093.
38 Hornberger JC, Chernew M, Petersen J, Garber AM: A multivariate analysis of mortality and hospital admission with high-flux dialysis. J Am Soc Nephrol 1992;3:1227–1237.
39 Locatelli F, Marcelli D, Conte F, Limido A, Malberti F, Spotti D: Comparison of mortality in ESRD patients on convective and diffusive extracorporeal treatments. The Registro Lombardo Dialisi e Trapianto. Kidney Int 1999;55:286–293.
40 Panichi V, Rizza GM, Paoletti S, Bigazzi R, Aloisi M, Barsotti G, Rindi P, Donati G, Antonelli A, Panicucci E, Tripepi C, Tetta C, Palla R: Chronic inflammation and mortality in haemodialysis: effect of different renal replacement therapies. Results from the RISCAVID study. Nephrol Dial Transplant 2008;23:2337–2343.
41 Rabindranath KS, Strippoli GF, Roderick P, Wallace SA, MacLeod AM, Daly C: Comparison of hemodialysis, hemofiltration and acetate-free biofiltration for ESRD: systematic review. Am J Kidney Dis 2005;45:437–447.
42 Locatelli F: Comparison of hemodialysis, hemodiafiltration and hemofiltration: systematic review or systematic error? Am J Kidney Dis 2005;46:787–788.

43 Bolasco P, Altieri P, Andrulli S, Basile C, Di Filippo S, Feriani M, Pedrini L, Santoro A, Zoccali C, Sau G, Locatelli F: Convection versus diffusion in dialysis: an Italian prospective multicentre study. Nephrol Dial Transplant 2003;18(suppl 7):50–54.
44 Locatelli F, Altieri P, Andrulli S, Bolasco P, Sau G, Pedrini LA, Basile C, David S, Feriani M, Montagna G, Di Iorio BR, Memoli B, Cravero R, Battaglia G, Zoccali C: Cardiovascular stability in pre-dilution hemofiltration and hemodiafiltration versus low-flux hemodialysis. J Am Soc Nephrol 2010 (submitted).
45 Penne EL, Blankestijn PJ, Bots ML, Van den Dorpel MA, Grooteman MPC, Nubé MJ, Ter Wee PM, on behalf of the CONTRAST Group: Resolving controversies regarding hemodiafiltration versus hemodialysis: The Dutch Convective Transport Study. Semin Dial 2005;18:47–51.

Francesco Locatelli, MD
Department of Nephrology, Dialysis and Renal Transplant
Alessandro Manzoni Hospital
Via dell'Eremo 9/11, IT–23900 Lecco (Italy)
Tel. +39 341 489850, Fax +39 341 489860, E-Mail f.locatelli@ospedale.lecco.it

Kawanishi H, Yamashita AC (eds): Hemodiafiltration – A New Era.
Contrib Nephrol. Basel, Karger, 2011, vol 168, pp 19–27

# Hemodiafiltration: Evolution of a Technique towards Better Dialysis Care

Claudio Ronco

Department of Nephrology, St. Bortolo Hospital, and International Renal Research Institute Vicenza, Vicenza, Italy

**Abstract**

Technological developments in the fields of membranes, machines and fluids have contributed to making hemodiafiltration (HDF) a safe and effective technique. Synthetic membranes with combined hydrophilic-hydrophobic structure and reduced wall thickness allowed to combine diffusion and convection into a unique technique. Accurate volumetric ultrafiltration control systems in dialysis machines reduce the risk for fluid balance errors and allow to perform safe and efficient online HDF. In fact, modern dialysis machines are equipped with specific balancing systems to manage fluid reinfusion and ultrafiltration simultaneously. Online preparation of sterile and pyrogen-free solutions for infusion is today possible, allowing the safe infusion of large fluid volumes during a HDF session. Dedicated software and enhanced user interfaces of modern dialysis machines simplify the procedures and reduce both operator workload and error. Emerging evidence suggests that these therapies may be superior to classic diffusive hemodialysis in terms of morbidity, and perhaps even mortality. There is a need for better understanding of the mechanisms involved, as well as further confirmation of these encouraging findings with prospective controlled trials. Nevertheless, HDF appears a promising therapy that likely will improve patient outcomes. Based on these considerations, HDF has the potential to become the new gold standard for dialysis in the years to come.



## Hemodiafiltration: From Origin to Today

Hemodiafiltration (HDF) is a renal replacement technique combining diffusion and convection to enhance solute removal in a wide spectrum of molecular weights, first introduced by Henderson [1] in 1967. In this modality, ultrafiltration exceeds the desired fluid loss in the patient, and replacement fluid is administered to achieve the target fluid balance. The relative contribution of

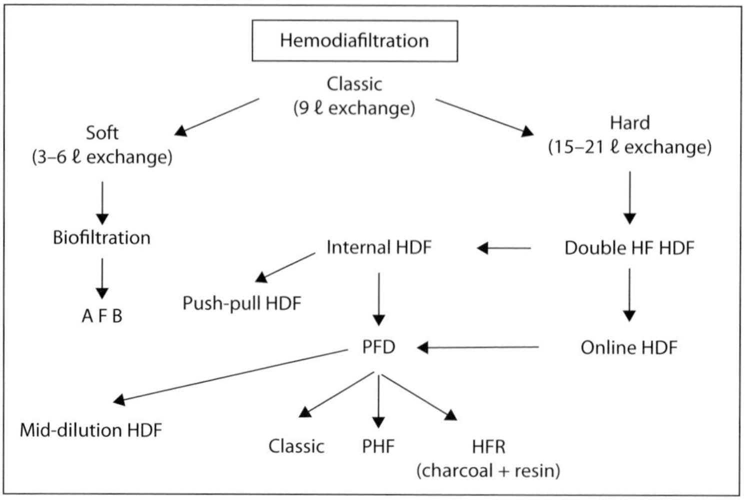


**Fig. 1.** Classic HDF and variants.

convection to overall solute removal increases progressively with increasing molecular weight.

Technological developments in the fields of membranes, machines and fluids have contributed to making HDF a safe and effective technique. First, synthetic polymer membranes with combined hydrophilic-hydrophobic structure and reduced wall thickness allowed a combination of diffusive-convective techniques. Second, the development of accurate volumetric ultrafiltration control systems in dialysis machines reduced the risk for fluid balance errors. Third, dialysis machines became equipped with specific balancing systems to manage fluid reinfusion and ultrafiltration simultaneously. Then, online preparation of sterile and pyrogen-free solutions for infusion became possible, allowing the safe infusion of large fluid volumes during a HDF session [2]. Lastly, significant improvements in dedicated software and machine-user interface simplified the procedure and reduced both operator workload and error. Nevertheless, at present, it remains a renal replacement modality used sporadically in Europe, and not at all in North America.

## Techniques of Hemodiafiltration

HDF has different aspects and a wide spectrum of technical configurations. The technique has evolved a great deal and today we have a variety of techniques that can be included under the general term of hemodiafiltration (fig. 1). Since its original conception, various forms of HDF have evolved through the years, from 'classic' HDF to the more commonly utilized online HDF, to variants using multicompartment filters such as mid-dilution HDF. A brief description of different techniques is presented here whilst a more detailed review has been previously published elsewhere [3].

*Classic HDF*: This technique uses an average reinfusion rate of 9 l/session (fluids contained in bags) in post-dilution (fig. 2a). A blood flow over 300 ml/min is required for sufficient rates of ultrafiltration at acceptable transmembrane pressure gradients. The equipment includes an ultrafiltration control system, a reinfusion pump and a scale to weigh reinfusion bags [4]. The amount of reinfusion varied from 3 l/session (fig. 2b, 'soft' HDF, e.g. biofiltration) to >15 l/session (fig. 2c, 'hard' HDF, discussed below).

*Acetate-Free Biofiltration:* This special form of HDF eliminates even small traces of acetate from both dialysate and replacement fluid, which is titrated based on blood bicarbonate level, varying from 6 to 9 l/session [4].

*High-Volume HDF ('Hard' HDF)*: A specific form of classic HDF, using fluid exchange of minimum 15 l/session. High ultrafiltration rate requires a high blood flow and replacement solution often infused in pre-dilution mode. While pre-dilution partially decreases the efficiency of the therapy, it optimizes blood flow distribution in the hemodialyzer and a lower protein concentration polarization at the blood-membrane interface [5].

*Online HDF (OLHDF)*: The high cost of commercial replacement fluids (bags) stimulated the development of this novel technique (fig. 2d). Fresh ultrapure dialysate from the dialysate inlet line is processed with multiple filtration steps and reinfused as replacement fluid. Large amounts of inexpensive replacement solution are generated and HDF can be performed with very high fluid turnover (up to 30–40 l/session). Fluid can be reinfused in either pre- or post-dilution mode, or both, in different proportions.

*Internal Filtration HDF:* The water flux in hollow-fiber hemodialyzers is characterized by a proximal filtration and a distal backfiltration. Proximal water flux can be enhanced by applying a constriction in the middle of the fiber bundle (fig 2e). Placing an obstruction to dialysate flow in the dialysate compartment or by reducing the inner diameter of the fibers, internal filtration can reach values of 40–50 ml/min in a 1.8-$m^2$ dialyzer. The ultrafiltration control system of the machine operates a fluid balance increasing the relative amount of backfiltration [6].

*Paired Filtration Dialysis (PFD):* This technique is based on two filters placed in series: first, a hemofilter (convection) and second, a hemodialyzer (predominantly diffusion) (fig. 2f). Replacement fluid is infused between the two units. This therapy minimizes interactions between convection and diffusion and prevents backfiltration in the hemodialyzer. Modifications of PFD are OLHDF with endogenous reinfusion (HFR) and PFD with exogenous reinfusion techniques. In HFR (fig. 2g) the ultrafiltrate produced is purified by adsorption through a resin/charcoal unit and utilized subsequently as a replacement fluid. In PFD with exogenous reinfusion, the first unit is used to backfilter some fresh dialysate which then acts as ultrapure online filtered replacement fluid [7].

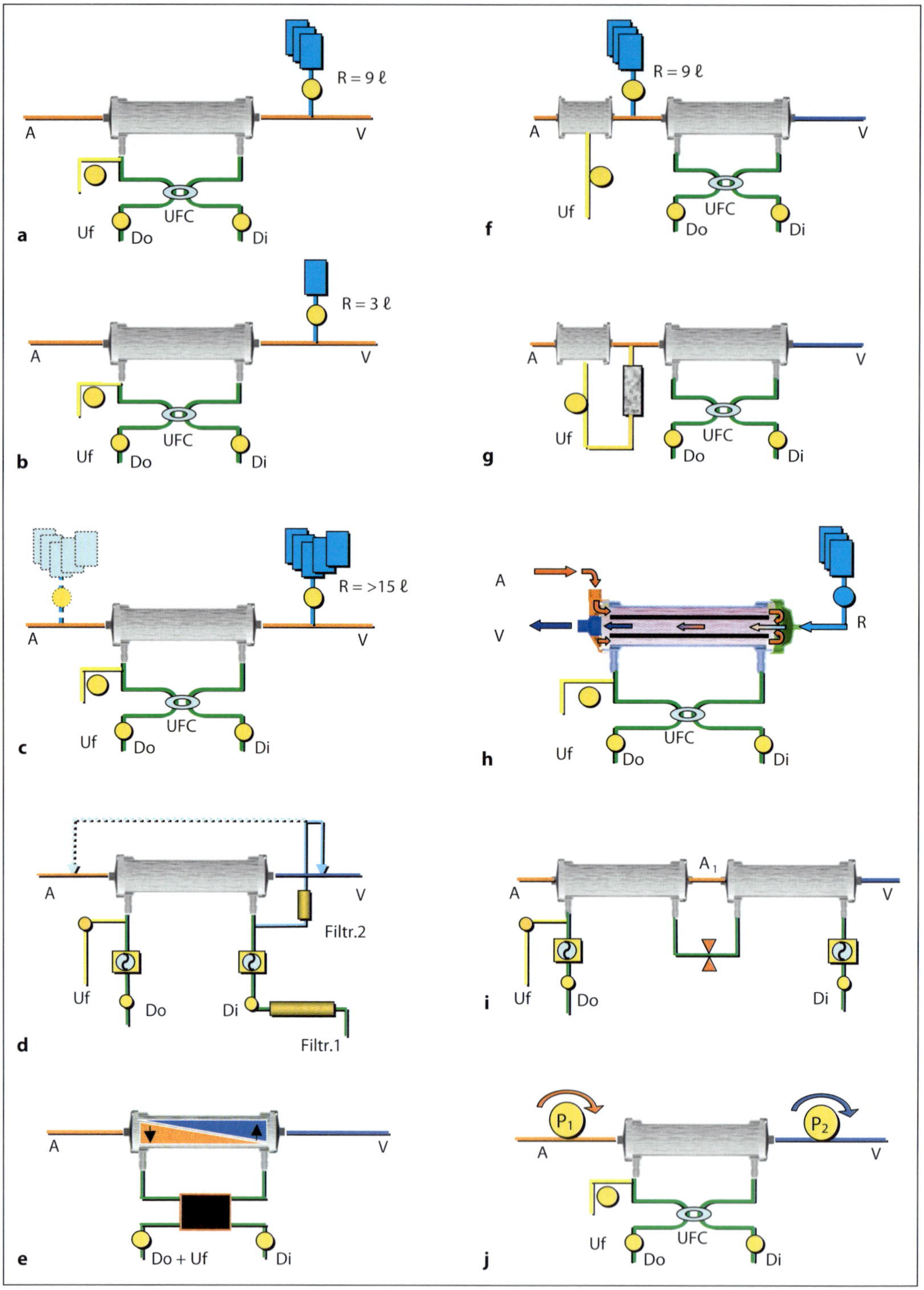

a
R = 9 ℓ
A
V
Uf
UFC
Do
Di
b
R = 3 ℓ
A
V
Uf
UFC
Do
Di
c
R = >15 ℓ
A
V
Uf
UFC
Do
Di
d
A
V
Filtr.2
Uf
Do
Di
Filtr.1
e
A
V
Do + Uf
Di
f
R = 9 ℓ
A
V
Uf
UFC
Do
Di
g
A
V
Uf
UFC
Do
Di
h
A
V
R
Uf
UFC
Do
Di
i
A
A1
V
Uf
Do
Di
j
P1
P2
A
V
Uf
UFC
Do
Di

*Mid-Dilution HDF:* This novel set-up consists of special filters with two longitudinal compartments (fig. 2h). Blood flow in the first compartment produces ultrafiltration, and at the end of the compartment, blood is redirected countercurrent into the second blood compartment. Blood leaves the dialyzer alongside the arterial entry. On the venous end of the dialyzer is a chamber designed to receive replacement fluid infusion and to reconstitute blood composition. Dialysate flows 50% countercurrent to blood, and 50% concurrent with blood [8].

*Double High-Flux HDF:* Also a technique utilizing two high-flux dialyzers in series: filtration in the proximal filter, backfiltration in the distal unit (fig. 2i). High blood flows and high efficiency enable treatments under 2 h/session [9].

*Push-Pull HDF:* Alternating filtration and backfiltration, produced by alternating pre- and post-filter pumps, are used. When the post-filter pump is stopped the filtration occurs, and when the pre-filter pump is stopped the negative pressure induced in the blood compartment produces backfiltration (fig. 2j) [10].

## Mechanism of Hemodiafiltration

Dialysis adequacy is a strong independent factor associated with various outcomes in end-stage renal disease (ESRD), including mortality, anemia, nutrition and cardiovascular disease. European data from the DOPPS study showed that patients on HDF achieved significantly higher Kt/V urea values compared to patients receiving hemodialysis (HD) [11]. Other studies have also demonstrated that urea and creatinine removal are increased in high-efficiency OLHDF by 10–15%, and maintained over time compared with high-efficiency HD [12–14].

HDF has also been shown to compare favorably with HD in terms of removal of various larger solutes. With the addition of convective solute clearance, HDF enhances phosphate removal, reaching up to 30–35 mM/session [15]. Patients on low-efficiency HDF had lower serum phosphate levels compared to those on low-flux HD [11]. In randomized cross-over studies, phosphate levels were significantly lower with HDF [14, 16]. Since the calcium-phosphate product and vitamin D-parathyroid hormone axis have been recently implicated as important factors associated with cardiovascular disease in ESRD patients, better phosphate removal achieved with HDF may contribute to cardioprotection in this population. Controlled trials have also shown a 20–30% greater reduction of $\beta_2$-microglobulin per session with OLHDF than with high-flux HD, resulting in lower serum $\beta_2$-microglobulin levels sustained over time [14, 17, 18]. This may be relevant in reducing dialysis-related amyloidosis (DRA). Other larger solutes

**Fig. 2.** Different techniques of HDF graphically depicted (explanation of the mechanisms in the text): (**a**) classic HDF, (**b**) 'soft' HDF, (**c**) 'hard' HDF, (**d**) online HDF, (**e**) internal filtration HDF, (**f**) paired filtration dialysis, (**g**) online HDF with endogenous reinfusion, (**h**) mid-dilution HDF, (**i**) double high-flux HDF, and (**j**) push-pull HDF.

which HDF appears to clear more efficiently include myoglobin and retinal-binding protein [19], protein-bound solutes such as *p*-cresol [20], homocysteine [21], and leptin [22]. HDF is hypothesized to remove protein-bound forms or inhibitors of homocysteine metabolism [21]. Leptin is also removed efficiently by HDF, and lower blood leptin levels have been reported in long-term HDF patients [22]. OLHDF also reduces circulating levels of advanced glycosylation end products which have been implicated in the pathogenesis of both DRA and atherosclerosis [23]. These may all potentially favor the improvement of nutritional and cardiovascular status, although these clinical endpoints have not yet been evaluated in a rigorous manner.

## Clinical Outcomes Achieved by HDF

Although HDF was first introduced decades ago, early evidence was not sufficient to substantiate its widespread use. More recently, several comparative studies, using one or more of the above techniques, have yielded promising results. A brief summary of the clinical effects of HDF variants is presented.

Intradialytic hypotension is the most common acute complication of HD, and has been associated with poor patient outcomes [24, 25]. 20–30% of dialysis sessions are complicated by dialysis hypotension [17, 26]. This is believed to be due to rapid removal of solutes and fluids, particularly in patients at increased risk. These include the elderly, diabetics, and those with autonomic insufficiency and structural heart disease. Reduction in the frequency of this complication could contribute significantly to improve the quality of life of patients, and possibly even improve outcome. Several observational studies suggest better intradialytic hemodynamic stability when patients were treated by convective therapies, including HDF [14, 26]. A meta-analysis of randomized controlled studies confirmed that systolic blood pressure during dialysis was significantly higher, and maximal drop in systolic pressure was less with convective modalities as compared to HD [18]. The precise mechanisms by which HDF maintains the arterial pressure during dialysis are not completely understood. One possible factor is an increase in peripheral vascular tone and vascular refilling rate due to neutral thermal balance, particularly with high volume exchange [26]. Other factors which have been speculated include the high sodium concentration of the replacement fluid, release of vasoconstrictor mediators, clearance of vasodilator mediators, and improvement of sympathetic activity.

DRA is a disorder caused by tissue deposition of $\beta_2$-microglobulin as amyloid fibrils. A registry study by Locatelli et al. [27] concluded that convective modalities, including HDF and hemofiltration, reduced the need for carpal tunnel surgery. However, the beneficial effect of convective clearances per se in this study may have been partly confounded by the simultaneous improvement of other factors. DRA is a difficult clinical endpoint to evaluate adequately through randomized studies, since it takes years for the clinical and radiologic manifestations of amyloidosis to appear. Moreover, there is a great deal of variability in the clinical assessment of DRA. Clinical symptoms, electroneurography, and X-rays have all been used to assess manifestations of DRA making it difficult to combine results from different studies looking at this outcome [18].

Anemia is an independent risk factor for left ventricular hypertrophy, cardiovascular and overall mortality in dialysis patients, and also impacts quality of life. A number of studies suggest that anemia was improved and recombinant human erythropoietin doses reduced in patients treated by HDF [11, 16, 28], and anemia correction was also associated with reduced inflammation [28]. These suggest that HDF may remove some specific receptor antagonists of erythropoietin, or, through the use of superior quality dialysate fluid, reduce the inflammatory state of patients, thereby increasing the sensitivity of erythroblasts to the drug.

Despite several technological improvements in both dialysis and overall patient care, mortality of ESRD patients remains unacceptably high. The quest to improve dialysis patient outcomes has led investigators to look towards convective therapies such as HDF, with their superior clearance for larger solutes. Data from initial small randomized studies have yielded disappointing results. A systematic review of 20 randomized studies on HDF, HF and HD for ESRD examined various endpoints, including mortality [18]. The meta-analysis for mortality included 6 studies (pooled sample size = 388) with follow-up ranging from 12 to 48 months, and showed that mortality was not significantly different for convective modalities compared to HD (RR 1.68, 95% CI, 0.23–12.13). However, the authors cautioned that there were no deaths in four of the analyzed studies and there was significant inter-trial heterogeneity. In addition, many of these studies were performed prior to the era of online production of replacement fluid, and had relatively low fluid exchange rates, falling into the category of 'soft' HDF.

More recently, analysis of 2,165 patients from the DOPPS study showed that patients receiving HDF treatment had a reduced risk of death compared to those treated by conventional HD, even though HDF patients had more co-morbid and cardiovascular conditions [11]. This mortality difference persisted after correction for demographic factors, co-morbid conditions, and several potentially confounding therapy-related factors, including dialysis vintage and Kt/V urea (RR 0.65, $p = 0.01$). Likewise, an analysis of 2,564 patients from a dialysis provider database also showed a 42.7% reduction in mortality risk with HDF [29]. These observational studies suggest that HDF may improve patient survival independently of its higher small solute clearance. A potential explanation for the apparent decrease in mortality is the enhancement of both the removal of middle molecular toxins as well as the biocompatibility of the dialysis system, through the use of ultrapure dialysate and highly permeable synthetic membranes. This hypothesis is strengthened by the finding that the relative reduction in mortality risk appears to be proportional to the intensity of the convective clearance, which itself is linearly related to the amount of fluid exchanged during the sessions [11]. Putative beneficial effects of HDF on inflammatory stress, as well as intermediate endpoints such as calcium-phosphate balance, lipid and homocysteine profile and anemia, as have been discussed above, may also contribute to this apparent reduction in mortality.

## Conclusion

In summary, the evolution of technology has made HDF simpler, safer and more effective. Emerging evidence suggests that these therapies may be superior to classic diffusive HD in terms of morbidity, and perhaps even mortality. There is a need for better understanding of the mechanisms involved, as well as further confirmation of these encouraging findings with prospective controlled trials. Nevertheless, HDF appears a promising alterative to improve dialysis patient outcomes, and may become the new gold standard in the years to come.

## References


1 Henderson LW: Biophysics of UF and hemofiltration; in Maher JF (ed): Replacement of Renal Function by Dialysis. A Textbook of Dialysis, ed 3. Dordrecht, Kluwer Academic, 1989, pp 300–326.

2 Ledebo I: Online preparation of solutions for dialysis: practical aspects versus safety and regulations. J Am Soc Nephrol 2002; 13(suppl 1):S78–S83.

3 Ronco C, Cruz D: Hemodiafiltration history, technology, and clinical results. Adv Chronic Kidney Dis 2007;14:231–243.

4 Maduell F: Hemodiafiltration. Hemodial Int 2005;9:47–55.

5 Pedrini LA, Cozzi G, Faranna P, Mercieri A, Ruggiero P, Zerbi S, Feliciani A, Riva A: Transmembrane pressure modulation in high-volume mixed hemodiafiltration to optimize efficiency and minimize protein loss. Kidney Int 2006;69:573–579.

6 Fiore GB, Guadagni G, Lupi A, Ricci Z, Ronco C: A new semiempirical mathematical model for prediction of internal filtration in hollow fiber hemodialyzers. Blood Purif 2006;24:555–568.

7 Mandolfo S, Corsi A, Wratten ML, Sereni L, Imbasciati E: Evaluation of hygiene and safety controls for online paired hemodiafiltration. Int J Artif Organs 2006;29:160–165.

8 Santoro A, Conz PA, De Cristofaro V, Acquistapace I, Gaggi R, Ferramosca E, Renaux JL, Rizzioli E, Wratten ML: Middilution: the perfect balance between convection and diffusion. Contrib Nephrol. Basel, Karger, 2005, vol 149, pp 107–114.

9 Miller J, von Albertini B, Gardner B, Shinaberger J: Technical aspects of high-flux hemodiafiltration for adequate short (under 2 hours) treatment. Trans Am Soc Artif Intern Organs 1984;30:377–379.

10 Miwa M, Shinzato T: Push-pull hemodiafiltration: technical aspects and clinical effectiveness. Artif Organs 1999;23:1123–1126.

11 Canaud B, Bragg-Gresham JL, Marshall MR, et al: Mortality risk for patients receiving hemodiafiltration versus hemodialysis: European results from the DOPPS. Kidney Int 2006;69:2087–2093.

12 Kerr PB, Argiles A, Flavier JL, et al: Comparison of hemodialysis and hemodiafiltration: a long-term longitudinal study. Kidney Int 1992;41:1035–1040.

13 Canaud B, Morena M, Leray-Moragues H, Chalabi L, Cristol JP: Overview of clinical studies in hemodiafiltration: what do we need now? Hemodial Int 2006; 10(suppl 1):S5–S12.

14 Schiffl H: Prospective randomized cross-over long-term comparison of online haemodiafiltration and ultrapure high-flux haemodialysis. Eur J Med Res 2007;12:26–33.
15 Lornoy W, De Meester J, Becaus I, et al: Impact of convective flow on phosphorus removal in maintenance hemodialysis patients. J Ren Nutr 2006;16:47–53.
16 Vaslaki L, Major L, Berta K, Karatson A, Misz M, Pethoe F, Ladanyi E, Fodor B, Stein G, Pischetsrieder M, Zima T, Wojke R, Gauly A, Passlick-Deetjen J: Online haemodiafiltration versus haemodialysis: stable haematocrit with less erythropoietin and improvement of other relevant blood parameters. Blood Purif 2006;24:163–173.
17 Lin CL, Yang CW, Chiang CC, et al: Long-term online hemodiafiltration reduces predialysis $\beta_2$-microglobulin levels in chronic hemodialysis patients. Blood Purif 2001;19:301–307.
18 Rabindranath KS, Strippoli GF, Roderick P, et al: Comparison of hemodialysis, hemofiltration, and acetate-free biofiltration for ESRD: systematic review. Am J Kidney Dis 2005;45:437–447.
19 Maduell F, Navarro V, Cruz MC, et al: Osteocalcin and myoglobin removal in online hemodiafiltration versus low- and high-flux hemodialysis. Am J Kidney Dis 2002;40:582–589.
20 Bammens B, Evenepoel P, Verbeke K, et al: Removal of the protein-bound solute *p*-cresol by convective transport: a randomized crossover study. Am J Kidney Dis 2004;44:278–285.
21 Gonella M, Calabrese G, Mengozzi A, et al: The achievement of normal homocysteinemia in regular extracorporeal dialysis patients. J Nephrol 2004;17:411–413.
22 Wiesholzer M, Harm F, Hauser AC, et al: Inappropriately high plasma leptin levels in obese haemodialysis patients can be reduced by high-flux haemodialysis and haemodiafiltration. Clin Sci (Lond) 1998;94:431–435.
23 Lin CL, Huang CC, Yu CC, Yang HY, et al: Reduction of advanced glycation end product levels by online hemodiafiltration in long-term hemodialysis patients. Am J Kidney Dis 2003;42:524–531.
24 Sasaki O, Nakahama H, Nakamura S, Yoshihara F, Inenaga T, Yoshii M, Kohno S, Kawano Y: Orthostatic hypotension at the introductory phase of haemodialysis predicts all-cause mortality. Nephrol Dial Transplant 2005;20:377–381.
25 Shoji T, Tsubakihara Y, Fujii M, Imai E: Hemodialysis-associated hypotension as an independent risk factor for two-year mortality in hemodialysis patients. Kidney Int 2004;66:1212–1220.
26 Donauer J, Schweiger C, Rumberger B, et al: Reduction of hypotensive side effects during online-haemodiafiltration and low temperature haemodialysis. Nephrol Dial Transplant 2003;18:1616–1622.
27 Locatelli F, Marcelli D, Conte F, et al: Comparison of mortality in ESRD patients on convective and diffusive extracorporeal treatments. The Registro Lombardo Dialisi E Trapianto. Kidney Int 1999;55:286–293.
28 Sitter T, Bergner A, Schiffl H: Dialysate related cytokine induction and response to recombinant human erythropoietin in haemodialysis patients. Nephrol Dial Transplant 2000;15:1207–1211.
29 Jirka T, Cesare S, Di Benedetto A, Perera Chang M, Ponce P, Richards N, Tetta C, Vaslaky L: Mortality risk for patients receiving hemodiafiltration versus hemodialysis. Kidney Int 2006;70:1524.

Claudio Ronco, MD, Director
Department of Nephrology, San Bortolo Hospital
Viale Rodolfi 37, IT–36100 Vicenza (Italy)
Tel. +39 0 444 753650, Fax +39 0 444 753973
E-Mail cronco@goldnet.it

Kawanishi H, Yamashita AC (eds): Hemodiafiltration – A New Era.
Contrib Nephrol. Basel, Karger, 2011, vol 168, pp 28–38

# Optimal Therapeutic Conditions for Online Hemodiafiltration

Bernard Canaud[a,b] · Leila Chenine[a] · Sophie Renaud[a] · Hélène Leray[a]

[a]Lapeyronie Hospital, Nephrology, Montpellier, and [b]Renal Research and Training Institute, Montpellier, France

**Abstract**

The safety of online hemodiafiltration (ol-HDF) relies on very strict rules of use. The use of ultrapure water to feed an ol-HDF machine is a basic requirement for ol-HDF. Technical aspects and microbial monitoring have been precisely described in the European Best Practice Guidelines. Specifically designed and certified ol-HDF machines are needed. All these machines share the production of substitution fluid by the cold sterilization process of fresh dialysate based on ultrafilters. Hygiene handling is a crucial measure to ensure permanent safety of the ol-HDF system. Frequent disinfection of the water treatment system and dialysis machine, destruction of biofilm by chemical agents and/or thermochemical disinfection, change of filters at regular intervals, and maintenance of a permanent circulation of water are among the basic measures required to ensure ultrapurity of water and dialysis fluid. Optimal performances of ol-HDF require the use of high blood flow (300–400 ml/min), highly permeable and adequately sized hemodiafilters, a high volume of substitution (5–6 l/h) and high dialysate flow (500 ml/min). The site and type of substitution (pre-, post-, mixed, and mid-dilution) should be customized to each patient according to its blood hemorheology and its filtration fraction limitation (transmembrane pressure). All attempts should be made to maximize the fluid volume exchange per session (convective dose) in any cases. The treatment schedule in terms of session duration and weekly frequency need to be adjusted individually to improve hemodynamic tolerance, to facilitate correction of fluid overload and to increase dialysis dose (for middle-sized solutes) in order to reduce circulating levels of major uremic toxins. ol-HDF is the more advanced form of renal replacement therapy offering high efficiency over a large spectrum of toxins, high biocompatibility profile and high flexible modality. ol-HDF may help to improve global care of chronic kidney disease patients and may be considered the renal replacement therapy of the future.

Today, online hemodiafiltration (ol-HDF) provides the more efficient and the most biocompatible modality of renal replacement therapy for chronic kidney disease (CKD) patients. By combining diffusive and enhanced convective clearances, ol-HDF offers the highest instantaneous solute clearances over a wide molecular weight range of uremic toxins [1–4]. By reducing the hemoincompatible profile of the dialysis system, ol-HDF reduces exposure to the chronic microinflammation state of CKD patients [5, 6]. High-efficient ol-HDF is now a well-established treatment modality with an increased prevalent use in CKD patients [7–9].

Online production of substitution fluid by 'cold sterilization' of dialysis fluid gives access to a virtually unlimited amount of sterile and non-pyrogenic solution permitting to optimize the treatment modality to the patient's needs [10–12]. Implementing ol-HDF module onto the hemodialysis machine has several advantages: it simplifies the handling procedure for nursing staff and technician; it secures the technical process by coupling the infusion/ultrafiltration module to the safety monitoring of the ol-HDF machine, and it permits online ultrafilter integrity monitoring by pressure test [13]. ol-HDF provides a multipurpose platform that permits to develop and customize ol-HDF options (HDF with post-, pre- mixed, and mid-dilution) to patient's metabolic needs and hemorheologic conditions [14–17].

## Technical Prerequisite and Basic Hygienic Rules for ol-HDF

The safety of ol-HDF relies on strict rules of use. Strict compliance with usual guidelines is the only to warranty success of the ol-HDF therapy program. The use of ultrapure water to feed the ol-HDF machine is a basic requirement for ol-HDF [18]. Ultrapure water is high-grade quality water which has been developed mainly to satisfy the needs of the semiconductor industry. For ol-HDF purposes, ultrapure water refers to reverse osmosis-treated water (two stages of reverse osmosis in series) with a resistivity in the range of 10–20 MΩ with a very low level of bacterial and endotoxin contamination (≥100 CFU/l, endotoxin LAL <0.03 EU/ml). Distribution pipes must be adequately designed to prevent stagnation, to eliminate dead arms and other recontamination sites. Permanent recirculation of treated water through a closed loop circuit with a microfiltration system is required particularly when a buffer tank is used [19].

The use of specifically designed ol-HDF and European Community (EC)-certified machine is necessary. Several ol-HDF-certified machines are presently available on the European market (fig. 1). Basically, these ol-HDF machines share common features including an infusion pump with a flow-measuring system, a dialysate ultrafilter module (usually two ultrafilters in series) placed onto the hydraulic circuit of the machine and controlled by the dialysis machine's monitoring system (fig. 2, 3). The infusate module consists in an adjustable

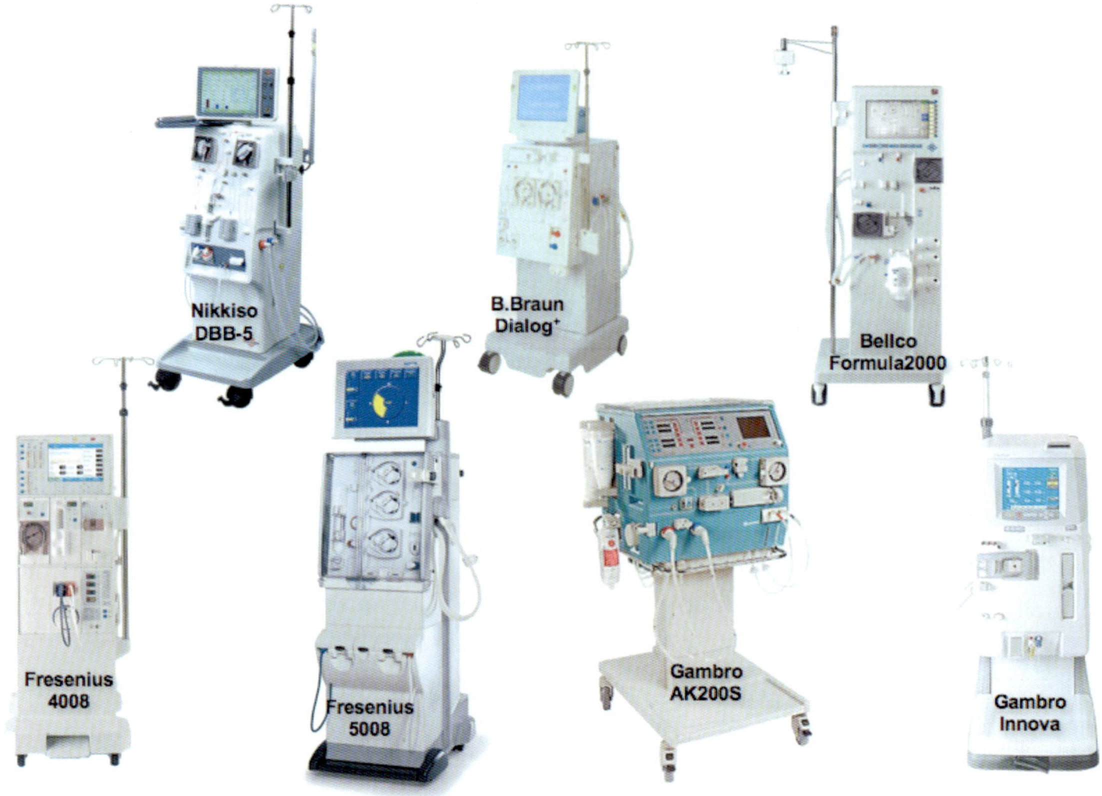


**Fig. 1.** Certified ol-HDF machines available on the European market.

pump running up to 200 ml/min with a counter calculating the total amount of fluid infused into the patient. The pump segment is a disposable plastic tubing replaced after each session. The built-in tubing part of the infusate module is disinfected simultaneously with each process of the disinfection process of the ol-HDF machine. Ultrapure dialysate flowing through the dialysate compartment of the hemodiafilter pass through an ultrafilter (UF1) placed at the exit site of the dialysate. A fraction of the fresh dialysate (100–200 ml/min) produced by the proportioning ol-HDF system is diverted by the infusion pump and infused directly into the patient's bloodstream (either post-, pre- or pre- and post-filter through mixing chambers). Ultrapurity of the infusate is then secured by a second ultrafilter (UF2) placed just before the patient's infusion site [20, 21]. Infusate diverted from the inlet dialysate is compensated by an equivalent ultrafiltration flow dragged from the patient, thanks to the fluid-balancing module. Ultrafilters are a captive part of the machine being disinfected after each ol-HDF run and changed periodically.

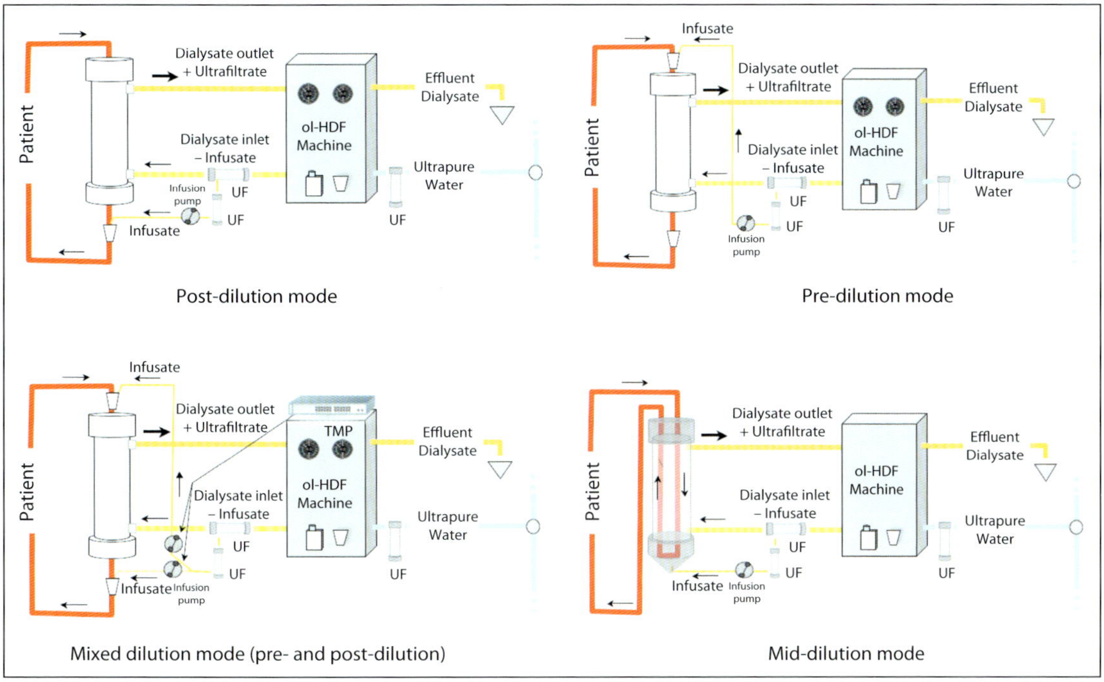


**Fig. 2.** Schematic representation of conventional ol-HDF machines (post-, pre-, mixed, and mid-dilution modality).

Hygiene handling is a crucial measure to ensure permanent safety of the ol-HDF system. Frequent disinfection of the water treatment system and dialysis machine, destruction of biofilm by chemical agents and/or thermochemical disinfection, change of filters at regular intervals, and maintenance of a permanent circulation of water are among the basic measures required to ensure ultrapurity of water and dialysis fluid [22].

Quality monitoring of the dialysate and the infusate is mandatory to detect early microbiologic contamination of the system. A microbiologic inventory of water, dialysate and infusate should be performed according to best practice guidelines and pharmacopeia regulation [23].

## Prerequisite and Technical Options of ol-HDF

### *Vascular Access*

Patients treated with ol-HDF require a vascular access capable of delivering regularly a blood flow of 350–400 ml/min. High blood flow facilitates ultrafiltration rate and reduces the transmembrane pressure regime during the session.

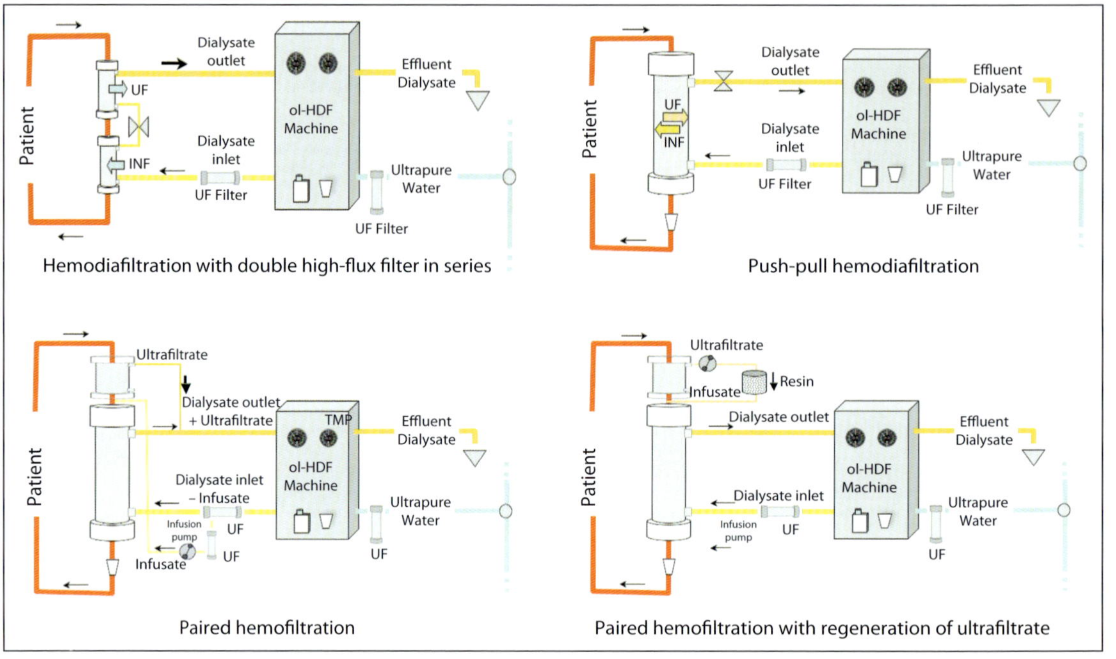


**Fig. 3.** Schematic representation of alternative ol-HDF machines (push-pull, double high-flux, PHF, and PHF with regeneration).

It must be acknowledged that based on new technical options and filter design, ol-HDF may be performed with reduced blood flow or catheters [24].

*Hemodiafilter*

The use of highly permeable hemodiafilters is mandatory. High hydraulic permeability ($K_{UF}$ ≥50 ml/h/mm Hg) and high solute permeability ($K_oA$ urea >600 and $\beta_2$-microglobulin ($\beta_2$-MG) >60 ml/min) with large surface area (1.50–2.10 $m^2$) dialyzers are needed. The size and design of hemodiafilters must be selected according to the blood flow regime and targeted performances [25, 26].

*Conventional ol-HDF* relies on the combination of diffusive and forced convective clearances in the same hemodiafilter module (see fig. 2). Basically, the substitution fluid (infusate) is a sterile non-pyrogenic solution produced extemporaneously from fresh dialysate and infused directly into the patient's blood at the venous site. Infusate diverted from the inlet dialysate is isovolumetrically compensated by ultrafiltering the patient via the fluid-balancing system of the dialysis machine. The ultrafiltration rate is coupled to infusion flow by adapting continuously the transmembrane pressure regime. Weight loss required to correct patient fluid overload is taken out in addition to this coupled infusion/ultrafiltration flow.

Depending on the infusion site of fluid substitution, several ol-HDF modalities have been described [27]: *postdilution ol-HDF* (infusion after the hemodiafilter); *predilution ol-HDF* (infusion before the hemodiafilter) [28]; *mid-dilution ol-HDF* (infusion between the ultrafiltration and diffusion compartment) [29, 30], and *mixed ol-HDF* (simultaneous infusion pre- and post-hemodiafilter) [31].

ol-HDF requires preferably the use of high blood flow rates (blood flow 350–450 and dialysate 600–800 ml/min). It is recommended to couple the infusion rate to effective blood flow for optimizing filtration fraction (20–30% maximum) and prevent filter fouling. In order to achieve equivalent small molecules clearances, recommended infusion flow rates are 100 ml/min (24 l for a 4-hour session) in postdilution mode and 200 ml/min (48 l for a 4-hour session) in predilution mode. Mid-dilution ol-HDF options (conventional of reversed configuration) have been proposed to enhance solute clearance performances [32, 33]. Mixed pre- and postdilution ol-HDF represents a recently introduced technical option for optimizing hemorheological conditions and for enhancing performances [34]. Pre- to postinfusion flow ratio is feedback-controlled by an ol-HDF monitor for maintaining the transmembrane pressure in a safe and optimal filtration regime [35].

*Alternative ol-HDF methods* have been described over the last decade. They are briefly described in the next section and presented in figure 3.

Push-pull hemodiafiltration is based on a double-cylinder piston pump (push-pull pump) implemented on the effluent dialysate line of the dialysis machine. Based on this alternate pump device, 25 alternate cycles of 20 ml of ultrafiltration (pull) and backfiltration (push) are performed through the hemodialyzer per minute meaning that 120 l of ultrafiltered plasma water are backfiltered from the fresh inlet dialysate in a 4-hour treatment [36, 37].

Double high-flux HD consists in two high-flux dialyzers assembled in series while the dialysis fluid irrigates countercurrently the two dialyzers [38, 39]. By means of an adjustable clamp restriction placed on the dialysis fluid pathway between the two dialyzers, ultrafiltration is promoted in the first dialyzer and backfiltration in the second dialyzer [40, 41].

Paired hemofiltration (PHF) is a double chamber ol-HDF technique that was initially proposed to separate convective and diffusive solute fluxes in two modules [42]. This method is based on the association of two high-flux dialyzers in series, one with a small surface (0.4 $m^2$) that permits the infusion of substitution fluid (backfiltration) and the second a high-flux hemodialyzer (1.8 $m^2$) that allows convective and diffusive exchange from dialysate. The substitution fluid produced by cold sterilization from the fresh dialysis fluid is infused either on predilution mode or on postdilution mode according to the position of the dialyzer [43].

Hemodiafiltration with endogenous reinfusion (HFR) derives from PHF. The main feature of HFR is the online regeneration of the ultrafiltrate by an adsorbing device [44]. The regenerated ultrafiltrate is then reinfused as an endogenous substitution fluid [45]. HFR has been evaluated in several clinical trials and appears to be beneficial on inflammatory, oxidative stress and nutritional markers [46–48].

## ol-HDF Prescription in Practice

A conventional ol-HDF treatment schedule based on three dialysis sessions per week of 4 h (12 h/week) requires a high blood flow (400 ml/min) coupled with a high dialysate and/or infusate flow to optimize solute exchange [49]. Increasing the frequency and/or duration of ol-HDF sessions may help to enhance effectiveness and physiological profile of intermittent dialysis [50, 51].

ol-HDF-treated patients should be observed and monitored as those treated by conventional hemodialysis methods. Dialysis adequacy targets are equivalents: extracellular fluid volume control, blood pressure control, minimum dialysis dose delivered (urea Kt/V >1.4), uremia control, acidosis and hyperkalemia correction, bone and mineral disorder correction, and anemia correction.

ol-HDF provides a higher solute removal rate for middle-size uremic toxins including $\beta_2$-MG. Blood $\beta_2$-MG concentrations, considered a surrogate of middle molecules, should be part of long-term surveillance. It is usually recommended to target predialysis $\beta_2$-MG concentrations <25 mg/l. Inflammation (CRP) and nutritional markers (albumin and transthyretin) should be monitored on a monthly basis in ol-HDF patients targeting normal values.

## Handling and Microbial Monitoring of ol-HDF

Regular disinfection procedures and water and dialysis fluid monitoring are mandatory for conducting ol-HDF therapies. A complete disinfection of the ol-HDF machine (chemical, heat or mixed) is recommended after each ol-HDF run. Periodical changes of ultrafilters installed on inlet dialysate and infusate lines should be performed according to the manufacturer's instructions. Disinfection of the water treatment system and water distribution circuit should be performed at a minimum on a monthly basis. Disinfection modality (chemical, heat or mixed) and periodicity may vary from one dialysis center to another according to practices and results, but should comply in all circumstances with the manufacturer's recommendations and microbiological and clinical results. Daily disinfection procedures of the water distribution pipe using heat or mixed heat/chemical procedures appear to be the best way to prevent bacterial contamination and biofilm formation [52].

Microbiological monitoring of the water treatment chain and ol-HDF machines should comply with best practices and country specificities [53]. The basic principles of these good clinical practices have been detailed in the ERA-EDTA best practices recommendations [54]. Today, virtually all international recommendations related to water and dialysis fluid purity tend to converge on the same targets and very close monitoring procedures [55]. Microbiological monitoring should include the culture of water and/or dialysate and the determination of endotoxin content. Sampling method, culture media and delay for observation have been published elsewhere. Membrane filtration and culture on a poor nutrient media ($R_2A$) are strongly recommended [56, 57]. Cultures are maintained at room temperature (20–22°C) and observed for 7 days. Endotoxin content (infusate and dialysate) should be performed with a sensitive LAL assay with a threshold detection limit of 0.03 EU/ml. Some divergences may occur according to country specificities on frequency of water and dialysate monitoring and reporting. Water-feeding ol-HDF machines should be performed more frequently during the validation phase and at least monthly during the maintenance period. Dialysis fluid produced by proportioning ol-HDF machines should be performed at least quarterly and frequency needs to be adjusted according to the results.

## Conclusions

At the present time, ol-HDF modalities offer the most effective renal replacement modality for CKD-5 patients [58–60]. By enhancing the convective fluxes, ol-HDF enlarges the spectrum and increases the uremic toxin mass removed. ol-HDF improves the hemocompatibility profile, reduces the cost of treatment and simplifies the technical aspect of the method. With these unique features, ol-HDF should be considered a dialysis platform permitting to develop new options such as feedback-controlled volemia and automation of priming and restitution. Currently, ol-HDF offers the best technical options for enhancing dialysis efficacy and improving global care of dialysis patients and finally profiling the renal replacement therapy of the future [61].

## References


1 Sprenger KB: Haemodiafiltration. Life Support Syst 1983;1:127–136.
2 Ofsthun NJ, Leypoldt JK: Ultrafiltration and backfiltration during hemodialysis. Artif Organs 1995;19:1143–1161.
3 Leypoldt JK: Solute fluxes in different treatment modalities. Nephrol Dial Transplant 2000;1:3–9.
4 Ledebo I: On-line hemodiafiltration: technique and therapy. Adv Ren Replace Ther 1999;6:195–208.
5 Canaud B, Bosc JY, Leray H, Stec F, Argiles A, Leblanc M, Mion C: On-line haemodiafiltration: state of the art. Nephrol Dial Transplant 1998;5:3–11.

6 Canaud B, Wizemann V, Pizzarelli F, Greenwood R, Schultze G, Weber C, Falkenhagen D: Cellular interleukin-1 receptor antagonist production in patients receiving on-line haemodiafiltration therapy. Nephrol Dial Transplant 2001;16:2181–2187.
7 Leber HW, Wizemann V, Goubeaud G, Rawer P, Schutterle G: Hemodiafiltration: a new alternative to hemofiltration and conventional hemodialysis. Artif Organs 1978;2:150–153.
8 Passlick-Deetjen J, Pohlmeier R: On-line hemodiafiltration. Gold standard or top therapy? Contrib Nephrol. Basel, Karger, 2002, vol 137, pp 201–211.
9 Van Laecke S, De Wilde K, Vanholder R: Online hemodiafiltration. Artif Organs 2006;30:579–585.
10 Henderson LW, Sanfelippo ML, Beans E: On-line preparation of sterile pyrogen-free electrolyte solution. Trans Am Soc Artif Intern Organs 1978;24:465–467.
11 Shinzato T, Sezaki R, Usuda M, Maeda K, Ohbayashi S, Toyota T: Infusion-free hemodiafiltration: simultaneous hemofiltration and dialysis with no need for infusion fluid. Artif Organs 1982;4:453–456.
12 Canaud B, Flavier JL, Argilés A, Stec F, Nguyen QV, Bouloux C, Garred LJ, Mion C: Hemodiafiltration with on-line production of substitution fluid: long-term safety and quantitative assessment of efficacy. Contrib Nephrol. Basel, Karger, 1994, vol 108, pp 12–22.
13 Canaud B, Nguyen QV, Argilés A, Polito C, Polaschegg HD, Mion C: Hemodiafiltration using dialysate as substitution fluid. Artif Organs 1987;11:188–190.
14 Sterby J: A decade of experience with on-line hemofiltration/hemodiafiltration. Contrib Nephrol. Basel, Karger, 1994, vol 108, pp 1–11.
15 Lonnemann G, Behme TC, Lenzner B, Floege J, Schulze M, Colton CK, Koch KM, Shaldon S: Permeability of dialyzer membranes to TNF-α-inducing substances derived from water bacteria. Kidney Int 1992;42:61–68.
16 Pedrini LA, De Cristofaro V, Pagliari B, Samà F: Mixed predilution and postdilution online hemodiafiltration compared with the traditional infusion modes. Kidney Int 2000;58:2155–2165.
17 Canaud B, Chenine L, Henriet D, Leray H: Online hemodiafiltration: a multipurpose therapy for improving quality of renal replacement therapy. Contrib Nephrol. Basel, Karger, 2008, vol 161, pp 191–198.
18 Canaud B, Peyronnet P, Armynot AM, et al: Ultrapure water: a need for future dialysis. Nephrol Dial Transplant 1986;1:110.
19 Canaud BJM, Mion CM: Water treatment for contemporary dialysis; in Jacob C, Kjellstrand KM, Koch KM, Winchester J (eds): Replacement of Renal Function by Dialysis. Section II. Berlin, Springer, 1996, pp 231–255.
20 Schindler R, Lonnemann G, Schaffer J, Shaldon S, Koch KM, Krautzig S: The effect of ultrafiltered dialysate on the cellular content of interleukin-1 receptor antagonist in patients on chronic hemodialysis. Nephron 1994;68:229–233.
21 Mion CM, Canaud B: Should hemodialysis fluid be sterile? Semin Dial 1993;6:28–30.
22 Cappelli G, Sereni L, Scialoja MG, Morselli M, Perrone S, Ciuffreda A, Bellesia M, Inguaggiato P, Albertazzi A, Tetta C: Effects of biofilm formation on haemodialysis monitor disinfection. Nephrol Dial Transplant 2003;18:2105–2111.
23 Pass T, Wright R, Sharp B, Harding GB: Culture of dialysis fluids on nutrient-rich media for short periods at elevated temperatures underestimate microbial contamination. Blood Purif 1996;14:136–145.
24 Mandolfo S, Borlandelli S, Imbasciati E, Badalamenti S, Graziani G, Sereni L, Varesani M, Wratten ML, Corsi A, Elli A: Pilot study to assess increased dialysis efficiency in patients with limited blood flow rates due to vascular access problems. Hemodial Int 2008;12:55–61.
25 Ronco C, Orlandini G, Brendolan A, Lupi A, La Greca G: Enhancement of convective transport by internal filtration in a modified experimental hemodialyzer: technical note. Kidney Int. 1998;54:979–985.
26 Hoenich NA: Membranes and filters for haemodiafiltration. Contrib Nephrol. Basel, Karger, 2007, vol 158, pp 57–67.
27 Canaud B: Online hemodiafiltration. Technical options and best clinical practices. Contrib Nephrol. Basel, Karger, 2007, vol 158, pp 110–122.

28 Canaud B, Lévesque R, Krieter D, Desmeules S, Chalabi L, Moragués H, Morena M, Cristol JP: On-line hemodiafiltration as routine treatment of end-stage renal failure: why pre- or mixed dilution mode is necessary in on-line hemodiafiltration today? Blood Purif 2004;22(suppl 2):40–48.
29 Feliciani A, Riva MA, Zerbi S, Ruggiero P, Plati AR, Cozzi G, Pedrini LA: New strategies in haemodiafiltration (HDF): prospective comparative analysis between on-line mixed HDF and mid-dilution HDF. Nephrol Dial Transplant. 2007;22:1672–1679.
30 Pedrini LA, Feliciani A, Zerbi S, Cozzi G, Ruggiero P: Optimization of mid-dilution haemodiafiltration: technique and performance. Nephrol Dial Transplant 2009;24:2816–2824.
31 Pedrini LA, De Cristofaro V, Pagliari B, et al: Mixed predilution and postdilution online hemodiafiltration compared with the traditional infusion modes. Kidney Int 2000;58:2155.
32 Krieter DH, Falkenhain S, Chalabi L, Collins G, Lemke HD, Canaud B: Clinical cross-over comparison of mid-dilution hemodiafiltration using a novel dialyzer concept and post-dilution hemodiafiltration. Kidney Int 2005;67:349–356.
33 Santoro A, Ferramosca E, Mancini E, Monari C, Varasani M, Sereni L, Wratten M: Reverse mid-dilution: new way to remove small and middle molecules as well as phosphate with high intrafilter convective clearance. Nephrol Dial Transplant 2007;22:2000–2005.
34 Pedrini LA, Zerbi S: Mixed dilution hemodiafiltration. Contrib Nephrol. Basel, Karger, 2007, vol 158, pp 123–130.
35 Joyeux V, Sijpkens Y, Haddj-Elmrabet A, Bijvoet AJ, Nilsson LG: Optimized convective transport with automated pressure control in on-line postdilution hemodiafiltration. Int J Artif Organs 2008;31:928–936.
36 Miwa M, Shinzato T: Push-pull hemodiafiltration: technical aspects and clinical effectiveness. Artif Organs 1999;23:1123.
37 Shinzato T, Maeda K: Push/pull hemodiafiltration. Contrib Nephrol Basel, Karger, 2007;158:169–176.
38 Von Albertini B, Miller JH, Gardner PW, Shinaberger JH: Performance characteristics of the hemoflow F-60 in high-flux hemodiafiltration. Contrib Nephrol. Basel, Karger, 1985;46:169–173.
39 Tiranathanagul K, Yossundharakul C, Techawathanawanna N, Katavetin P, Hanvivatvong O, Praditpornsilp K, Tungsanga K, Eiam-Ong S: Comparison of middle-molecule clearance between convective control double high-flux hemodiafiltration and on-line hemodiafiltration. Int J Artif Organs 2007;30:1090–1097.
40 Pisitkun T, Eiam-Ong S, Tiranathanagul K, Sakunsrijinda C, Manotham K, Hanvivatvong O, Suntaranuson P, Praditpornsilpa K, Chusil S, Tungsanga K: Convective-controlled double high-flux hemodiafiltration: a novel blood purification modality. Int J Artif Organs 2004;27:195–204.
41 Von Albertini B: Double high-flux hemodiafiltration. Contrib Nephrol. Basel, Karger, 2007, vol 158, pp 161–168.
42 Ghezzi PM, Botella J, Sartoris AM, et al: Use of the ultrafiltrate obtained in two-chamber (PFD) hemodiafiltration as replacement fluid. Experimental ex vivo and in vitro study. Int J Artif Organs 14:327, 1991
43 Pizzarelli F: Paired hemodiafiltration. Contrib Nephrol. Basel, Karger, 2007, vol 158, pp 131–137.
44 De Francisco AL, Pinera C, Heras M, Rodrigo E, Fernandez G, Ruiz JC, Tetta C, Arias M: Hemodafiltration with on-line endogenous reinfusion. Blood Purif 2000;18:231–236.
45 Marinez de Francisco AL, Ghezzi PM, Brendolan A, Fiorini F, La Greca G, Ronco C, Arias M, Gervasio R, Tetta C: Hemodiafiltration with online regeneration of the ultrafiltrate. Kidney Int Suppl 2000;76:S66–S71.
46 Panichi V, Manca-Rizza G, Paoletti S, Taccola D, Consani C, Filippi C, Mantuano E, Sidoti A, Grazi G, Antonelli A, Angelini D, Petrone I, Mura C, Tolaini P, Saloi F, Ghezzi PM, Barsotti G, Palla R: Effects on inflammatory and nutritional markers of haemodiafiltration with online regeneration of ultrafiltrate (HFR) vs. online haemodiafiltration: a cross-over randomized multicentre trial. Nephrol Dial Transplant 2006;21:756–762.

47 Calò LA, Naso A, Carraro G, Wratten ML, Pagnin E, Bertipaglia L, Rebeschini M, Davis PA, Piccoli A, Cascone C: Effect of haemodiafiltration with online regeneration of ultrafiltrate on oxidative stress in dialysis patients. Nephrol Dial Transplant. 2007;22:1413–1419.
48 Kim S, Oh KH, Chin HJ, Na KY, Kim YS, Chae DW, Ahn C, Han JS, Kim S, Joo KW: Effective removal of leptin via hemodiafiltration with on-line endogenous reinfusion therapy. Clin Nephrol 2009;72:442–448.
49 Maduell F: Optimizing the prescription of hemodiafiltration. Contrib Nephrol. Basel, Karger, 2007, vol 158, pp 225–231.
50 Maduell F, Navarro V, Torregrosa E, Rius A, Dicenta F, Cruz MC, Ferrero JA: Change from three times a week on-line hemodiafiltration to short daily on-line hemodiafiltration. Kidney Int 2003;64:305–313.
51 Fischbach M, Terzic J, Menouer S, Dheu C, Seuge L, Zalosczic A: Daily online haemodiafiltration promotes catch-up growth in children on chronic dialysis. Nephrol Dial Transplant 2010;25:867–873.
52 Cappelli G, Tetta C, Canaud B: Is biofilm a cause of silent chronic inflammation in haemodialysis patients? A fascinating working hypothesis. Nephrol Dial Transplant 2005;20:266–270.
53 Nystrand R: Official recommendations for quality of fluids in dialysis: the need for standardisation. J Ren Care 2009;35:74–81.
54 European Best Practice Guidelines for Haemodialysis – Part 1. Section IV. Dialysis fluid purity. Nephrol Dial Transplant 2002;1(suppl 7):45–62.
55 Kawanishi H, Masakane I, Tomo T: The new standard of fluids for hemodialysis in Japan. Blood Purif 2009;27(suppl 1):5–10.
56 Ward RA, Luehmann DA, Klein E: Are current standards for the microbiological purity of hemodialysate adequate? Semin Dial 1989;2:69–72.
57 Pass T, Wright R, Sharp B, Harding GB: Culture of dialysis fluids on nutrient-rich media for short periods at elevated temperatures underestimate microbial contamination. Blood Purif 1996;14:136–145.
58 Golper TA: What technological advances will significantly alter the future care of dialysis patients? Semin Dial 1994;7:323–324.
59 Canaud B, Kerr P, Argilés A, Flavier JL, Stec F, Mion C: Is hemodiafiltration the dialysis modality of choice for the next decade? Kidney Int 1993;43(suppl 41):S296–S299.
60 Van der Weerd NC, Penne EL, van den Dorpel MA, Grooteman MP, Nube MJ, Bots ML, Ter Wee PM, Blankestijn PJ: Haemodiafiltration: promise for the future? Nephrol Dial Transplant 2008;23:438–443.
61 Henderson LW: Dialysis in the 21st century. Am J Kidney Dis 1996;28;6:951–957.



Prof. Bernard Canaud
Nephrology, Dialysis and Intensive Care, Hôpital Lapeyronie, CHU Montpellier
371, Avenue du Doyen G. Giraud, FR–34925 Montpellier Cedex 05 (France)
Tel. +33 467 338955, Fax +33 467 603783, E-Mail b-canaud@chu-montpellier.fr

Kawanishi H, Yamashita AC (eds): Hemodiafiltration – A New Era.
Contrib Nephrol. Basel, Karger, 2011, vol 168, pp 39–52

# Effect of Hemodiafiltration on Mortality, Inflammation and Quality of Life

Claire H. den Hoedt[a,b] · Albert H.A. Mazairac[a] · Marinus A. van den Dorpel[b] · Muriel P.C. Grooteman[c,d] · Peter J. Blankestijn[a]

[a]Department of Nephrology, University Medical Center Utrecht, Utrecht, [b]Department of Internal Medicine, Maasstad Hospital, Rotterdam, [c]Department of Nephrology, VU Medical Center, Amsterdam, and [d]Institute for Cardiovascular Research VU Medical Center (ICaR-VU), VU Medical Center, Amsterdam, The Netherlands

**Abstract**

Online hemodiafiltration may improve clinical outcome in end-stage kidney disease. The supposed mechanism is the improved clearance of uremic toxins by the convective transport which is added to the standard diffusive transport. This review summarizes the effects of hemodiafiltration on mortality, inflammation and health-related quality of life.



Online hemodiafiltration ((ol)-HDF) is an increasingly applied dialysis modality, especially in Europe [1]. This is most likely caused by the fact that sterile dialysis fluids can now be produced online. HDF has the advantage of combining clearance of small molecular weight substances by diffusion, with clearance of middle and large molecular weight substances by convection [2]. HDF requires the use of synthetic high-flux membranes and ultrapure dialysate and sterile substitution fluids. Several studies suggest a potential benefit for patients treated with HDF [3–6]. It is hypothesized that increased clearance of a broader range of uremic substances leads to less inflammation, oxidative stress and endothelial dysfunction, which will result in less morbidity and mortality. We have previously reviewed several aspects of HDF [7–12].

C.H.d.H and A.H.A.M. contributed equally.

This review provides an overview on studies on the effects of HDF on mortality, inflammatory state and health-related quality of life (HRQOL). The importance of several practical issues, such as water quality and different convection volumes, will be discussed as well.

## Mortality

Several large observational studies suggest a survival benefit of HDF as compared to standard hemodialysis (HD) (summarized in table 1). Locatelli et al. [13] compared convective (HDF or hemofiltration (HF)) and diffusive dialysis modalities (HD) using data from the Lombardy registry and found no significant survival benefit of HDF. In contrast, in the observational Dialysis Outcomes and Practice Patterns Study (DOPPS) the adjusted mortality risk was 35% lower in high-efficiency HDF (i.e. HDF with a convection volume of ≥15 l per treatment session, in practice meaning ol-HDF) as compared to low-flux HD [3]. In addition, Jirka et al. [4] published data of the European Clinical Database (EuCliD) network, showing that the use of ol-HDF was associated with a 35% lower adjusted mortality risk as compared to HD, so results very similar to DOPPS data. The RISchio CArdiovascolare nei pazienti afferenti all' Area Vasta In Dialisi (RISCAVID) study compared ol-HDF, HDF with sterile fluid in bags and low-flux HD [5]. After several adjustments, both HDF modalities had a 22% lower all-cause mortality compared with HD, which was significant. However, the results were not adjusted for previous cardiovascular disease or residual renal function [14]. Recently, a retrospective analysis over an 18-year period of patients receiving predominantly ol-HDF (>50% of sessions) as compared to high-flux HD in the United Kingdom was published [6]. A total of almost 450,000 treatment sessions was analyzed. After adjustments for confounders, a 55% lower hazard rate for mortality was found for HDF.

An important limitation of these studies is the lack of information on censored events. Most studies did not properly discuss the various reasons for loss to follow-up. Differences in drop-out rates and reasons for drop-out between groups may bias study outcome. The most important problem with the interpretation of these observational studies is confounding (by indication) due to the non-randomized design. There may be clinically important differences between patients treated with HD or HDF. Although adjustments were made for observed confounding in the applied regression models, this does not eliminate unobserved confounding due to (un)known risk factors. This limits the validity. Properly designed randomized clinical trials (RCTs) do not have these methodological limitations, because patient characteristics, as well as known and unknown confounders, will be equally distributed over study groups. Up till now, two small RCTs on the effect of HDF have been carried out with 44 patients (23 on HDF) and 208 patients (50 on HDF) both with a follow-up of 24 months [15, 16]. These studies showed no survival benefit for patients treated by HDF as compared to HD, but were inadequately powered.

Finally, there may be important differences in convection volumes and water quality in the available studies. Convection volumes vary greatly between studies or are not mentioned. In table 1, convection volumes and results of water quality monitoring are depicted. Results on water quality are difficult to compare, because cultures of the dialysis fluids were taken at different locations of the purification system. Nevertheless, there are differences in water quality within and between studies. We analyzed microbiological results of infusate in 8 centers during 12 months and showed that in over 99% of cases the results met the reference quality levels with respect to colony-forming unit count and endotoxin level [17].

The need for RCT is further emphasized by the fact that sometimes cohort analyses show a considerable benefit, which is not confirmed by a RCT: an example is the use of statins in patients with end-stage kidney disease (ESKD) [18].

Several prospective randomized trials are now ongoing (cf. table 3). In three, mortality is the primary endpoint (CONTRAST, the Turkish HDF study and ESHOL) [19–21]. CONTRAST and the Turkish study have ended inclusion and results on primary endpoints are expected soon. Inclusion into the ESHOL study was ended September 2008, the study runs to September 2011. Two studies mainly focus on intradialytic morbidity (the French and Italian study) [22, 23]. The Italian study shows that indeed the use of convective therapies is associated with less intradialytic morbidity [pers. commun.]. An Australian study (FINESSE) is of particular interest because the effect on neuropathy is the primary endpoint [24]. Neuropathy affects the majority of ESKD patients, which results in function loss and discomfort.

In conclusion, most observational studies suggest a (substantial) survival benefit for patients receiving a therapy which also allows convective transport (table 1). Prospective randomized trials will hopefully provide definite answers in the near future (cf. table 3).

## Inflammation

A persistent low-grade inflammation is commonly observed in patients with chronic kidney disease [25]. Convective and diffusive therapies may differ in their effects on this inflammatory state. Therefore, it seems appropriate to focus on this issue. Especially in ESKD, the systemic concentrations of both pro-, but also anti-inflammatory cytokines are severalfold higher due to decreased renal clearance and/or increased production. Several factors, both dialysis-related (e.g. microbiological quality of the dialysate or membrane bioincompatibility) and non-dialysis-related (e.g. retention of uremic toxins, infection, comorbidity),

**Table 1.** Effect of HDF on mortality and inflammation

| Reference (first author or study) | Design and Intervention | Patients n | Water quality | |
|---|---|---|---|---|
| | | | CFU | EU |
| Locatelli [13] | observational: HD ↔ HDF/HF | 6,444 HDF/HF 1,082 | | |
| DOPPS [3] | observational: LF-HD ↔ HDF | 2,165 HDF: 97 | | |
| Jirka [4] | observational: LF-HD ↔ olHDF | 2,564 olHDF: 394 | | |
| RISCAVID [5] | observational: LF-HD ↔ olHDF ↔ HDF sterile bags | 757 olHDF: 129 | sdf | up |
| Vilar [6] | observational: HF-HD ↔ olHDF[2] | 858 olHDF: 233 | up | up |
| Vaslaki [32] | cross-over: LF-HD ↔ postdilution olHDF | 27 | up | |
| Carracedo [43] | cross-over: HF-HD ↔ olHDF | 31 | sdf | up |
| Panichi [38] | cross-over: HD ↔ postdilution olHDF/HFR | 25 | | |
| Vaslaki [36] | cross-over: LF-HD ↔ postdilution olHDF | 70 | sdf | |
| Schiffl [37] | cross-over: LF-HD ↔ HF-HD/postdilution olHDF | 76 | * → up | up |
| Filiopoulos [35] | observational: HD ↔ postdilution HDF | 9 | * | |
| Kuo [33] | observational: HD ↔ postdilution olHDF | 17 | sdf | sdf |
| Tiranathanagul [34] | observational: HF-HD ↔ predilution olHDF | 22 | up | up |

CRP = C-reactive protein; IL-6 = interleukin-6, $\beta_2$-MG = $\beta_2$-microglobulin; HD = hemodialysis (LF = low-flux, HF = high-flux); ol = online; HDF = hemodiafiltration; HF = hemofiltration; HFR = hemodiafiltration with regeneration of ultrafiltrate; CFU = colony-forming units per ml; EU = endotoxin units per ml; up = ultrapure (<0.1 CFU/ml; <0.03 EU/ml), sdf = standard dialysis fluid <100 CFU/ml; <0.25 EU/ml), * = worse.
[1] Assumption of convection volume. [2] >50% of the sessions HDF. [3] Ultrafiltration volume or rate. [4] Flow rate substitution fluid. [5] Only in the group that started on HD. [6] In HF-HD vs. olHDF. [7] In LF-HD vs. HF-HD or HDF.

| Convection volume | Mortality | Inflammation | | Remarks | |
|---|---|---|---|---|---|
| | | CRP | IL-6 | Kt/V | $\beta_2$-MG |
| | ns. 10% ↓ | | | | |
| 15–25 l | 35% ↓ | | | ↑ | |
| [1] | 35% ↓ | | | | |
| 23±3 l | 22% ↓ | = | ↓ | = | |
| 15 ± 4 l[3] | 55% ↓ | ↓ | ↓ | = | |
| 5.6±0.1 l/h[4] | | = | = | | |
| 20 l (16–24) | | | n.s. ↓ | = | = |
| 4.5 ± 0.3 l/h[4] | | ↓ | n.s. ↓ | | = |
| 20 ± 3 l | | ↓ [5] | ↓ [5] | | = / ↓ |
| 4.5 l/h | = [6] | ↓ [7] | | ↑ | ↓ |
| 10 l | | ↓ | n.s. ↓ | = | |
| 20 l | | = | = | | |
| 9.6 l/h[1] | | n.s. ↓ | | = | ↓ |

may contribute to a state of persistent inflammation [26]. Inflammation has been shown to play a major role in the pathogenesis of atherosclerosis [27] and to predict cardiovascular disease and mortality in ESKD [25, 28]. HDF might exert a beneficial effect on outcome by removing and/or reducing the production of pro-inflammatory factors.

*C-Reactive Protein (CRP)*

CRP (±107 kDa) is a reliable plasma marker of systemic inflammation and predicts cardiovascular risk and mortality in ESKD patients [28, 29]. Whether CRP is only a marker of, or a causal factor in atherosclerosis remains a matter of debate [30]. Single CRP measurements can predict mortality in ESKD patients, however CRP levels fluctuate over time and are greatly influenced by transient infections and comorbidity. So, repeated measurements may give additional information about the actual inflammatory state as compared to a single measurement [31].

The association of CRP with treatment modality was investigated in two observational studies. In the RISCAVID study, no significant difference in hs-CRP levels (single measurement) was observed between HD, HDF (with sterile bags) and ol-HDF [5]. In the study by Vilar et al. [6], CRP levels were lower in patients predominantly treated with HDF (median (IQR) 7.0 (12.5) vs. 10.0 (16.2) mg/l at 12 months).

The influence of HDF on hs-CRP has been studied in small interventional studies, with number of patients ranging from 9 to 76. Whereas some studies found no (significant) reductions in CRP levels [32–34], possibly due to small sample size, others described a significant decrease [35–38]. In one study, there was only a decrease in CRP levels after 9 months (mean ± SD 16.3 ± 11.4 → 6.0 ± 5.1 mg/l) with a substitution volume of 10 l [35]. The decreased CRP levels described by Vaslaki et al. [36] might be influenced by different dialysis membranes or a different distribution of residual kidney function across groups. In the study of Schiffl [37], CRP levels were significantly decreased when patients were shifted from LF-HD to HF-HD or ol-HDF (mean ± SD 10.5 (3) → 5.0 (3) mg/l), with no difference between the two latter groups. These results might be explained by differences in water quality. Finally, Panichi et al. [38] showed a significant decrease in CRP after 4 months of therapy with ol-HDF (mean ± SE 9.4 ± 4.3 → 5.9 ± 3.9 mg/l), with no difference between ol-HDF and HFR (HDF with regeneration of ultrafiltrate). It is interesting to note that Panichi et al. [39] showed that HDF with substitution volumes of <10 l resulted in an increase in CRP levels as compared to HD and HDF with substitution volumes >20 l.

*Interleukin 6 (IL-6)*

IL-6 is a major pro-inflammatory cytokine. It plays a key role in the inflammatory response, regulating the hepatic synthesis of acute phase proteins. Furthermore, it may contribute to atherosclerosis. IL-6 mRNA is present in atherosclerotic arteries at a 10- to 40-fold higher level than in non-atherosclerotic vessels [40] and IL-6 gene polymorphisms have been described to influence cardiovascular disease risk in dialysis patients [41]. With regard to prognosis, IL-6 has been shown to be one of the strongest predictors of inflammation, cardiovascular disease and mortality in ESKD [28, 42]. It is attractive to hypothesize that IL-6, with a molecular weight of approximately 25 kDa, can be lowered by HDF. However, there is very limited evidence available.

In an observational setting, the RISCAVID study found lower IL-6 levels in HDF as compared HD [5]. Interventional studies however showed no significant differences [32, 33, 35, 38]. In a very elegant cross-over study, Carracedo et al. [43] showed that the percentage of pro-inflammatory CD14+CD16+ monocytes lowered during ol-HDF. Also a trend towards lower IL-6 levels in ol-HDF was described (mean (min-max) 18.9 (10.6–17.8) → 13.2 (5–19) pg/ml).

So, some (but not all) studies suggest that there might be a difference between diffusive and convective therapies in their effect on inflammatory state. As mentioned earlier, water quality may act as an effect modifier, if less pure water is used in LF-HD as compared to HDF. In the available studies, it is not always clear if water of the same quality was applied. In addition, cultures of dialysis fluids were taken at different locations. So, differences in inflammatory state may be a result of differences in water quality and/or monitoring procedures.

## Health-Related Quality of Life

Patients on HD not only face the physical, mental and social burden of their disease, but also the limitations caused by the time-consuming nature of the therapy. As a result, it has been shown that the HRQOL of HD patients is even less than that of patients with cancer [44]. Although an important outcome, HRQOL is difficult to measure and interpret [45, 46]. It is not a single entity like mortality, nor is it assessable by measuring for instance biomarkers. Measuring HRQOL means assessing multiple domains of physical, psychological and social status taken from the patients' perspective [45, 47].

With the now available standardized and validated questionnaires [48, 49], HRQOL is increasingly investigated in dialysis care [50]. In an understanding that survival is not all that counts, cost-utility studies on new interventions combine mortality and HRQOL as their effect measure [51]. As HRQOL is a key outcome in HD patients, we evaluated the literature not only with regard to mortality and inflammation, but also on perceived health status (table 2). Do high-flux or convective therapies lead to a better HRQOL? The HEMO study found no differences in HRQOL between patients treated with low- or high-flux HD [52]. However, an increased dialysis dose (eKt/V 1.05 vs. 1.45) was associated with minor improvements in HRQOL, i.e. better physical health and less bodily pain. Two small studies compared the effects of HD with online HF on

**Table 2.** Hemodialysis modality and HRQOL

| Reference (first author or study) | Design | Intervention | Patients, n | Effect on HRQOL |
|---|---|---|---|---|
| HEMO [52] | RCT | high-flux ↔ low-flux HD | 1,846<br>921 on high-flux | no difference |
| Altieri [53] | cross-over | olHF ↔ high-flux HD | 24 | no difference |
| Beerenhout [54] | RCT | olHF ↔ low-flux HD | 27<br>13 on HF | no difference [note: p = 0.06 for better HRQOL in HF (14%)] |
| Moreno [55] | cross-sectional | HDF ↔ HD ↔ PD | 1,013<br>71 on HDF | no difference |
| Ward [56] | RCT | olHDF ↔high-flux HD | 44<br>24 on HDF | no difference |
| Lin [57] | RCT | olHDF ↔ high-flux HD | 111* | better physical well-being in HDF (32%) |
| Schiffl [58] | cross-over | olHDF ↔high-flux HD | 76 | better perception of physical symptoms in HDF (26%) |
| DOPPS [3] | observational | HDF ↔ high- ↔ low-flux HD | 2,165<br>253 on HDF | no difference |

HRQOL = Health-related quality of life; RCT = randomized clinical trial; ol = online; HD = hemodialysis; HF = hemofiltration; HDF = hemodialfiltration.
* Randomization into four groups: 3×/week HD, 3×/week HDF, and 2 intermediate versions with a 2 × vs. 1×/week distribution of HD or HDF.

HRQOL [53, 54]. Although no significant differences were found, both studies describe a trend towards an improved HRQOL in patients on HF, especially in patients' assessed physical symptoms. With regard to HDF, the results are inconclusive: three studies found no differences between HD or HDF [3, 55, 56], but two other describe a significant improvement in physical well-being [57, 58]. Further studies are warranted to provide definite results. It is important to note that if HDF does not lead to an improved survival, the dialysis modality may still be the treatment of choice if it is associated with a better HRQOL. Three of the ongoing trials depicted in table 3 will evaluate HDF with regard to HRQOL: CONTRAST, the Turkish HDF study and FINESSE [19, 20, 24].

**Table 3.** HDF and ongoing RCTs

| Reference | Modality control group | Patients, n | Primary endpoint |
|---|---|---|---|
| CONTRAST [7, 19] | low-flux HD | 715 | mortality |
| French study [22] | high-flux HD | target ± 600 | intradialytic morbidity |
| Italian study [23] | low-flux HD and olHF | 146 | hemodynamic stability |
| Turkish study [20] | high-flux HD | 782 | cardiovascular morbidity and mortality |
| ESHOL [21] | HD (94% high-flux) | 939 | mortality |
| FINESSE [24] | high-flux HD | target ± 120 | neuropathy |

HD = Hemodialysis; ol = online; HF = hemofiltration.

Finally, the additional costs of HDF should be taken into account. Medical resources are limited and current dialysis modalities are already among the most expensive therapies [59]. In CONTRAST, a formal cost-utility analysis will be performed to compare the additional costs with a possible difference in quality-adjusted life-years (QALYs). QALYs combine survival with HRQOL in one effect measure. At present, there is no scientific literature on HDF costs or QALYs available.

## Treatment Optimization Parameters

In everyday clinical practice, there is a clear need for clinical and/or laboratory parameters to guide or to 'dose' the HDF treatment. This parameter should be sensitive, valid, and be related to meaningful clinical outcome variables. Given the considerations outlined above on the results of inflammatory markers, it is questionable if these can be used to guide therapy. The levels of these substances are determined by many factors other than the treatment.

$\beta_2$-Microglobulin ($\beta_2$-MG, 11.8 kDa) could also be used as a variable to guide treatment, as it is one of the middle-sized molecules. However, the plasma levels of $\beta_2$-MG are determined substantially by factors other than the extracorporeal clearance, i.e. residual kidney function and inflammatory state. Further, there is a relative resistance of $\beta_2$-MG transfer between body compartments [60], so plasma levels decrease more rapidly than interstitial levels during HDF. This phenomenon limits enhanced $\beta_2$-MG clearance by increasing convection volumes. We recently showed that change in $\beta_2$-MG after 6 months of therapy was not related to applied convection volumes [61]. Therefore, assessment of $\beta_2$-MG levels does not seem appropriate.

It seems reasonable to assume that there is a dose-effect relationship when applying HDF, i.e. that a certain minimum amount of convection volume needs to be applied in order to obtain the beneficial effect. The results of the DOPPS suggest that this volume should be ≥15 l [3]. This is the only set of data relating treatment-related factors with meaningful clinical endpoints. Further studies on this subject are clearly needed.

## Conclusion

Results of observational studies suggest an improved survival of patients on HDF as compared to HD. Furthermore, some (but not all) studies suggest that there might be a difference between diffusive and convective therapies in their effect on inflammatory state. At present, the effect of HDF on HRQOL is unclear, and there is no scientific literature on HDF costs or QALYs.

RCTs are needed in nephrology [62]. Well-designed RCTs are now underway to (hopefully) provide an answer, whether HDF is associated with any survival benefit (table 3). In addition, meta-analysis of the individual trials may also help to define an evidence-based approach towards HDF. Apart from survival, differences in other clinical endpoints, including non-fatal cardiovascular morbidity and HRQOL, are important as well and are studied in (some of) these trials. Differences between HDF and standard HD in these endpoints seem reason enough to choose for ol-HDF as a standard treatment, especially now it has been shown that ol-HDF can be applied safely. Finally, the ongoing trials may help to define variables such as biomarkers or levels of convection volumes, which can be used to guide and optimize the therapy.

## References


1 Stel VS, Kramer A, Zoccali C, Jager KJ: The 2007 ERA-EDTA Registry Annual Report – a precis. NDT Plus 2009;2:514–521.

2 Vanholder R, Van LS, Glorieux G: The middle-molecule hypothesis 30 years after: lost and rediscovered in the universe of uremic toxicity? J Nephrol 2008;21:146–160.

3 Canaud B, Bragg-Gresham JL, Marshall MR, Desmeules S, Gillespie BW, Depner T, Klassen P, Port FK: Mortality risk for patients receiving hemodiafiltration versus hemodialysis: European results from the DOPPS. Kidney Int 2006;69:2087–2093.

4 Jirka T, Cesare S, Di BA, Perera CM, Ponce P, Richards N, Tetta C, Vaslaky L: Mortality risk for patients receiving hemodiafiltration versus hemodialysis. Kidney Int 2006;70:1524–1525.

5 Panichi V, Rizza GM, Paoletti S, Bigazzi R, Aloisi M, Barsotti G, Rindi P, Donati G, Antonelli A, Panicucci E, Tripepi G, Tetta C, Palla R: Chronic inflammation and mortality in haemodialysis: effect of different renal replacement therapies. Results from the RISCAVID study. Nephrol Dial Transplant 2008;23:2337–2343.
6 Vilar E, Fry AC, Wellsted D, Tattersall JE, Greenwood RN, Farrington K: Long-term outcomes in online hemodiafiltration and high-flux hemodialysis: a comparative analysis. Clin J Am Soc Nephrol 2009;4:1944–1953.
7 Penne EL, Blankestijn PJ, Bots ML, van den Dorpel MA, Grooteman MP, Nube MJ, Ter Wee PM: Resolving controversies regarding hemodiafiltration versus hemodialysis: the Dutch Convective Transport Study. Semin Dial 2005;18:47–51.
8 Van der Weerd NC, Penne EL, van den Dorpel MA, Grooteman MP, Nube MJ, Bots ML, Ter Wee PM, Blankestijn PJ: Haemodiafiltration: promise for the future? Nephrol Dial Transplant 2008;23:438–443.
9 Penne EL, van BT, van der Weerd NC, Grooteman MP, Blankestijn PJ: Optimizing haemodiafiltration: tools, strategy and remaining questions. Nephrol Dial Transplant 2009;24:3579–3581.
10 Ledebo I, Blankestijn PJ: Haemodiafiltration – optimal efficiency and safety. NDT Plus 2010;3:8–16.
11 Blankestijn PJ, Ledebo I, Canaud B: Hemodiafiltration: clinical evidence and remaining questions. Kidney Int 2010;77:581–587.
12 Grooteman MP, Ter Wee PM, Blankestijn PJ, Bots ML, Dorpel MA, Nube MJ: Haemodiafiltration: an update. Eur Nephrol 2010 (in press).
13 Locatelli F, Marcelli D, Conte F, Limido A, Malberti F, Spotti D: Comparison of mortality in ESRD patients on convective and diffusive extracorporeal treatments. The Registro Lombardo Dialisi E Trapianto. Kidney Int 1999;55:286–293.
14 Penne EL, van der Weerd NC, Grooteman MP, Blankestijn PJ: Results from the RISCAVID study: is haemodiafiltration associated with improved survival? Nephrol Dial Transplant 2008;23:3034.
15 Wizemann V, Lotz C, Techert F, Uthoff S: On-line haemodiafiltration versus low-flux haemodialysis. A prospective randomized study. Nephrol Dial Transplant 2000;15(suppl 1):43–48.
16 Locatelli F, Mastrangelo F, Redaelli B, Ronco C, Marcelli D, La GG, Orlandini G: Effects of different membranes and dialysis technologies on patient treatment tolerance and nutritional parameters. The Italian Cooperative Dialysis Study Group. Kidney Int 1996;50:1293–1302.
17 Penne EL, Visser L, van den Dorpel MA, van der Weerd NC, Mazairac AH, van Jaarsveld BC, Koopman MG, Vos P, Feith GW, Kremer Hovinga TK, van Hamersvelt HW, Wauters IM, Bots ML, Nube MJ, Ter Wee PM, Blankestijn PJ, Grooteman MP: Microbiological quality and quality control of purified water and ultrapure dialysis fluids for online hemodiafiltration in routine clinical practice. Kidney Int 2009;76:665–672.
18 Fellstrom BC, Jardine AG, Schmieder RE, Holdaas H, Bannister K, Beutler J, Chae DW, Chevaile A, Cobbe SM, Gronhagen-Riska C, De Lima JJ, Lins R, Mayer G, McMahon AW, Parving HH, Remuzzi G, Samuelsson O, Sonkodi S, Sci D, Suleymanlar G, Tsakiris D, Tesar V, Todorov V, Wiecek A, Wuthrich RP, Gottlow M, Johnsson E, Zannad F: Rosuvastatin and cardiovascular events in patients undergoing hemodialysis. N Engl J Med 2009;360:1395–1407.
19 Penne EL, Blankestijn PJ, Bots ML, van den Dorpel MA, Grooteman MP, Nube MJ, van der Tweel, I, Ter Wee PM: Effect of increased convective clearance by on-line hemodiafiltration on all-cause and cardiovascular mortality in chronic hemodialysis patients – the Dutch CONvective TRAnsport STudy (CONTRAST): rationale and design of a randomised controlled trial [ISRCTN38365125]. Curr Control Trials Cardiovasc Med 2005;6:8.
20 Turkish HDF Study: Comparison of post-dilution on-line hemodiafiltration and hemodialysis (http://clinicaltrials.gov/ct2/show/nct00411177), 2006.
21 Maduell F: Convection versus diffusion: Is it time to make a change? (in Spanish) Nefrologia 2009;29:589–593.

22 Canaud B, Morena M, Leray-Moragues H, Chalabi L, Cristol JP: Overview of clinical studies in hemodiafiltration: what do we need now ? Hemodial Int 2006;10(suppl 1):S5–S12.
23 Bolasco P, Altieri P, Andrulli S, Basile C, Di FS, Feriani M, Pedrini L, Santoro A, Zoccali C, Sau G, Locatelli F: Convection versus diffusion in dialysis: an Italian prospective multicentre study. Nephrol Dial Transplant 2003;18(suppl 7):vii50–vii54.
24 FINESSE Trial: Filtration in the neuropathy of end-stage kidney disease symptom evolution (http://www.anzctr.org.au/trial_view.aspx?ID = 308240), 2009.
25 Stenvinkel P, Carrero JJ, Axelsson J, Lindholm B, Heimburger O, Massy Z: Emerging biomarkers for evaluating cardiovascular risk in the chronic kidney disease patient: how do new pieces fit into the uremic puzzle? Clin J Am Soc Nephrol 2008;3:505–521.
26 Carrero JJ, Yilmaz MI, Lindholm B, Stenvinkel P: Cytokine dysregulation in chronic kidney disease: how can we treat it? Blood Purif 2008;26:291–299.
27 Carrero JJ, Stenvinkel P: Persistent inflammation as a catalyst for other risk factors in chronic kidney disease: a hypothesis proposal. Clin J Am Soc Nephrol 2009;4(suppl 1):S49–S55.
28 Tripepi G, Mallamaci F, Zoccali C: Inflammation markers, adhesion molecules, and all-cause and cardiovascular mortality in patients with ESRD: searching for the best risk marker by multivariate modeling. J Am Soc Nephrol 2005;16(suppl 1): S83–S88.
29 Qureshi AR, Alvestrand A, Vino-Filho JC, Gutierrez A, Heimburger O, Lindholm B, Bergstrom J: Inflammation, malnutrition, and cardiac disease as predictors of mortality in hemodialysis patients. J Am Soc Nephrol 2002;13(suppl 1):S28–S36.
30 Calabro P, Golia E, Yeh ET: CRP and the risk of atherosclerotic events. Semin Immunopathol 2009;31:79–94.
31 Snaedal S, Heimburger O, Qureshi AR, Danielsson A, Wikstrom B, Fellstrom B, Fehrman-Ekholm I, Carrero JJ, Alvestrand A, Stenvinkel P, Barany P: Comorbidity and acute clinical events as determinants of C-reactive protein variation in hemodialysis patients: implications for patient survival. Am J Kidney Dis 2009;53:1024–1033.
32 Vaslaki LR, Berta K, Major L, Weber V, Weber C, Wojke R, Passlick-Deetjen J, Falkenhagen D: On-line hemodiafiltration does not induce inflammatory response in end-stage renal disease patients: results from a multicenter cross-over study. Artif Organs 2005;29:406–412.
33 Kuo HL, Chou CY, Liu YL, Yang YF, Huang CC, Lin HH: Reduction of pro-inflammatory cytokines through hemodiafiltration. Ren Fail 2008;30:796–800.
34 Tiranathanagul K, Praditpornsilpa K, Katavetin P, Srisawat N, Townamchai N, Susantitaphong P, Tungsanga K, Eiam-Ong S: On-line hemodiafiltration in Southeast Asia: a three-year prospective study of a single center. Ther Apher Dial 2009;13:56–62.
35 Filiopoulos V, Hadjiyannakos D, Metaxaki P, Sideris V, Takouli L, Anogiati A, Vlassopoulos D: Inflammation and oxidative stress in patients on hemodiafiltration. Am J Nephrol 2008;28:949–957.
36 Vaslaki L, Major L, Berta K, Karatson A, Misz M, Pethoe F, Ladanyi E, Fodor B, Stein G, Pischetsrieder M, Zima T, Wojke R, Gauly A, Passlick-Deetjen J: On-line haemodiafiltration versus haemodialysis: stable haematocrit with less erythropoietin and improvement of other relevant blood parameters. Blood Purif 2006;24:163–173.
37 Schiffl H: Prospective randomized cross-over long-term comparison of online haemodiafiltration and ultrapure high-flux haemodialysis. Eur J Med Res 2007;12:26–33.
38 Panichi V, Manca-Rizza G, Paoletti S, Taccola D, Consani C, Filippi C, Mantuano E, Sidoti A, Grazi G, Antonelli A, Angelini D, Petrone I, Mura C, Tolaini P, Saloi F, Ghezzi PM, Barsotti G, Palla R: Effects on inflammatory and nutritional markers of haemodiafiltration with online regeneration of ultrafiltrate (HFR) vs. online haemodiafiltration: a cross-over randomized multicentre trial. Nephrol Dial Transplant 2006;21:756–762.

39 Panichi V, Rizza GM, Taccola D, Paoletti S, Mantuano E, Migliori M, Frangioni S, Filippi C, Carpi A: C-reactive protein in patients on chronic hemodialysis with different techniques and different membranes. Biomed Pharmacother 2006;60:14–17.
40 Seino Y, Ikeda U, Ikeda M, Yamamoto K, Misawa Y, Hasegawa T, Kano S, Shimada K: Interleukin-6 gene transcripts are expressed in human atherosclerotic lesions. Cytokine 1994;6:87–91.
41 Liu Y, Berthier-Schaad Y, Fallin MD, Fink NE, Tracy RP, Klag MJ, Smith MW, Coresh J: IL-6 haplotypes, inflammation, and risk for cardiovascular disease in a multiethnic dialysis cohort. J Am Soc Nephrol 2006;17:863–870.
42 Zoccali C, Tripepi G, Mallamaci F: Dissecting inflammation in ESRD: do cytokines and C-reactive protein have a complementary prognostic value for mortality in dialysis patients? J Am Soc Nephrol 2006;17:S169–S173.
43 Carracedo J, Merino A, Nogueras S, Carretero D, Berdud I, Ramirez R, Tetta C, Rodriguez M, Martin-Malo A, Aljama P: On-line hemodiafiltration reduces the proinflammatory CD14+CD16+ monocyte-derived dendritic cells: a prospective, crossover study. J Am Soc Nephrol 2006;17:2315–2321.
44 Mittal SK, Ahern L, Flaster E, Maesaka JK, Fishbane S: Self-assessed physical and mental function of haemodialysis patients. Nephrol Dial Transplant 2001;16:1387–1394.
45 Unruh ML, Weisbord SD, Kimmel PL: Health-related quality of life in nephrology research and clinical practice. Semin Dial 2005;18:82–90.
46 King MT, Fayers PM: Making quality-of-life results more meaningful for clinicians. Lancet 2008,371:709–710.
47 Testa MA, Simonson DC: Assessment of quality-of-life outcomes. N Engl J Med 1996;334:835–840.
48 Ware JE, Snow KK, Kosinski M, Gandek B: SF-36 Health Survey-Manual and Interpretation Guide. Boston, The Health Institute, New England Medical Center, 1993.
49 Hays RD, Kallich JD, Mapes DL, Coons SJ, Carter WB: Development of the kidney disease quality of life (KDQOL) instrument. Qual Life Res 1994;3:329–338.
50 Liem YS, Bosch JL, Arends LR, Heijenbrok-Kal MH, Hunink MG: Quality of life assessed with the Medical Outcomes Study Short Form 36-Item Health Survey of patients on renal replacement therapy: a systematic review and meta-analysis. Value Health 2007;10:390–397.
51 Drummond MF, Sculpher MJ, Torrance GW, O'Brien BJ, Stoddart GL: Methods for the Economic Evaluation of Health Care Programmes, ed 3. Oxford, Oxford University Press, 2005.
52 Unruh M, Benz R, Greene T, Yan G, Beddhu S, DeVita M, Dwyer JT, Kimmel PL, Kusek JW, Martin A, Rehm-McGillicuddy J, Teehan BP, Meyer KB: Effects of hemodialysis dose and membrane flux on health-related quality of life in the HEMO Study. Kidney Int 2004;66:355–366.
53 Altieri P, Sorba G, Bolasco P, Asproni E, Ledebo I, Cossu M, Ferrara R, Ganadu M, Cadinu F, Serra G, Cabiddu G, Sau G, Casu D, Passaghe M, Bolasco F, Pistis R, Ghisu T: Predilution haemofiltration – the Second Sardinian Multicentre Study: comparisons between haemofiltration and haemodialysis during identical Kt/V and session times in a long-term cross-over study. Nephrol Dial Transplant 2001;16:1207–1213.
54 Beerenhout CH, Luik AJ, Jeuken-Mertens SG, Bekers O, Menheere P, Hover L, Klaassen L, van der Sande FM, Cheriex EC, Meert N, Leunissen KM, Kooman JP: Pre-dilution on-line haemofiltration vs. low-flux haemodialysis: a randomized prospective study. Nephrol Dial Transplant 2005;20:1155–1163.
55 Moreno F, Lopez Gomez JM, Sanz-Guajardo D, Jofre R, Valderrabano F: Quality of life in dialysis patients. A Spanish multicentre study. Spanish Cooperative Renal Patients Quality of Life Study Group. Nephrol Dial Transplant 1996;11(suppl 2):125–129.
56 Ward RA, Schmidt B, Hullin J, Hillebrand GF, Samtleben W: A comparison of on-line hemodiafiltration and high-flux hemodialysis: a prospective clinical study. J Am Soc Nephrol 2000;11:2344–2350.
57 Lin CL, Huang CC, Chang CT, Wu MS, Hung CC, Chien CC, Yang CW: Clinical improvement by increased frequency of on-line hemodialfiltration. Ren Fail 2001;23:193–206.

58 Schiffl H: Prospective randomized cross-over long-term comparison of online haemodiafiltration and ultrapure high-flux haemodialysis. Eur J Med Res 2007;12:26–33.
59 De Wit GA, Ramsteijn PG, de Charro FT: Economic evaluation of end stage renal disease treatment. Health Policy 1998;44:215–232.
60 Ward RA, Greene T, Hartmann B, Samtleben W: Resistance to intercompartmental mass transfer limits $\beta_2$-microglobulin removal by post-dilution hemodiafiltration. Kidney Int 2006;69:1431–1437.
61 Penne EL, van der Weerd NC, Blankestijn PJ, van den Dorpel MA, Grooteman MP, Nube MJ, Ter Wee PM, Levesque R, Bots ML: Role of residual kidney function and convective volume on change in $\beta_2$-microglobulin levels in hemodiafiltration patients. Clin J Am Soc Nephrol 2010;5:80–86.
62 Himmelfarb J: Chronic kidney disease and the public health: gaps in evidence from interventional trials. JAMA 2007;297:2630–2633.

Peter J. Blankestijn
Department of Nephrology, University Medical Center Utrecht
Heidelberglaan 100, NL–3584 CX Utrecht (The Netherlands)
Tel. +31 88 7557336, Fax +31 30 2543492, E-Mail P.J.Blankestijn@umcutrecht.nl

Kawanishi H, Yamashita AC (eds): Hemodiafiltration – A New Era.
Contrib Nephrol. Basel, Karger, 2011, vol 168, pp 53–63

# How to Prescribe Hemodialysis or Hemodiafiltration in Order to Ameliorate Dialysis-Related Symptoms and Complications

Ikuto Masakane

Yabuki Shima Clinic, Yamagata, Japan

## Abstract

The golden target for dialysis therapy should guarantee longer survival and a higher quality of life without dialysis-related complications. In order to achieve this target, dialysis prescriptions have been modified by increasing the efficiency of uremic solute removal and improving biocompatibility of dialysis membranes. Chronic dialysis patients frequently complain about uncomfortable symptoms such as insomnia, itchy skin, and irritability. Some of these symptoms are well known as independent mortality risk factors. Although these symptoms are serious problems for the patients, they have not yet been a parameter for prescribing a dialysis modality. In our recent experience, dialysis patients had preferences or some feelings concerning their dialysis therapy, for example they favored dialysis membranes which were composed of polymethylmethacrylate, ethylene vinyl alcohol copolymer, and polyacrylnitrate (AN69), and also preferred predilution online HDF. The common characteristics of these modalities are the nutritional advantage, fewer uremic symptoms and a higher survival rate. The mechanisms of these favorable effects were supposed to be caused by well-balanced removal of small solute and low-molecular-weight protein, and by being free from the influence of chemical compositions of dialysis membrane material. The patients' preferences were surely proven to have a scientific basis and could be a useful parameter to prescribe a dialysis modality.



The golden target for dialysis therapy should guarantee longer survival and a higher quality of life without dialysis-related complications. In order to achieve the target, various dialysis equipments, prescriptions and programs have been developed such as high-performance membrane (HPM), hemodiafiltration

(HDF), and daily dialysis. The qualities of these therapeutic modalities are evaluated according to various points – patient survival rate and quality of life in dialysis patients, solute removal property of the treatment and biocompatibility. We have various parameters to assess the dialysis qualities such as Kt/V, serum levels of $\beta_2$-microglobulin ($\beta_2$-MG) for the solute removal property, white blood cell counts, complement system, C-reactive protein and other biological assays for the biocompatibility of dialysis treatment. In the last two decades there has been a trend in dialysis therapy – the more efficiently uremic solutes are removed, the better the survival and quality of life the patients have.

Chronic dialysis patients frequently complain about the sense of itching, irritability, depression, disturbed sleep and other uncomfortable symptoms. These symptoms are a serious problem for the patient because they deteriorate their quality of life. Some of these symptoms have been known as significant predictors for patient mortality [1, 2]. These symptoms are evaluated by some questionnaires to study the relationship between the quality of life and survival in dialysis patients, however the symptoms have never been adopted as a parameter to prescribe dialysis modality. With this issue we would like to clarify that patients' symptoms can be a useful parameter to prescribe a dialysis modality, and introduce how it is done in daily practice.

## Classical Parameters for Prescribing a Dialysis Modality

The dialysis dose is the first issue to be considered for a better outcome in dialysis patients. Kt/V is one of the most frequently used parameters for dialysis adequacy because it is simple to calculate and gives some insight into the assessment of dialysis patient survival. If we wish to get a higher Kt/V, we have to increase the blood flow rate, the dialysis fluid flow rate, the size of the dialyzer, and the frequency and time of the dialysis treatment. Kt/V has been composed as a dialysis dose standardized by body size, however Kt/V is still dependent on body mass. If we evaluate a dialysis dose only by Kt/V it would be contradictory to the report which concluded that smaller-sized women or older patients are easily undertreated [3]. The Dialysis Outcomes and Practice Pattern Study (DOPPS) has not yet clarified the reason why patient survival in Japan has been so excellent even though the mean Kt/V is markedly lower in Japan [4]. These issues suggest that high Kt/V does not always lead to good patient survival and cannot be the golden target of a dialysis prescription.

$\beta_2$-MG is an important low-molecular-weight protein (LMWP) that has been proven to be a uremic toxin leading to dialysis-related complications [5]. In the last two decades, various types of HPM and HDF have been produced to remove $\beta_2$-MG effectively and prevent dialysis-related amyloidosis (DRA). In order to remove $\beta_2$-MG efficiently, a highly efficient and postdilution HDF is desirable, however it is still controversial whether or not more $\beta_2$-MG removal could result in longer patient survival. Furthermore, ultrapure dialysis fluid and HPM have been reducing the risk of DRA, and dialysis patients have become older and older. Therefore, DRA has been recognized as a diminishing complication [6].

Biocompatibility of dialysis therapy is another important issue for a dialysis prescription [7]. Various types of synthetic dialysis membranes have been developed to improve the bioincompatibility which was observed in the original cellulosic membrane. Biocompatible membrane and purified dialysis fluid are generally desirable for all dialysis patients in order to achieve longer patient survival. Dialysis membrane is usually only focused on the property of solute removal but is rarely concerned with a dialysis prescription for each individual patient.

## New Concept for Prescribing a Dialysis Modality

Body mass has been recognized as one of the most powerful predictors for patient survival in dialysis patients [8–10]. It is generally accepted because comorbidity and inflammatory complications will make patients lose their body mass which then shortens their survival. In dialysis patients, uremic retention solutes and bioincompatibility of the dialysis therapy itself have been known to lead microinflammation in dialysis patients, and it would be a common pathogenesis of various dialysis-related complications [7]. Malnutrition inflammation atherosclerosis (MIA) syndrome is the most important issue among these complications [11]. If we could prevent the sustained muscle loss completely, we could ensure longer patient survival without complications. In these lines of evidence, to maintain body mass is a solo and indispensable parameter to assess the quality of dialysis and to prescribe a dialysis modality.

As previously addressed, chronic dialysis patients have various uncomfortable symptoms related to their dialysis, among them are pruritus, irritability, depression, insomnia and intradialytic hypotension. Although some of these symptoms have been clarified as a risk for death and deterioration of life quality in patients, we have not yet had any parameters concerning the patients' symptoms for evaluation of the dialysis quality and strategies for prescribing a dialysis in order to improve their symptoms. Uremic pruritus is one of the most frequent symptoms in dialysis patients and well known as an independent prognostic factor [1]. In the DOPPS-1 and other previous reports, the prevalence of pruritus was reported to be 45% in all dialysis patients [1, 12]. In our facilities we have focused uremic pruritus as the most representative therapeutic target.

In our recent experience, many patients in our facilities have favored dialyzers made of polymethylmethacrylate (PMMA), ethylene vinyl alcohol copolymer (EVAL), polyacrylnitrate (PAN, AN69) or a predilution online HDF mode [13]. We found that these dialysis modes could relieve patients' dialysis-related

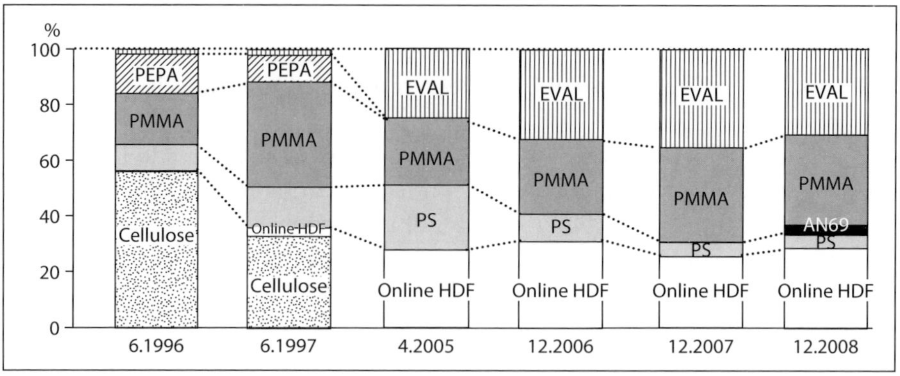


**Fig. 1.** Changes in the selection of dialysis membranes (in HD mode) or HDF mode (with PS membrane) in our facilities. PMMA, EVAL and online HDF have been the most commonly used recently.

symptoms, maintain their muscle volume and provide them a longer and higher quality of life. In other words, patients' preferences or feelings could be a new parameter for prescribing a dialysis modality. We have named this therapeutic concept the *patient-oriented dialysis system*, or POD system [13].

### Results of the Dialysis Prescription Based on the POD System

We have two basic tests which we perform twice a year with the POD system. The POD sheet has 36 questions about quality of life and dialysis-related symptoms. The malnutrition inflammation score sheet is an assessment tool used to screen the nutritional status originally composed by Kalantar-Zadeh et al. [9]. If the patients have any problems with the POD sheet and the malnutrition inflammation score sheet, dialysis therapies and nutritional approaches will be reconsidered and changed to solve the problems. In this therapeutic concept, the choice of dialysis membranes and online HDF mode are a major key to achieve a good dialysis. Over 90% of our patients have been treated by EVAL, PMMA, AN69 membranes and predilution online HDF mode; EVAL in particular was used in all new patients starting dialysis (fig. 1).

Uremic pruritus is one of the most frequent symptoms we confront and has been recognized to be associated with a higher mortality risk and sleep disturbance. The prevalence of more than moderate itching was reported to be relatively high, 40–50% [1, 13], but only 15% of patients complained about itchiness in our facilities (fig. 2). The prevalence of sleep disturbance as 'poor' or 'bad' was 18% and it was less frequent than that of DOPPS by one third [14].

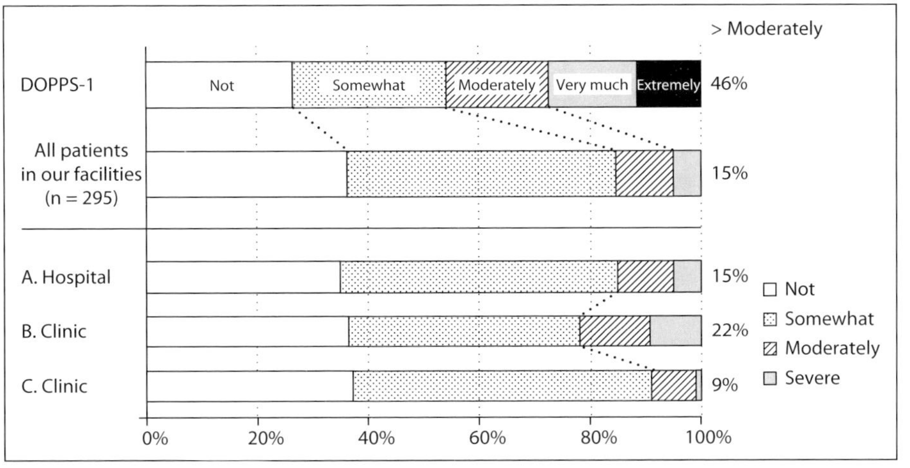


**Fig. 2.** Prevalence of pruritus in dialysis patients. In our facilities it is less than that of DOPPS-1.

In order to evaluate the advantage of the POD system, a 5-year survival rate in our facilities was compared with that of the Japanese Society for Dialysis Therapy (JSDT). The accumulated 5-year survival rate was 77% in our facilities compared to 57% in JSDT, although the mean age of the patients was 69 years and was 3 years older than that of JSDT [13]. The 5-year survival rate of the older patients was 52% in our facilities compared to 27% in JSDT. The POD system enables chronic dialysis patients to live longer without uncomfortable dialysis-related symptoms [13].

## Rationale of the New Concept for a Dialysis Prescription

### *Solute Removal Pattern and Nutritional Advantage*

In the preliminary study we found that online HDF could maintain the muscle volume of dialysis patients [13] (fig. 3). Muscle volume calculated by bioelectrical impedance analysis gradually reduced for 2 years in HD patients but was well preserved in online HDF patients. Those patients who switched from HD to online HDF had an increase in muscle volume just after the switch. Almost all online HDFs were performed by the predilution method. We compared the muscle volume change between pre- and postdilution and the muscle volume was better preserved in predilution than in postdilution (data not shown). The same effect on maintaining body mass has been reported in hemodialysis performed by EVAL, PMMA, and AN69. Muta et al. [15] reported that body mass reduction observed in HD with PS membrane dramatically improved with

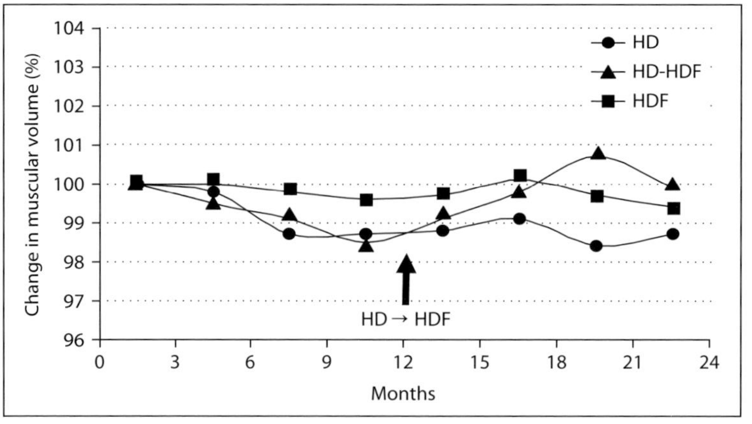


**Fig. 3.** Changes of muscular volume in HD and online HDF patients. The muscular volumes of HD patients have gradually reduced for 2 years, but those of online HDF patients are well preserved. Those patients who switched from HD to online HDF had an increase in muscle volume just after the switch.

the change of the dialysis membrane to EVAL in older dialysis patients. Their hypothesis for the advantage of EVAL membrane in maintaining muscle volume was that the loss of amino acids during a dialysis session was milder in HD with EVAL membrane.

In order to clarify why predilution HDF and the other modalities have a nutritional advantage, we compared the solute removal pattern between HD, predilution online HDF and postdilution online HDF modes. All therapies were performed using PS membrane at a blood flow rate of 270–300 ml/min, and the total volume of substitution fluid per session was 48–72 l in the predilution mode and 12–18 l in the postdilution mode. In the predilution online HDF mode it has widely been taken for granted that small solute removal is lower than in the HD mode because of the osmotic pressure gradient decreased by diluted plasma and slower dialysis fluid flow rate. In our study, small solute removal was reduced but amino acids were better preserved in the predilution online HDF mode than in the HD or postdilution HDF modes. On the other hand, LMWPs such as $\beta_2$-MG (MW: 12 kDa) or leptin (MW: 16 kDa) were effectively removed in the HDF mode, especially in the predilution HDF mode of our therapeutic prescription [13]. Albumin loss per session was 0.8 g in the HD mode, 1.3 g in the predilution HDF mode and 3.1 g in the postdilution HDF mode [13]. LMWPs or some albumin are effectively removed by convection in HDF, large pore size in EVAL membrane, or the protein adsorptive property in PMMA or PAN membrane. This broad removal pattern of dialysis membranes or predilution online HDF mode might be similar to the native kidneys and have an advantage in keeping body mass in the dialysis patients.

In the native kidney, the clearance of urea is around 60 ml/min and it is smaller than that of most dialysis membranes (i.e. almost 200 ml/min). A lot of nutrients such as amino acids or carnitine are also filtered by glomeruli, but almost all of them are retrieved by the proximal tubules. The more efficiently we would try to remove small solute, the more we would lose small solute nutrients. The small solute clearance of EVAL, PMMA and PAN membranes or predilution online HDF mode is rather lower than that of the HD mode with PS. LMWP and some albumin are also filtered by glomeruli and reabsorbed and catabolized by the proximal renal tubules. The molecular weight of inflammatory cytokines related to MIA syndrome is around 15–30 kDa and that of leptin which is recognized as a uremic substance is 16 kDa. It is reported that albumin is partially deteriorated in the uremic milieu because oxidative stress and uremic toxins deteriorate the nature of albumin [16]. If renal failure progresses, inflammatory cytokines and deteriorated albumin would be accumulated inside the body. The accumulation of inflammatory elements is the key concept behind MIA syndrome and chronic kidney disease. Large-molecular-weight uremic toxins or protein-conjugated uremic toxins were supposed to suppress erythropoiesis. It was reported that protein-permeable dialysis by EVAL and PMMA membranes reduced the resistance to erythropoietic-stimulating agents [17, 18]. Native kidneys act not only as a filter of small-molecular-weight substances but also play an important role as a metabolic organ for LMWPs or some albumin.

*Biocompatibility of Dialyzers*

Polyvinylpyrrolidone (PVP) is a chemical agent which gives hydrophilicity to hydrophobic products so it is widely used to make many products such as beverages, soft contact lenses, povidone iodide – which is most frequently used as a bactericidal agent, and many synthetic dialysis membranes. PVP is an indispensable component to make PS, polyethersulfone and many other synthetic membranes. Bisphenol-A is an essential element used in making plastics and polycarbonate, which is widely used for dialyzer-housing material. However, bisphenol-A is also well known as an environmental hormone or endocrine disrupter. There are many dialysis membranes which contain PVP or bisphenol-A, but some membranes do not have them. PS is most widely used as a dialysis membrane material throughout the world but some recent studies have suggested that PS has some uncomfortable side effects such as anaphylaxis, skin lesions and thrombocytopenia, which are supposed to be caused by PVP. Just after they changed PS to the dialysis membranes which did not contain PVP or bisphenol-A, these symptoms disappeared. That is why PVP or bisphenol-A was believed to be related to these complications. Surprisingly, our patients choose the therapies with PMMA, EVAL, AN69 membranes and predilution online HDF mode surely without the knowledge of chemical components of dialysis membranes. These therapies are free from the influence of PVP or Bisphenol-A [13].

*Dialysis Fluid Quality and Clinical Effects of Online HDF*

Online HDF has been developed concomitantly with the purification of dialysis fluid and both of them have actually delayed the onset of DRA. Bioincompatibility of dialysis therapy is supposed to cause the chronic inflammatory response in dialysis patients and lead to various dialysis-related complications, like MIA syndrome and DRA. Bacteriological contamination of dialysis fluid is one of the important factors deteriorating biocompatibility of dialysis therapy [19]. Endotoxin fragments, peptide glycan and bacterial DNA can easily pass through the dialysis membrane from dialysis fluid to blood and they cause the inflammatory response. The more permeable the dialysis membrane becomes, the higher the risk of the contaminations. Many clinical effects of purified dialysis fluid have been reported, such as the retardation of the onset of DRA, the improvement of erythropoietin-resistant anemia, and the improvement of inflammation and nutritional status [19]. Purified dialysis fluid quality has become known as an indispensable factor in the prevention of the MIA syndrome, so we should purify the dialysis fluid when we use HPM. We have kept the bacteriological quality of dialysis fluid at a ultrapure level since 1996 in our facilities.

*The Advantage of Predilution HDF*

In 2003 the Japanese Society for Hemodiafiltration held an international symposium on HDF and had a debate session entitled 'Predilution vs. Postdilution'. In the session the dilution method in HDF was debated only by the point of solute removal efficiency, and it was assumed that small solute removal and LMWP removal was better in postdilution than predilution [20]. Not according to the results of the debate, postdilution HDF had been a major method in Europe and the USA but predilution had been a major method in Japan. Why has predilution HDF been a major method in Japan?

It is well known that small solute removal by diffusion in predilution online HDF is lower than that of HD or postdilution HDF because some dialysis fluid is used for substitution fluid. From the viewpoint of solute removal, it is a drawback of predilution HDF; however, as previously addressed, the suppressed removal of small solute prevents excessive loss of amino acid or other small molecular nutrients during the dialysis session. Leptin is a well-known uremic toxin which deteriorates the appetite of dialysis patients and has been classified into two uremic toxin groups – protein-bound solutes and middle molecules [21]. One of the most typical protein-bound solutes is *p*-cresol and it was effectively removed by predilution online HDF advantageously based on the dilution of serum in predilution [22]. The same mechanism is supposed to enhance more removal of leptin in predilution than HD and postdilution HDF. These characteristics of predilution HDF, well-balanced removal of small solute and LMWP, suggest its nutritional advantage.

One more advantage of predilution HDF is an issue concerning its biocompatibility. As previously addressed, the influence of PVP or other chemical

**Table 1.** Example for prescribing dialysis modalities in a 43-year-old male with chronic glomerulonephritis

| Date | Event or symptom | Dialysis prescription |
|---|---|---|
| 2002.08 | starting dialysis | EVAL 18 $m^2$, QB 250 ml/min, DT: 4 h |
| 2003.08 | insomnia | high-flux PS 1.8 $m^2$, QB 250 ml/min, DT: 5 h |
| 2003.12 | itchy skin | super-flux PS 1.8 $m^2$, QB 250 ml/min, DT: 5 h |
| 2004.05 | severe itchy skin<br>skin eruption on the face | super-flux PS 2.1 $m^2$, QB 250 ml/min, DT: 5 h |
| 2004.10 | severe insomnia | super-flux PS 2.1 $m^2$, predilution HDF, DT: 5 h<br>QB 250 ml/min, QF 200 ml/min |
| 2004.11 | fatigue, nausea<br>sense of 'underdialysis' | high-flux PS 2.1 $m^2$, postdilution HDF, DT: 5 h<br>QB 250 ml/min, QF 50 ml/min |
| 2005.01 | excessive hemoconcentration at the dialyzer | super-flux PS 2.1 $m^2$, predilution HDF, DT: 5 h<br>QB 300 ml/min, QF 200 ml/min |
| | no symptom<br>discontinuance of EPO | continuing the same prescription |

compositions of dialysis membrane has become a new problem which deteriorates the quality of life in dialysis patients. In predilution HDF the blood is much more diluted before the dialyzer, and a large amount of fluid is filtered from the blood side to the dialysis fluid side. If the elution of PVP or other chemical components from dialyzer occur, a large amount of fluid could wash these substances out of the dialysis fluid side. Much diluted blood in predilution HDF would enable the reduction of a close contact between blood cells and the dialysis membrane. It was also reported that the dilution of the serum reduced the hydroxyl radical production in an vitro experiment [pers. commun.]. Shear stress for blood cells would also be milder in predilution than postdilution, so we could decide that the predilution online HDF is more biocompatible than HD and postdilution HDF.

## Practice Pattern for Prescribing Online HDF from a Case Study (table 1)

A 43-year-old male subject started to receive maintenance hemodialysis using EVAL membrane in August 2002. One year after the initiation when he realized his daily urine volume was almost zero, he had been suffering from insomnia and pruritus. PS membrane was adopted and the 4-hour dialysis time was extended 5 h. Seven months after the prescription change, pruritus and skin eruption became worse again so online predilution HDF was inducted. In the first months on predilution HDF he told us that he felt being underdialyzed, so we changed the modality from predilution to postdilution. We could not continue the postdilution HDF because an excessive concentration of the blood was observed in the dialyzer. Therefore we changed it again to predilution at a higher blood flow rate of 300 ml/min. Two months after the prescription change, all symptoms disappeared and erythropoietin administration was discontinued. As we learned from this case, the dialyzer should be changed from a low permeable membrane to a higher permeable membrane according to the status of the target symptom.

## Conclusion

The golden target of chronic dialysis should guarantee longer survival and higher quality of life in dialysis patients. To achieve this target it is very important to prescribe a dialysis modality based on the nutritional status and the symptoms of dialysis patients. Our patients have preferences concerning their dialysis treatments such as PMMA, EVAL, AN69 membranes and predilution online HDF mode. Our experience has revealed that these prescriptions ameliorate the various symptoms, nutritional status and survival rate in dialysis patients. In conclusion, patients' symptoms could be a useful parameter to prescribe a dialysis modality.

## References


1 Pisoni R, Wikström B, Elder SJ, Akizawa T, Asano Y, Keen ML, Saran R, Mendelssohn DC, Young EW, Port FK: Pruiritus in haemodialysis patients: international results from the Dialysis Outcomes and Practice Patterns Study (DOPPS). Nephrol Dial Transplant 2006;21:3495–3505.

2 Lopes AA, Albert JM, Young EW, Satayathum S, Pisoni RL, Andreucci VE, Mapes DL, Mason NA, Fukuhara S, Wikström B, Saito A, Port FK: Screening for depression in hemodialysis patients: associations with diagnosis, treatment, and outcomes in the DOPPS. Kidney Int 2004;66:2047–2053.

3 Lowrie EG, Zhu X, Lew NL: Primary associates of mortality among dialysis patients: trends and reassessment of Kt/V and urea reduction ratio as outcome-based measures of dialysis dose. Am J Kidney Dis 1998;32:S16–S31.

4 Goodkin DA, Bragg-Gresham JL, Koenig KG, Wolfe RA, Akiba T, Andreucci VE, Saito A, Rayner HC, Kurokawa K, Port FK, Held PJ, Young EW. Association of comorbid conditions and mortality in hemodialysis patients in Europe, Japan, and the United States: the Dialysis Outcomes and Practice Patterns Study (DOPPS). J Am Soc Nephrol 2003;14:3270–3277.

5 Gejyo F, Odani S, Yamada T, Honma N, Saito H, Suzuki Y, Nakagawa Y, Kobayashi H, Maruyama Y, Hirasawa Y, et al: Beta-2-microglobulin: a new form of amyloid protein associated with chronic hemodialysis. Kidney Int 1986;30:385–390.

6 Schwalbe S, Holzhauer M, Schaeffer J, Galanski M, Koch KM, Floege J: Beta-2-microglobulin associated amyloidosis: a vanishing complication of long-term hemodialysis? Kidney Int 1997;52:1077–1083.

7 Colton CK, Ward RA, Shaldon S: Scientific basis for assessment of biocompatibility in extracorporeal blood treatment. Nephrol Dial Transplant 1994;9(suppl 2):11–7.
8 Kopple JD, Zhu X, Lew NL, Lowrie EG: Body weight-for-height relationships predict mortality in maintenance hemodialysis patients. Kidney Int 1999;56:1136–1148.
9 Kalantar-Zadeh K, Kopple JD, Block G, Humphreys MH: A malnutrition-inflammation score is correlated with morbidity and mortality in maintenance hemodialysis patients. Am J Kidney Dis 2001;38:1251–1263.
10 Port FK, Ashby VB, Dhingra RK, Roys EC, Wolfe RA: Dialysis dose and body mass index are strongly associated with survival in hemodialysis patients. J Am Soc Nephrol 2002;13:1061–1066.
11 Stenvinkel P, Heimburger O, Paultre F, Diczfalusy U, Wang T, Berglund L, Jogestrand T: Strong association between malnutrition, inflammation, and atherosclerosis in chronic renal failure. Kidney Int 1999;55:1899–1911.
12 Narita I, Alchi B, Omori K, Sato F, Ajiro J, Saga D, Kondo D, Skatsume M, Maruyama S, Kazama JJ, Akazawa K, Gejyo F: Etiology and prognostic significance of severe uremic pruritus in chronic hemodialysis patients. Kidney Int 2006;69:1626–1632.
13 Masakane I: High-quality dialysis: a lesson from the Japanese experience. Nephrol Dial Transplant 2010;3(suppl 1):i28–i35,
14 Elder SJ, Pisoni RL, Akizawa T, Fissell R, Andreucci VE, Fukuhara S, Kurokawa K, Rayner HC, Furniss AL, Port FK, Saran R: Sleep quality predicts quality of life and mortality risk in haemodialysis patients: results from the Dialysis Outcomes and Practice Patterns Study (DOPPS). Nephrol Dial Transplant 2008;23:998–1004.
15 Muta T, Fujimoto T, Harada Y, et al: Are there any differences on amino acid loss during dialysis session by the dialysis membrane material? (in Japanese) Kidney Dial 2005;59(suppl):241–244.
16 Himmelfarb J, McMonagle E: Albumin is the major plasma protein target of oxidant stress in uremia. Kidney Int 2001;60:358–363.
17 Saito A, Suzuki I, Chung TG, Okamoto T, Hotta T: Separation of an inhibitor of erythropoiesis in ‘middle molecules’ from hemodialysate from patients with chronic renal failure. Clin Chem 1986;32:1938–1941.
18 Yamada S, Kataoka H, Kobayashi H, Ono T, Minakuchi J, Kawano Y: Identification of erythropoietic inhibitor from the dialysate collected in the hemodialysis with PMMA membrane (BK-F) and its clinical effects. Contrib Nephrol. Basel, Karger, 1998, vol 125, pp 159–172.
19 Masakane I: Clinical usefulness of ultrapure dialysate – recent evidence and perspectives. Ther Apher Dial 2006;10:348–354.
20 Masakane, I.: Selection of dilutional method for on-line HDF, pre- or post-dilution. Blood Purif 2004;22(suppl 2):49–54.
21 Vanholder R, De Smet R, Glorieux G, Argilés A, Baurmeister U, Brunet P, Clark W, Cohen G, De Deyn PP, Deppisch R, Descamps-Latscha B, Henle T, Jorres A, Lemke HD, Massy ZA, Passlick-Deetjen J, Rodriguez M, Stegmayr B, Stenvinkel P, Tetta C, Wanner C, Zidek W: Review on uremic toxins: classification, concentration, and interindividual variability. Kidney Int 2003;63:1934–1943.
22 Bammens B, Evenepoel P, Verbeke K, Vanrenterghem Y: Removal of the protein-bound solute *p*-cresol by convective transport: a randomized crossover study. Am J Kidney Dis 2004;44:278–285.

Ikuto Masakane
Yabuki Shima Clinic
4-5-5 Shima Kita, Yamagata 990-0885 (Japan)
Tel. +81 23 682 8566, Fax +81 23 682 8567, E-Mail imasakan.aipod@seieig.or.jp

Kawanishi H, Yamashita AC (eds): Hemodiafiltration – A New Era.
Contrib Nephrol. Basel, Karger, 2011, vol 168, pp 64–77

# Optimizing Home Dialysis: Role of Hemodiafiltration

Enric Vilar[a,b] · Ken Farrington[a,b] · Chris Bates[a] · Carol Mumford[a] · Roger Greenwood[a]

[a]Lister Renal Unit, Lister Hospital, Stevenage, and [b]University of Hertfordshire, Hatfield, UK

**Abstract**

Over the last 40 years the technical obstacles which prevented a convective contribution to diffusive dialysis have been overcome. Hemodiafiltration represents a natural evolution of intermittent extracorporeal blood purification and the technology is now available to offer this as standard treatment in-center. The first randomized control trial of dialysis dose (National Cooperative Dialysis Study) showed that for three times weekly dialysis a critical level of urea clearance was necessary to ensure complication-free survival, the effect being noticeable by 3 months. Following this, observational studies suggested that higher doses improved longer term outcome. In a second large randomized controlled study (HEMO), higher small molecule clearance did not further improve outcome, but high-flux membranes, which permitted enhanced clearance of middle molecules, appeared to confer survival benefit in patients who had already been on dialysis >3.7 years. Recently, outcomes from the Membrane Permeability Outcome study confirmed a survival benefit of high-flux membranes in high-risk patients. These studies indicate that in the medium term survival is critically dependent on achieving a minimum level of small solute removal. However, longer term survival (measured in years or decades) not only requires better small solute clearance but also enhanced clearance of middle molecules, the toxicity of which manifest over longer time scales. The rationale for convective treatment is strongest, therefore in those patients who have the greatest potential for long-term survival. Patients who opt for self-care at home to allow frequent dialysis generally are constituents of this group. Hemodiafiltration is likely to become standard therapy in-center and in the home. 

The goal of renal replacement therapy is to replicate the various functions of the native kidney. Over millions of years the kidney has developed into an extraordinary remover of solutes by predominantly convection, aided by active secretion and reabsorption mechanisms. When intermittent dialysis became established as a long-term treatment for kidney failure the process was based around diffusive clearance of solutes. There were formidable obstacles to convective removal including lack of suitable membranes and the expense of producing large volume of sterile 'replacement fluid'. The unmodified cellulosic membranes which were employed delivered excellent small molecule clearances, including urea. Their relatively low permeability to water was convenient in that it allowed a simple 'negative pressure' hydraulic circuit to be used to control ultrafiltration (UF). While high urea clearances were achieved, the removal of middle molecules by diffusion was poor. The term 'low flux' has been coined for such dialyser membranes whose UF rate is typically limited to 5–6 ml/h/mm $Hg/m^2$.

In the late 1970s, 'high-flux' modified cellulosic and synthetic membranes appeared in hollow-fiber dialysers which favored convection. For these dialysers water permeability is much higher, typically around 20 ml/h/mm $Hg/m^2$, while the membrane remains thin enough to permit diffusion. Control of UF was achieved using balanced volumetric chambers in the dialysis fluid circuit. In addition to clearing small molecules, such membranes permit middle molecule removal. Compared to low-flux, high-flux membranes may also have improved biocompatibility characteristics because a protein cake develops on the membrane surface as a result of high UF forces [1]. It has been suggested that this may reduce the inflammatory response to the membrane [2] and limit backdiffusion of dialysate [3].

Although a limited number of dialysis centers still perform low-flux dialysis, many now routinely favor hemodialysis (HD) with high-flux membranes for all patients. Although the HEMO study [4] demonstrated no overall survival benefit in patients treated with low- and high-flux membranes, for those surviving >3.7 years a benefit was seen [5]. The probability that long survivors on HD may benefit from high-flux membranes has fuelled the move to high-flux HD.

Development of hemofiltration (HF) provided a purely convective therapy where large volumes of ultrafiltrate are balanced by infusing replacement solution. HF was successfully applied as a continuous therapy in the intensive care setting but its application in intermittent maintenance dialysis was impractical. The limited time available in a single session was insufficient to permit the large volume of blood filtration necessary to equal the urea clearances being achieved in diffusive dialysis. However, interest in convective blood purification was rekindled by the first reports of dialysis-related amyloid in 1984–1985 [6] and the recognition that $\beta_2$-microglobulin, a middle molecule which accumulated in renal failure and was not removed in diffusive dialysis, was a key building block [7]. The possibility of adding a convective component to diffusive dialysis was therefore pursued. The main technical challenge in so-called, hemodiafiltration (HDF) was the purification of dialysis fluid so that it could be used as a cheap source of replacement fluid. Online HDF whereby 15–20 l of convective exchange takes place over a typical 4-hour diffusive dialysis session was the

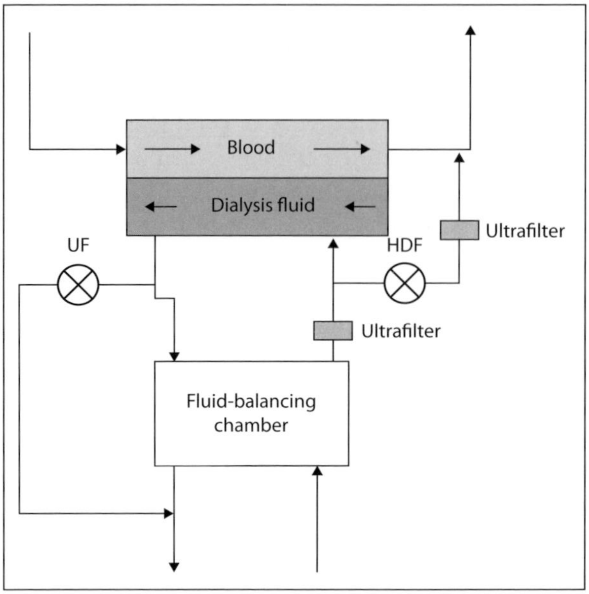


**Fig. 1.** Schematic diagram of a postdilutional online HDF circuit. As in standard dialysis the ultrafiltration pump (UF) removes fluid from the return limb of the dialyser, which requires an equal volume of ultrafiltrate to be drawn from the blood across the dialyser membrane. In contrast to HD, an additional HDF pump (HDF) draws fluid from the input to the dialyser and passes it through an extra ultrafilter and into the venous return circuit. A substitution fluid flow rate between 80 and 100 ml/min would be typical. A volumetric fluid-balancing chamber ensures that the flow rate to and from the dialyser is equal, typically between 500 and 800 ml/min.

result. While small molecule clearance is little affected, significant middle molecule clearances are achieved.

HDF, first described in mid-1970s [8], adds convection to the dialysis process which is largely uninterrupted. There are two pumps, one controlling the rate of UF and the other the rate of HDF, as shown in figure 1. Both pumps vary the transmembrane pressure and draw ultrafiltrate across the dialyser membrane. The balancing chamber ensures volumetric control. The UF pump discharges a set volume into the dialysate waste according to prescribed UF requirements. The HDF pump feeds via an ultrafilter into the venous return limb from the dialyser (postdilutional HDF) or into the arterial limb (predilutional HDF, not shown) ensuring balanced fluid substitution.

Although the provision of HDF has until recently been for dialysis aficionados, there is now growing evidence that it may benefit certain groups of patients and it is now becoming more widely used. It is increasingly recognized that conventional three times weekly HD, which most often totals 12 h/week, replaces only 10–15% of lost kidney function and has limited impact on quality of life. More frequent treatments not only allow for a relaxation of dietary and fluid restrictions, but can also deliver a much higher dialysis dose. Impressive improvements in well-being and measureable clinical outcomes are being reported with enhanced, frequent HD. In practice, this therapy is best carried out in the home or in a community setting by patients trained in self-care. The usual modality to date has been high- or low-flux HD.

Some authors have suggested that a progression to delivery of home HDF is logical, and may improve outcomes for certain patients by increasing middle molecule clearance.

In this article we will review the benefits offered by HDF, and which patients stand to benefit most from this form of renal replacement therapy. Factors which might be taken into consideration in targeting this dialysis modality are discussed. We will review the potential advantages of providing HDF at home, and also the technical barriers to this at present.

### Benefits of HDF over Low-Flux and High-Flux Hemodialysis

Despite the growing adoption of HDF, there is a relative lack of outcome data when compared to conventional HD and high-flux HD. In comparison to low-flux HD with conventional membranes, middle molecules exemplified by $\beta_2$-microglobulin are cleared to a greater degree by high-flux HD [4, 9, 10]. Dialysis-related amyloidosis is also remarkably less frequent in patients on high-flux HD [9, 10]. Strong evidence now exists that HDF, when compared with high-flux HD, provides increased $\beta_2$-microglobulin clearance and is associated with a lower frequency of dialysis-related amyloid [11, 12].

This leads to the question of whether increased middle molecule clearance in high-flux HD and HDF impacts on survival. Although the HEMO study [4] did not find overall survival differences in those randomized to high-flux over conventional HD, it was subsequently noted that mortality was lower in a subset of those dialysed for >3.7 years [5]. More recently the Membrane Permeability Outcome study [13] has demonstrated a survival benefit for high-flux HD over conventional (low-flux) HD at least for those with a low albumin.

Does HDF confer a survival benefit compared to low-flux HD and high-flux HD? The prospective, observational but non-randomized RISCAVID study [14] found evidence for a survival benefit of HDF over and above low-flux HD. In a retrospective analysis of Dialysis Outcomes and Practice Patterns Study data, Canaud et al. [15] found a lower mortality in those receiving HDF compared to those on low-flux HD. Furthermore, this study reports a benefit of HDF over and above a group dialysed by a mixture of high-flux and low-flux HD. A retrospective observational study by Jirka et al. [16] of data collected in EuCliD found a 35.3% reduced mortality associated with HDF, although this report did not describe the proportion of patients using high-flux membranes. Two randomized control trials may provide confirmatory evidence for these findings which indicate a potential benefit of convective therapies of HDF over low-flux HD. An Italian study will randomize patients to conventional low-flux HD or a convective therapy (HDF or HF) [17]. The Dutch CONTRAST study [18] will randomize 800 subjects to HDF or low-flux HD. Even without data from randomized control trials, many nephrologists have already concluded, however, that high-flux HD provides survival benefits over low-flux HD.

Data comparing high-flux HD with HDF are even more scarce. A recent large retrospective observational study by our own unit found that in a group of patients who had exclusively high-flux HD or HDF (i.e. no conventional low-flux dialysis) the proportion of time spent on HDF predicted survival, even after correcting for confounding factors including dialysis dose and comorbidities. The only published randomized control trial directly comparing HDF to high-flux HD (n = 76) was too small for comparison of survival outcomes [19]. In this study, hypotensive episodes were less frequent in those treated by HDF which matches findings from the large retrospective study conducted at our renal unit [20] and other studies [21, 22]. It has been postulated that the apparent hemodynamic benefits of HDF may in fact be related to the cooling effect of the replacement fluid [23, 24].

Evidence for benefits of HDF over other treatment modalities in terms of bone metabolism parameters is variable. Although a randomized cross-over control trial of online HDF versus high-flux HD by Schiffl [19] found lower serum phosphate during HDF treatment, this finding has not been confirmed in our much larger, though retrospective analysis [20]. Similarly, data from Schiffl's study found evidence for lower erythropoietin requirements during HDF treatment, but this may be due to a higher Kt/V as our own data did not confirm this finding. Infusion of replacement fluid does not seem to have any adverse consequences in terms of inflammation, and indeed there is a suggestion of marginal benefit associated with HDF compared to high-flux HD [20].

To conclude, therefore, it seems that HDF may provide a survival benefit both over and above conventional low-flux HD, and also above high-flux HD. The explanation for this remains elusive, but may be related to enhanced clearance of middle molecules, reflected in $\beta_2$-microglobulin levels. Deciding which patients are likely to benefit most from HDF is crucial both for designing randomized control trials, and for targeting this therapy. Particular consideration needs to be given to the effect of residual renal function which has an overriding effect on middle molecule clearance [25]. We hypothesize that the maximal benefit of convective therapies is likely to be in those with low middle molecule clearance due to limited residual renal function. Additionally, the benefit is more likely to be found in those who are likely to remain dependent on dialysis for survival for a prolonged period of time.

### Individualizing Choice of Renal Replacement Therapy

Selection of ideal treatment modality for renal replacement therapy is highly individualized and should take into account factors that include cardiac status, physical frailty, estimated survival time, level of residual renal function, and whether a home-based therapy is feasible. Experience of home-based therapies has now expanded in many centers so that both peritoneal dialysis and HD can be offered as alternative home choices. Although renal transplant will remain the ideal method of renal replacement therapy for many patients, a substantial proportion will require peritoneal dialysis or HD for many years.

There is a paucity of outcome studies comparing outcomes between three times weekly home dialysis versus in-hospital HD. Excellent results have been obtained for patients treated by frequent home HD although there may be substantial bias in outcome data due to patient selection. Frequent dialysis regimes show particular benefits in terms of quality-of-life measures, blood pressure [26, 27], anemia parameters [27, 28], bone mineral metabolism [28, 29] and left ventricular hypertrophy [26, 30]. Two randomized trials by the Frequent Hemodialysis Network will look at differences in outcomes where clearance is substantially increased [31, 32] but may not have sufficient differences to demonstrate mortality differences [33].

Many nephrologists already consider that for patients considered to be low-risk, a home-based therapy is the best treatment option, particularly if this allows more frequent dialysis than three times weekly. For this patient subset, where residual renal function is high, peritoneal dialysis may provide adequate clearance, but for low-risk patients without significant residual renal function, peritoneal dialysis may be insufficient [34]. Home-based HD performed frequently (or nocturnally) may benefit this group particularly and may be provided in the form of high-flux HD or HDF. Higher risk patients who are not considered safe for home-based HD may still be able to tolerate peritoneal dialysis, but alternatively may require hospital HD. For such patients, blood purification may be best performed by high-flux HD or HDF particularly if residual renal function is poor. In a small subset of patients who have renal replacement therapy with a palliative goal, the frequency of dialysis will depend not on long-term outcomes, but rather on symptom control. These treatment considerations are summarized in figure 2 which aims to demonstrate that the potential choices available to patients will depend on risk group and residual renal function, with the maximum benefit of convective therapies being obtained for those predicted to survive for a prolonged time on dialysis with low levels of residual renal function.

In summary, therefore, we suggest that for patients considered to be low-risk, until transplant is possible a home-based therapy should be first choice (either peritoneal dialysis or HD). Where HD is chosen, a frequent dialysis regime with a high-flux membrane is likely to provide the best outcome. Furthermore, it

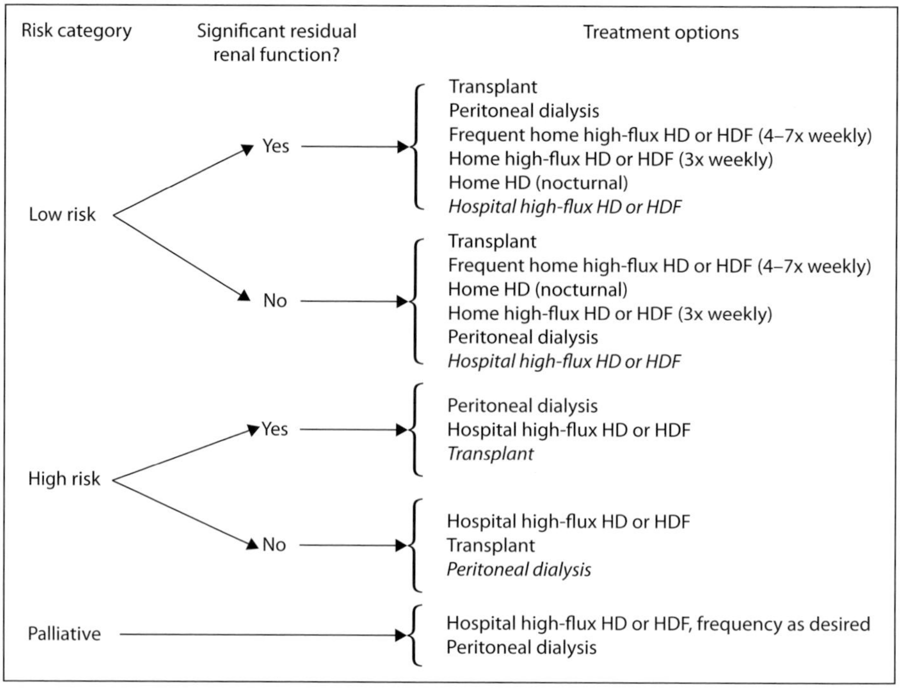


**Fig. 2.** Renal replacement therapy options which might be appropriate for patients of different overall risk categories, dependent on level of residual renal function. Options in italics are less likely to be suitable.

seems likely that HDF at home will provide the best outcomes, at least for those with low levels of residual renal function.

## Providing HDF at Home: Technical Considerations

A number of technical issues need to be considered when using HDF in the home. For home HDF it is necessary to have a supply of dialysis fluid/replacement solution in similar volume as for conventional HD, typically 150–200 liters per session. Additionally, the provision of ultrapure water is essential due to the potential risk of exposure to contaminants and endotoxin from replacement solution. Although HDF with commercially available sterile bags has been attempted, ultrapure water is now most commonly generated locally using online HDF. In this technique the excess fluid ultrafiltered using a high-flux membrane is replaced using substitution solution that has been generated from a process of stepwise UF of dialysis fluid. With the correct procedure, it is possible to produce fluid locally which can be considered both pyrogen-free and

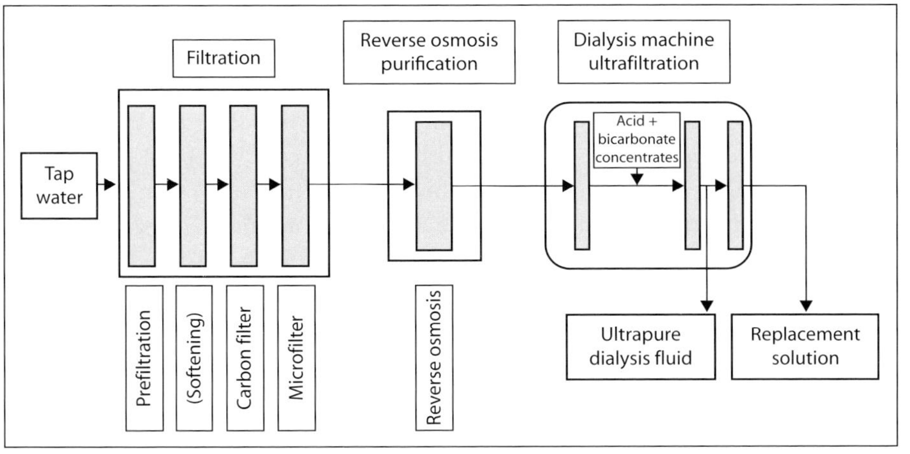


**Fig. 3.** Water purification system for use in home HD and home HDF. The system will produce ultrapure dialysis fluid and ultrapure replacement solution for online HDF. The home water pretreats water using microfilters, softeners (optional) and carbon filters prior to reverse osmosis. The reverse osmosis step softens water by removing most ions and removes organic material and large particles. Hospital dialysis unit purification systems may include two reverse osmosis modules in series. Purified water is then transferred to the dialysis machine where it is passed through an ultrafilter and concentrates of acid and bicarbonate are added to produce ultrapure dialysis fluid. To generate replacement solution the ultrapure dialysis fluid is passed through a final ultrafilter.

sterile. Although online HDF carries an additional cost in water purification and use of ultrafilters, the cost increment is small and generally affordable [35, 36]. Portable home water filters now available are able, using stepwise ultrafilters, to produce ultrapure water. This makes home HDF technically feasible. In fact, the exposure to high volumes of water by HD patients measured in hundreds of liters per week makes it difficult to justify the use of non-ultrapure water even for low-flux HD. The European Best Practice Guidelines and Japanese Society for Dialysis guidelines reflect this in their recommendations that ultrapure water be used for all forms of dialysis [37, 38].

Figure 3 shows a diagram of a typical system used to produce dialysis water for home HD. Municipal water is subjected to a process of pretreatment followed by purification by reverse osmosis, and finally stepwise UF [39]. The pretreatment consists of downsizing microfilters, water softening to remove calcium and magnesium, and carbon filtration which removes chlorine. The softening step is not always performed for home-based systems due to the potential increased risk of microbiological contamination but subsequent UF provides microbiological protection. Reverse osmosis, usually performed twice for in-hospital systems but once only for home purifiers, is a major purification step which will result in removal of large molecules and organic impurities including water-borne parasites, bacteria and viruses. Reverse osmosis is the term used to describe purification whereby a pressure is applied to fluid on one side of a semipermeable membrane, resulting in retention of solute on the pressurized side of the membrane. Ion removal by this process will have a softening effect. The final step is passage of water through an ultrafilter within the dialysis machine and the addition of bicarbonate and acid concentrates (fig. 3) to produce ultrapure dialysis fluid. Ultrapure dialysis fluid is then passed through a final ultrafilter to produce ultrapure replacement solution which is ready for infusion intravenously. Some systems have an alternative disposable ultrafilter with each HDF line set.

Guaranteeing the safety of ultrapure substitution fluid is crucial both for unit-delivered and home HDF. Reassurance on the safety of in-hospital online HDF is provided by an absence of studies demonstrating worse outcomes for HDF, and our own retrospective data has not demonstrated higher erythropioetin resistance or inflammatory markers in those treated by HDF [20]. However, there are at present no published studies demonstrating the safety of home-delivered online HDF. Regular and routine monitoring of water quality is now a well-established safety mechanism in water purification systems for dialysis units and it seems logical to conclude that monitoring of water quality in the home setting should be performed. Microbiological surveillance of water quality should ensure that dialysis fluid for HDF be ultrapure, defined by <0.1 colony-forming unit (CFU) per ml and <0.03 endotoxin unit (EU) per ml [40–42]. Substitution fluid produced from further UF of ultrapure dialysis fluid should be of substantially higher microbiological quality at $<1 \cdot 10^{-6}$ CFU/ml due to the high volumes infused intravenously, as described by Ledebo [43, 44]. In practice such microbiological quality is unmeasurable due to the high sampling volume required to detect such low CFU concentrations.

In addition to microbiological safety, potential contaminants should be monitored including chlorine, nitrogen and trace elements. Trace elements present in ultrapure water which have not been removed by reverse osmosis bind to plasma proteins, but the effect of potential long-term accumulation has yet to be established [45]. In the case of high-flux HD, the backfiltration effect that occurs across the dialyser membrane [46] also increases exposure. The protein cake which develops on the membrane may limit this [47, 48]. For HDF, there is no such protection as replacement fluid is infused intravenously.

Chemical water contamination needs to be carefully considered. Seasonal and regional variation of contaminant ions may occur in municipal water. Potentially significant contaminants include chlorine, chloramines, nitrates, calcium, copper, fluoride and sulphate. Typically, home dialysis water purifiers do not include a water-softening stage and this may result in insufficient nitrate removal, particularly during seasonal peaks in municipal water supply. It may be necessary to employ a mixed bed softener including a nitrate removal resin prior to the reverse osmosis step. Additionally, home dialysis water purifiers employ a single-pass reverse osmosis system which potentially may remove insufficient amounts of solutes, but whether a double-pass system would improve quality substantially remains to be seen. Microbiological water quality does not seem to be inferior in single-pass systems [39]. In our own experience, one of our dialysis units has provided HDF for more than 10 years with high incoming levels of nitrate (approx. 40 mg/l) using a single module reverse osmosis system, without any obvious deleterious effects on patients. For home HD patients, maintenance of the reverse osmosis system should include cleaning. In our unit, patients perform a chemical disinfect of their module weekly, but equipment is also available which allows heat cleaning without the need to store chemical disinfectants at home.

In our own dialysis unit, ultrapure dialysis water is checked for microbiological purity, chlorine and nitrate concentration monthly; full chemical assay including trace elements is performed 6 monthly. We suggest that for online HDF at home there is no reason to think that monitoring could be substantially less frequent which may create some logistical difficulties. Risk assessment should be performed based on local potable water quality which should include solutes such as nitrates with seasonal variation.

## Dialysis Adequacy for Home HDF

Measurement of dialysis adequacy is normally performed using urea clearance and the Kt/V model. Convective dialysis techniques do not substantially increase the removal of small molecules, provided that other variables which define clearance are kept constant [49]. HDF delivers greater elimination of middle molecules compared to both high- and low-flux HD [11, 50], but their elimination is not usually measured. In a complex, but retrospective, survival analysis at our own unit we have demonstrated that the survival benefit of HDF over high-flux HD seems to be independent of Kt/V urea [20]. It seems likely that the unmeasured and unquantified middle molecule clearance may be the underlying factor. There is now clear evidence that plasma concentration of $\beta_2$-microglobulin has a relationship with mortality [51, 52]. The benefit of measuring middle molecule clearance routinely has yet to be proven, but could be performed using $\beta_2$-microglobulin as a surrogate marker.

For patients who choose home HDF and dialyse more frequently than three times per week, the urea Kt/V model cannot be used as it has been validated for three times weekly dialysis only. Frequent HD or HDF dialysis adequacy can be measured using a variety of methods such as the standard Kt/V model proposed by Gotch [53], converting per-session clearance to a weekly equivalent.

Alternatively, the Casino-Lopez equivalent urea clearance can be used [54]. For those wishing to accurately model urea clearance for complex home dialysis regimes, Daugirdas et al. [55] have recently described SoluteSolver, a formal urea kinetic modelling program which can model HDF of varying session frequency.

## Equipment Portability

At present there are no technologies licensed to provide a portable HDF system, unless replacement solution is used with sterile bags. Online HDF requires large volumes of guaranteed water quality which is regularly tested, and for this reason it is unlikely that HDF in its current form develops into a portable technology.

## Conclusion

Evidence is now growing that HDF confers outcome benefits over and above both high-flux HD and low-flux (standard) HD. This evidence is predominantly retrospective and results of several prospective randomized studies are awaited [17, 18]. The development of online HDF has resulted in more widespread use of the HDF technique. The resurgence of home dialysis in recent years may result in improved outcomes and quality of life for selected patients. However, until recently, home dialysis has been provided mainly in the form of low- and high-flux HD. Home dialysis patients potentially might benefit from HDF, particularly if their expected career on dialysis is long or if their level of residual renal function is low. In order to test this hypothesis it is necessary to develop safe methods of delivering HDF at home. Online HDF can deliver higher convection volumes which maximize middle molecule clearance. However, providing online HDF at home requires water quality issues to be considered and overcome. Units wishing to develop home HDF programs will need to put in place systems of monitoring ultrapure water quality to ensure safety, although the frequency with which monitoring is required will vary depending on local potable water quality. The absence of published safety and outcome data for home HDF creates a knowledge gap which requires urgent filling. We are optimistic that increased interest in HDF will produce these data in the near future.

## Acknowledgement

E.V. is supported by a Kidney Research UK Fellowship.

## References


1 Birk HW, Kistner A, Wizemann V, Schutterle G: Protein adsorption by artificial membrane materials under filtration conditions. Artif Organs 1995;19:411–415.

2 Teruel JL, Pascual J, Serrano P, Ortuno J: ACE inhibitors and AN69 membranes: absence of anaphylactoid reactions in haemodiafiltration process. Nephrol Dial Transplant 1992;7:275.

3 Klinkmann H, Ebbighausen H, Uhlenbusch I, Vienken J: High-flux dialysis, dialysate quality and backtransport. Contrib Nephrol. Basel, Karger, 1993, vol 103, pp 89–97.

4 Eknoyan G, Beck GJ, Cheung AK, Daugirdas JT, Greene T, Kusek JW, Allon M, Bailey J, Delmez JA, Depner TA, Dwyer JT, Levey AS, Levin NW, Milford E, Ornt DB, Rocco MV, Schulman G, Schwab SJ, Teehan BP, Toto R: Effect of dialysis dose and membrane flux in maintenance hemodialysis. N Engl J Med 2002;347:2010–2019.

5 Cheung AK, Levin NW, Greene T, Agodoa L, Bailey J, Beck G, Clark W, Levey AS, Leypoldt JK, Ornt DB, Rocco MV, Schulman G, Schwab S, Teehan B, Eknoyan G: Effects of high-flux hemodialysis on clinical outcomes: results of the HEMO study. J Am Soc Nephrol 2003;14:3251–3263.

6 Kuntz D, Naveau B, Bardin T, Drueke T, Treves R, Dryll A: Destructive spondylarthropathy in hemodialyzed patients. A new syndrome. Arthritis Rheum 1984;27: 369–375.

7 Gejyo F, Yamada T, Odani S, Nakagawa Y, Arakawa M, Kunitomo T, Kataoka H, Suzuki M, Hirasawa Y, Shirahama T, et al: A new form of amyloid protein associated with chronic hemodialysis was identified as $\beta_2$-microglobulin. Biochem Biophys Res Commun 1985;129:701–706.

8 Henderson LW, Colton CK, Ford CA: Kinetics of hemodiafiltration. II. Clinical characterization of a new blood cleansing modality. J Lab Clin Med 1975;85:372–391.

9 Kuchle C, Fricke H, Held E, Schiffl H: High-flux hemodialysis postpones clinical manifestation of dialysis-related amyloidosis. Am J Nephrol 1996;16:484–488.

10 Van Ypersele de Strihou C, Jadoul M, Malghem J, Maldague B, Jamart J: Effect of dialysis membrane and patient's age on signs of dialysis-related amyloidosis. The Working Party on Dialysis Amyloidosis. Kidney Int 1991;39:1012–1019.

11 Lornoy W, Becaus I, Billiouw JM, Sierens L, Van Malderen P, D'Haenens P: On-line haemodiafiltration. Remarkable removal of $\beta_2$-microglobulin. Long-term clinical observations. Nephrol Dial Transplant 200;15(suppl 1):49–54.

12 Ward RA, Schmidt B, Hullin J, Hillebrand GF, Samtleben W: A comparison of on-line hemodiafiltration and high-flux hemodialysis: a prospective clinical study. J Am Soc Nephrol 2000;11:2344–2350.

13 Locatelli F, Martin-Malo A, Hannedouche T, Loureiro A, Papadimitriou M, Wizemann V, Jacobson SH, Czekalski S, Ronco C, Vanholder R: Effect of membrane permeability on survival of hemodialysis patients. J Am Soc Nephrol 2009;20:645–654.

14 Panichi V, Rizza GM, Paoletti S, Bigazzi R, Aloisi M, Barsotti G, Rindi P, Donati G, Antonelli A, Panicucci E, Tripepi G, Tetta C, Palla R: Chronic inflammation and mortality in haemodialysis: effect of different renal replacement therapies. Results from the RISCAVID study. Nephrol Dial Transplant 2008;23:2337–2343.

15 Canaud B, Bragg-Gresham JL, Marshall MR, Desmeules S, Gillespie BW, Depner T, Klassen P, Port FK: Mortality risk for patients receiving hemodiafiltration versus hemodialysis: European results from the DOPPS. Kidney Int 2006;69:2087–2093.

16 Jirka T, Cesare S, Di Benedetto A, Perera Chang M, Ponce P, Richards N, Tetta C, Vaslaky L: Mortality risk for patients receiving hemodiafiltration versus hemodialysis. Kidney Int 2006;70:1524–1525.

17 Bolasco P, Altieri P, Andrulli S, Basile C, Di Filippo S, Feriani M, Pedrini L, Santoro A, Zoccali C, Sau G, Locatelli F: Convection versus diffusion in dialysis: an Italian prospective multicentre study. Nephrol Dial Transplant 2003;18(suppl 7):vii50–vii54, vii59–vii62.

18 Penne EL, Blankestijn PJ, Bots ML, van den Dorpel MA, Grooteman MP, Nube MJ, ter Wee PM: Resolving controversies regarding hemodiafiltration versus hemodialysis: the Dutch Convective Transport Study. Semin Dial 2005;18:47–51.
19 Schiffl H: Prospective randomized cross-over long-term comparison of online haemodiafiltration and ultrapure high-flux haemodialysis. Eur J Med Res 2007;12:26–33.
20 Vilar E, Fry AC, Wellsted D, Tattersall JE, Greenwood RN, Farrington K: Long-term outcomes in online hemodiafiltration and high-flux hemodialysis: a comparative analysis. Clin J Am Soc Nephrol 2009;4: 1944–1953.
21 Munoz R, Gallardo I, Valladares E, Saracho R, Martinez I, Ocharan J, Montenegro J: Online hemodiafiltration: four years of clinical experience. Hemodial Int 2006;10(suppl 1):S28–S32.
22 Velasco N: Convection with conviction-online hemodiafiltration for all: single-center clinical observations. Hemodial Int 2006;10(suppl 1):S67–S71.
23 Karamperis N, Sloth E, Jensen JD: Predilution hemodiafiltration displays no hemodynamic advantage over low-flux hemodialysis under matched conditions. Kidney Int 2005;67:1601–1608.
24 Donauer J, Schweiger C, Rumberger B, Krumme B, Bohler J: Reduction of hypotensive side effects during online-haemodiafiltration and low temperature haemodialysis. Nephrol Dial Transplant 2003;18:1616–1622.
25 Fry AC, Singh DK, Chandna SM, Farrington K: Relative importance of residual renal function and convection in determining $\beta_2$-microglobulin levels in high-flux haemodialysis and on-line haemodiafiltration. Blood Purif 2007;25:295–302.
26 Suri RS, Nesrallah GE, Mainra R, Garg AX, Lindsay RM, Greene T, Daugirdas JT: Daily hemodialysis: a systematic review. Clin J Am Soc Nephrol 2006;1:33–42.
27 Walsh M, Culleton B, Tonelli M, Manns B: A systematic review of the effect of nocturnal hemodialysis on blood pressure, left ventricular hypertrophy, anemia, mineral metabolism, and health-related quality of life. Kidney Int 2005;67:1500–1508.
28 Lockridge RS Jr, Spencer M, Craft V, Pipkin M, Campbell D, McPhatter L, Albert J, Anderson H, Jennings F, Barger T: Nightly home hemodialysis: five and one-half years of experience in Lynchburg, Virginia. Hemodial Int 2004;8:61–69.
29 Ayus JC, Achinger SG, Mizani MR, Chertow GM, Furmaga W, Lee S, Rodriguez F: Phosphorus balance and mineral metabolism with 3 h daily hemodialysis. Kidney Int 2007;71:336–342.
30 Culleton BF, Walsh M, Klarenbach SW, Mortis G, Scott-Douglas N, Quinn RR, Tonelli M, Donnelly S, Friedrich MG, Kumar A, Mahallati H, Hemmelgarn BR, Manns BJ: Effect of frequent nocturnal hemodialysis vs. conventional hemodialysis on left ventricular mass and quality of life: a randomized controlled trial. JAMA 2007;298:1291–1299.
31 Suri RS, Garg AX, Chertow GM, Levin NW, Rocco MV, Greene T, Beck GJ, Gassman JJ, Eggers PW, Star RA, Ornt DB, Kliger AS: Frequent Hemodialysis Network (FHN) randomized trials: study design. Kidney Int 2007;71:349–359.
32 Greene T, Daugirdas JT, Depner TA, Gotch F, Kuhlman M: Solute clearances and fluid removal in the Frequent Hemodialysis Network trials. Am J Kidney Dis 2009;53:835–844.
33 Rocco MV: Short daily and nocturnal hemodialysis: new therapies for a new century? Saudi J Kidney Dis Transpl 2009;20:1–11.
34 Bargman JM, Thorpe KE, Churchill DN: Relative contribution of residual renal function and peritoneal clearance to adequacy of dialysis: a reanalysis of the CANUSA study. J Am Soc Nephrol 2001;12:2158–2162.
35 Canaud B, QV NG, Polito C, Stec F, Mion C: Hemodiafiltration with on-line production of bicarbonate infusate. A new standard for high-efficiency, low-cost dialysis in elderly and uncompliant patients. Contrib Nephrol. Basel, Karger, 1989, vol 74, pp 91–100.
36 Greenwood RN: An incremental high-flux dialysis/hemodiafiltration program based on urea kinetic modeling. Semin Dial 1999;12:S71–S75.
37 Section IV. Dialysis fluid purity. Nephrol Dial Transplant 2002;17(suppl 7):45–62.

38 Kawanishi H, Akiba T, Masakane I, Tomo T, Mineshima M, Kawasaki T, Hirakata H, Akizawa T: Standard on microbiological management of fluids for hemodialysis and related therapies by the Japanese Society for Dialysis Therapy 2008. Ther Apher Dial 2009;13:161–166.
39 Penne EL, Visser L, van den Dorpel MA, van der Weerd NC, Mazairac AH, van Jaarsveld BC, Koopman MG, Vos P, Feith GW, Kremer Hovinga TK, van Hamersvelt HW, Wauters IM, Bots ML, Nube MJ, Ter Wee PM, Blankestijn PJ, Grooteman MP: Microbiological quality and quality control of purified water and ultrapure dialysis fluids for online hemodiafiltration in routine clinical practice. Kidney Int 2009;76:665–672.
40 Lonnemann G: On-line fluid preparation. Contrib Nephrol. Basel, Karger, 2002, vol 137, pp 332–337.
41 Ledebo I, Nystrand R: Defining the microbiological quality of dialysis fluid. Artif Organs 1999;23:37–43.
42 Canaud B, Bosc JY, Leray H, Morena M, Stec F: Microbiologic purity of dialysate: rationale and technical aspects. Blood Purif 2000;18:200–213.
43 Ledebo I: On-line preparation of solutions for dialysis: practical aspects versus safety and regulations. J Am Soc Nephrol 2002;13(suppl 1):S78–S83.
44 Ledebo I, Blankestijn PJ: Haemodiafiltration – optimal efficiency and safety. NDT Plus 2010;3:8–16.
45 Vanholder R, Cornelis R, Dhondt A, Lameire N: The role of trace elements in uraemic toxicity. Nephrol Dial Transplant 2002;17(suppl 2):2–8.
46 Ronco C, Brendolan A, Feriani M, Milan M, Conz P, Lupi A, Berto P, Bettini M, La Greca G: A new scintigraphic method to characterize ultrafiltration in hollow fiber dialyzers. Kidney Int 1992;41:1383–1393.
47 Lonnemann G, Schindler R, Lufft V, Mahiout A, Shaldon S, Koch KM: The role of plasma coating on the permeation of cytokine-inducing substances through dialyser membranes. Nephrol Dial Transplant 1995;10:207–211.
48 Canaud B, Bosc JY, Leray H, Stec F: Microbiological purity of dialysate for online substitution fluid preparation. Nephrol Dial Transplant 2000;15:21–30.
49 Briones JL: Convection versus diffusion: is it time to make a change? (in Spanish) Nefrologia 2009;29:594–603.
50 Tattersall J: Clearance of $\beta_2$-microglobulin and middle molecules in haemodiafiltration. Contrib Nephrol. Basel, Karger, 2007, vol 158, pp 201–209.
51 Cheung AK, Rocco MV, Yan G, Leypoldt JK, Levin NW, Greene T, Agodoa L, Bailey J, Beck GJ, Clark W, Levey AS, Ornt DB, Schulman G, Schwab S, Teehan B, Eknoyan G: Serum $\beta_2$-microglobulin levels predict mortality in dialysis patients: results of the HEMO study. J Am Soc Nephrol 2006;17:546–555.
52 Okuno S, Ishimura E, Kohno K, Fujino-Katoh Y, Maeno Y, Yamakawa T, Inaba M, Nishizawa Y: Serum $\beta_2$-microglobulin level is a significant predictor of mortality in maintenance haemodialysis patients. Nephrol Dial Transplant 2009;24:571–577.
53 Gotch FA: The current place of urea kinetic modelling with respect to different dialysis modalities. Nephrol Dial Transplant 1998;13(suppl 6):10–14.
54 Casino FG, Lopez T: The equivalent renal urea clearance: a new parameter to assess dialysis dose. Nephrol Dial Transplant 1996;11:1574–1581.
55 Daugirdas JT, Depner TA, Greene T, Silisteanu P: Solute-solver: a web-based tool for modeling urea kinetics for a broad range of hemodialysis schedules in multiple patients. Am J Kidney Dis 2009;54:798–809.

E. Vilar
Lister Renal Unit, Lister Hospital
Corey's Mill Lane, Stevenage SG1 4AB (UK)
E-Mail evilar@doctors.org.uk

Kawanishi H, Yamashita AC (eds): Hemodiafiltration – A New Era.
Contrib Nephrol. Basel, Karger, 2011, vol 168, pp 78–88

# Quality Management of Dialysis Fluid for Online Convective Therapies

Richard A. Ward

Department of Medicine, University of Louisville, Louisville, Ky., USA

**Abstract**

Increasing evidence supports use of convective therapies, such as hemodiafiltration, to improve outcomes for hemodialysis patients. Maximizing convection requires large volumes of substitution solution, which is practical only if online technology is used for its preparation. Substitution solution must be sterile and non-pyrogenic. Since it is not practical to test solutions prepared online for sterility and non-pyrogenicity before use, they must be prepared using processes that have been validated to produce solutions of the required quality. Preparation of substitution solution begins with treatment of municipal water to produce dialysis water, followed by proportioning of that water with concentrates to provide dialysis fluid, and ends with sequential filtration of the dialysis fluid with bacteria- and endotoxin-retentive filters to provide substitution solution. Whether dialysis fluid is prepared centrally or using individual dialysis machines, production of sterile, non-pyrogenic substitution solution requires maintenance of a hygienic chain from the beginning to the end of the fluid-handling pathway. Maintaining the integrity of that hygienic chain under routine operating conditions requires a comprehensive quality management program involving the design, operation and maintenance of all fluid-handling systems and ongoing training of the staff responsible for all aspects of their use.



Secondary analysis of two recently completed large randomized clinical trials suggests that increased clearance of larger molecules is associated with improved outcomes in hemodialysis patients [1, 2]. However, diffusive clearance decreases rapidly with increasing molecular size making it difficult to improve the clearance of larger molecules by hemodialysis, even when highly permeable membranes are used. In contrast, convective clearance decreases more gradually than diffusive clearance as molecular size increases, thus allowing significant increases in clearance to be obtained by using therapies such as hemofiltration (HF) and hemodiafiltration (HDF).

HF and HDF provide convective clearance by ultrafiltering plasma water at a much greater rate than that required to achieve a patient's dry body weight and infusing an electrolyte solution, referred to as substitution solution, immediately before or after the dialyzer to maintain body volume. In HF, clearance occurs only through convection and substitution solution volumes in excess of 70 l/treatment can be required to achieve adequate clearance of small molecules for thrice weekly therapy. HDF avoids the need for such large volumes by combining convective and diffusive clearances in a single treatment; even then, substitution solution volumes >17 l are needed to achieve optimal clearances of large molecules. These volumes are not practical if prepackaged, terminally sterilized substitution fluid is used and this limitation initially slowed the uptake of convective therapies. However, in the 1990s, systems became available that prepared substitution solution by filtration of dialysis fluid through two or more bacteria- and endotoxin-retentive filters [3, 4]. These systems, referred to as online systems, removed the limitation on substitution solution volume and allowed the growth of convective therapies, particularly HDF. The results of several observational studies [5, 6] and one small randomized clinical trial [7] support the hypothesis that convective therapies provide superior outcomes than conventional hemodialysis and this hypothesis is currently being tested in a number of randomized clinical trials [8]. If these trials confirm an advantage for online convective therapies the production of large volumes of substitution solution will need to become routine in dialysis facilities.

## Online Preparation of Substitution Solution for Convective Therapies

Because they are introduced directly into the bloodstream in large volumes, substitution solutions for convective therapies must be sterile and non-pyrogenic. In the early days of convective therapy, this quality was assured by using bags of fluid that had been terminally sterilized by autoclaving. The process conditions for this form of sterilization are well defined and there is only one chance in a million that a bag of fluid prepared in this manner will be contaminated. However, there is a practical limit to the volume of substitution solution that can be used with prepackaged bags and the pioneers of convective therapies soon realized that alternative methods of producing sterile and non-pyrogenic substitution fluids were needed. Henderson et al. [9] were the first to apply filtration to prepare substitution solution online from dialysis fluid. After a lengthy period during which both technical and regulatory issues were resolved, dialysis machines that prepared substitution solution online by a process of sequential filtration through bacteria- and endotoxin-retentive filters finally became commercially available in the 1990s [3, 4].

Because substitution solution prepared online is used immediately, it is not possible to determine that it is sterile and non-pyrogenic by testing before it is infused into the patient. Rather, the substitution solution must be produced using a process that has been validated by the manufacturer to produce a sterile and non-pyrogenic solution [10]. Currently available HDF and HF systems use one of two approaches, both of which utilize series-connected filters capable of reducing the level of bacteria and endotoxin by factors of $>10^6–10^7$ and $10^3–10^4$, respectively [3, 4]. Use of such filters in series allows sterile, non-pyrogenic substitution fluid to be produced even if one of the filters was to fail [4].

The starting materials for the online preparation of substitution solution are municipal water and acid and bicarbonate concentrates. Municipal water must be treated to remove harmful contaminants before being combined with the acid and bicarbonate concentrates to produce dialysis fluid that is, in turn, used to prepare substitution solution. Chemical contaminants are removed from municipal water in a water treatment system usually centered on reverse osmosis. Once these contaminants are removed they will not re-enter the treated water, referred to as dialysis water, provided appropriate inert materials are used throughout the water distribution system. Acid and bicarbonate concentrates can be obtained ready to use from commercial sources that must meet applicable regulatory requirements in the manufacturing process. In some situations, however, concentrates are obtained as dry salts that are reconstituted with dialysis water at the dialysis facility to provide a batch of liquid concentrate sufficient for one or more treatment shifts. In this situation, the concentrate preparation system must also be fabricated from appropriate inert materials.

Reverse osmosis is a good barrier against microbiological as well as chemical contaminants. However, since the water treatment system removes antibacterial agents such as chlorine and chloramines from the water, there is nothing to prevent bacterial proliferation and recontamination of dialysis water as it passes through the distribution system. Therefore, the major challenge in routine production of substitution solution is to maintain a hygienic chain from the product water side of the reverse osmosis unit to the point at which substitution solution enters the patient's blood. This hygienic chain must encompass not only the dialysis water distribution system, including storage tanks, but also any concentrate preparation and handling systems, the combining of dialysis water and concentrates to produce dialysis fluid, and final production of substitution solution.

Although the final production of substitution solution from dialysis fluid is performed using a system validated by its manufacturer, that validation only applies if the system is operated under specified conditions. In particular, the incoming fluid quality must comply with maximum contaminant levels specified by the manufacturer of the dialysis machine. For example, one widely used online HDF machine requires that the incoming dialysis water meets current quality standards [3], while another requires that it contains <100 CFU/ml of bacteria and <0.25 EU/ml of endotoxin [4], which are the same as the levels currently set by ISO for dialysis water [11]. In other words, to safely produce

**Table 1.** Elements of system design that impact the quality of fluids used for the online preparation of substitution solution

| Favorable impact | Unfavorable impact |
|---|---|
| Two-stage reverse osmosis with full-fit membrane modules | Indirect-feed distribution systems with storage tanks |
| Direct-feed distribution systems configured as a loop | Batch preparation of bicarbonate concentrate |
| Online preparation of bicarbonate concentrate | Use of a conventional single-pass line to connect the dialysis machine to the dialysis water distribution loop |
| Construction materials that allow the use of hot water or ozone for disinfection | Use of conventional Hansen connectors to dialyzers and filters into fluid pathways |

substitution solution for online convective therapies with these machines, a dialysis facility must demonstrate that its water treatment and distribution system is capable of consistently providing the HDF machine with dialysis water and concentrates that meet the standards set by ISO, or other appropriate standards body. Achieving this goal on a routine basis requires that a dialysis facility establish a quality management system that covers the design, operation, and monitoring of all the systems used to prepare the dialysis fluid and serves to ensure that the hygienic chain remains intact.

## Components of a Quality Management System

### *System Design*

Good system design is an important prerequisite for successful quality management. It is clear from experience and studies of bacterial proliferation in systems used to produce and distribute fluids of high microbiological purity that certain design features help maintain the hygienic chain, while others present potential weaknesses that can be exploited by invading bacteria. Some of these design aspects are summarized in table 1.

The pretreatment section of a water treatment system is intended to produce the optimal feed water for the reverse osmosis unit in terms of levels of contaminants, such as oxidants and scale-forming substances that can damage reverse osmosis membranes, temperature, pH, and pressure. This is done by utilizing processes, such as carbon filtration, which predispose to bacterial proliferation. Therefore, the reverse osmosis unit must present a reliable barrier against those bacteria to prevent contamination of the dialysis water distribution system. Conventional spiral wound membrane modules use brine seals to separate the feed and product sides of the membrane in the pressure vessel. The use of brine seals creates stagnant areas which are difficult to disinfect adequately. Contamination of these areas can lead to bacteria bypassing the brine seals and contaminating the dialysis water distribution system. Use of membrane module designs (known as sanitary or full-fit membranes) that eliminate brine seals allows for much more effective cleaning and sanitization and reduces the likelihood of bacteria bypassing the reverse osmosis membrane. Additional protection can be obtained by operating a two-stage reverse osmosis system in which the product water from the first stage serves as the feed water to the second stage [12, 13].

As discussed later, effective disinfection of the water and concentrate distribution systems is the cornerstone to maintaining a high level of microbiological quality. Disinfection can be accomplished using traditional chemical germicides, such as bleach and peracetic acid/hydrogen peroxide solutions, ozone, or hot water. Ozone and hot water are generally preferred to traditional chemical germicides because they leave no chemical residuals that must be rinsed from the system before it can be used for patient treatments, thus allowing more frequent disinfection. However, the use of ozone or hot water requires that distribution systems be fabricated from appropriate materials. For example, use of hot water is possible only if these systems are fabricated from heat-tolerant materials, such as Teflon, cross-linked polyethylene, and certain stainless steels. Also, reverse osmosis membranes that tolerate hot water pasteurization are now available, and use of these membranes allows frequent disinfection of the entire dialysis water distribution system.

Direct-feed water distribution systems are advantageous because they do not have a storage tank that can act as a focus for bacterial proliferation. However, the use of a direct-feed system is often prevented by logistical considerations, such as when the length of the distribution system results in the pressure at the outlet of the reverse osmosis unit being inadequate to maintain the required pressure for dialysis machine operation at the most distal connections to the loop. In that situation, use of a storage tank and re-pressurizing pump might be unavoidable. If a storage tank is used, it should be no larger than necessary and should be capable of being easily and completely disinfected. When a direct-feed system is used, unused dialysis water is usually returned to the feed side of the reverse osmosis unit and this arrangement presents an opportunity for retrograde contamination of the dialysis water distribution system should there be a transient pressure fluctuation that results in the feed side of the reverse osmosis unit being at a higher pressure than the end of the dialysis water distribution loop. Direct-feed distribution systems should be fitted with a means of preventing retrograde flow and, in general, a single check valve is not sufficient for this purpose.

While the connection between the dialysis machine and the dialysis water distribution system is a simple piece of tubing, it can be difficult to adequately disinfect and is, therefore, a weak point in the hygienic chain. Disinfection of a dialysis machine according to the manufacturer's instructions does not result in disinfection of this tubing because it is upstream of the point where germicide is introduced into the dialysis machine in the case of chemical disinfection or where water is heated in the case of hot water pasteurization. Moreover, the tubing is not an integral part of the treated water distribution system. Thus, it is left to the dialysis facility to devise a means of disinfecting the tubing. Most frequently, this is done by allowing water to flow through the dialysis machine when the treated water distribution loop is disinfected. However, this approach can result in only a brief exposure of the tubing to germicide or hot water. A better solution could be to use a secondary loop to connect the treated water distribution loop to the back of the dialysis machine, such as the one available from Lauer Membran Wassertechnik GmbH, which is based on the Bernoulli principle.

Bicarbonate concentrate is a relatively good growth medium for bacteria and the practice of mixing batches of bicarbonate concentrate from dialysis water and powder at a dialysis facility and then distributing the concentrate over a period of hours either through a central distribution system or individual containers offers opportunity for bacteria to contaminate the bicarbonate concentrate, the dialysis machine, and the final dialysis fluid. This vulnerability can be minimized by utilizing systems that prepare bicarbonate concentrate online from dialysis water and powder, either at individual dialysis machines (bibag® or BiCart®) or as part of a central dialysis fluid delivery system [14]. Indeed, manufacturers of machines for online convective therapies require the use of such systems when the machines are used to prepare substitution solution.

Finally, the connectors used to incorporate dialyzers and bacteria- and endotoxin-retentive ultrafilters into the fluid pathways are a potential site of contamination. The design of standard Hansen connectors makes them very difficult to clean and disinfect. More advanced connectors are now available [4, 14] and these should always be used in preference to standard Hansen connectors in machines producing online substitution solution.

*System Installation and Operational Verification*

The operation of a facility's dialysis water and concentrate systems should be governed by a formal document covering validation, initial performance qualification, and routine monitoring of these systems. The document should clearly and concisely define responsibility for the systems, describe the systems and their operational status, provide detailed procedures to be followed in the event that changes to the systems are required, provide detailed procedures for ongoing maintenance and operational verification of the systems' performance, and establish a training program for all facility staff involved in any aspect of dialysis fluid preparation and use. When the dialysis fluid is to be used for the online preparation of substitution solution, the procedures set forth in the document should be consistent with the manufacturer's instructions for use of the system used to prepare the substitution solution.

Installation of new systems should be followed by formal verification that they have been installed according to preapproved plans, that they perform in accordance with the instructions for use, and that their performance meets the functional specifications of the systems, including operation of all safety systems. A complete analysis for the contaminants listed in the relevant dialysis water standard should be performed. This initial operational verification should be followed by a period of frequent data acquisition to demonstrate consistent performance under normal operating conditions. The length of this period will depend on the performance data. Generally, two consecutive months of satisfactory performance is adequate to demonstrate consistent performance and allow a shift to routine monitoring. Data obtained during the initial period of performance qualification should also be used to establish initial disinfection schedules, monitoring plans, and action levels for the various fluid-handling systems. In establishing a disinfection schedule, it is important to recognize that the results of cultures and endotoxin tests performed during the initial few weeks that follow installation of a new system might not accurately reflect the bacterial burden within that system, because bacterial biofilm takes some time to form and mature to the point where it begins to shed clusters of bacteria that lead to the establishment of new biofilm and widespread contamination of fluid pathways.

*System Maintenance*

Once the initial performance of the dialysis fluid preparation system has been verified, the challenge is to maintain that system so that it continues to provide dialysis fluid of the specified quality. In terms of providing dialysis fluid for the online production of substitution solution, the single most important aspect of maintenance is regular disinfection to suppress formation of mature biofilms on the surfaces of fluid pathways. Biofilms represent colonies of bacteria that form when a single organism or group of organisms adheres to a surface and produces an extracellular matrix that enables bacteria to proliferate and ultimately form a complex structure characterized by multiple bacterial species contained within a glycoprotein matrix. Biofilm is the preferred habitat for bacteria in fluid distribution systems and it is estimated that approximately 99% of the bacterial burden in a system resides within biofilm. Planktonic organisms, which are those detected by surveillance cultures, comprise only about 1% of the bacterial burden and occur when bacteria enter the system from the outside or when a portion of biofilm is shed from the surface of a pipe or other component of the system. Once biofilms are allowed to form and mature on surfaces in the fluid-handling system, they are extremely difficult to eliminate [15] and will continually reinfect fluids passing through the system. For these reasons, disinfection schedules must be proactive, that is they must be designed to suppress biofilm formation, not to eliminate biofilm after it has formed.

As mentioned previously, use of hot water or ozone is preferred to disinfection with traditional chemicals, such as bleach and peracetic acid/hydrogen peroxide solutions. Not only do the latter agents penetrate biofilm poorly [16, 17], but they leave chemical residuals that can require extensive rinsing to remove before the system can be safely used to prepare dialysis fluid. The time required for rinsing means that disinfection with bleach or peracetic acid/hydrogen peroxide solutions is generally limited to the one day of the week when the dialysis facility is not treating patients. Hot water and ozone are more effective against biofilm and leave no chemical residuals in the case of hot water or residuals with a very short half-life in the case of ozone, thus allowing more frequent disinfection. If the materials of construction of an existing system preclude the use of hot water or ozone, the effectiveness of bleach or peracetic acid/hydrogen peroxide solutions can be improved by first cleaning the system with an acid, such as citric acid [18].

*System Monitoring*

Monitoring of the performance of the dialysis water, concentrate, and dialysis fluid preparation systems is required to demonstrate the adequacy of system maintenance procedures and ensure that dialysis fluid routinely meets the input requirements of the manufacturer of the system used for online preparation of substitution fluid. Adequate removal of chemical contaminants from the water is usually ensured by monitoring the performance of the reverse osmosis unit, particularly the conductivity of the product water and the percent rejection of the membrane, together with measurement of the level of total chlorine. Separate testing for total chlorine is necessary because chlorine and chloramines are not removed by reverse osmosis. Monitoring is preferably performed continuously using online monitors. If continuous monitoring is not possible, monitoring should be at least daily, and if chloramine is present in the municipal water testing each treatment shift is recommended. Monitoring of the performance of the reverse osmosis unit is supplemented by periodic chemical analysis for the contaminants listed in the relevant standard for dialysis water quality [11] at least annually, or more frequently if there are significant seasonal changes in municipal water quality. The ability of a system to adequately remove chemical contaminants may change even with a well-functioning reverse osmosis unit if there is a change in the municipal water. For that reason, as part of its quality management system, a dialysis facility should endeavor to build a relationship with its municipal water supplier and request the establishment of a formal procedure to notify the dialysis facility of impending changes in municipal water quality.

Monitoring of the microbiological quality of the fluids via cultures and endotoxin testing is central to verifying good system performance. Cultures and endotoxin testing are not used to decide when disinfection is needed. Rather, they are intended to demonstrate that the disinfection schedules established during system validation are adequate to consistently yield levels of contamination in dialysis water, bicarbonate concentrate, or dialysis fluid less than the maximum allowable levels specified by the manufacturer of the system used to prepare substitution solution. If unacceptable bacterial counts of endotoxin concentrations are found, then the frequency of disinfection should be increased until acceptable test results are routinely obtained.

Meticulous sample collection and appropriately sensitive methods should always be used for cultures and endotoxin testing. Samples should be drawn directly from the fluid pathway using aseptic technique and cultures should be plated within 4 h of sample collection or immediately refrigerated and assayed within 24 h. The number of sampling points should be based on the complexity of the system. The culturing method and sample volume should be appropriate to detect bacteria at the level defined in the relevant quality standard. For example, a sample volume of 300–500 μl is required to yield 3–5 colonies for a spread plate culture of a sample containing 10 CFU/ml. If more sensitivity is required, such as would be the case if ultrapure quality was to be demonstrated, a much larger sample volume (30–50 ml) and use of the membrane filtration method of culturing is required. The culture medium and incubation conditions should also be appropriate for maximum recovery of bacteria. Typically, a low nutrient agar, such as tryptone glucose extract agar or Reasoner's number 2 agar, is used with incubation for 7 days at 22–25°C [11]. While no culturing method can provide an absolute measure of the microbial burden in a fluid-handling system, use of low nutrient agars and incubation at room temperature for longer periods has been demonstrated to produce a higher yield of organisms than more general-purpose agars, such as tryptic soy agar, incubated at body temperature for shorter periods [19]. Alternative methods based on dyes and fluorescence microscopy can provide information on both viable and non-viable organisms in 1–2 h [20]; however, the relationship between these methods and the maximum allowable levels for bacteria in current standards has yet to be established. Endotoxin levels should be determined using the *Limulus* amebocyte lysate assay. Different versions of the assay are commonly available. The turbidometric and chromogenic methods are preferred because they provide an absolute value of endotoxin concentration; while easier to perform, the gel clot method can only indicate if the concentration of endotoxin is greater or less than some preselected value. Whichever assays are used for bacteria and endotoxin, the data should be subjected to ongoing trend analysis to help provide an early indication of changes in the level of contamination.

In summary, the technology to perform online convective therapies is now widely available and has been shown to perform safely and effectively in studies involving multiple centers and large numbers of patients over long periods [5, 6, 13]. While the equipment used to perform online convective therapies incorporates a wide range of safety systems, certain residual risks remain the responsibility of the user. Chief among these is ensuring that the fluids delivered to the equipment routinely meet the quality requirements for which operation of the equipment has been validated. This responsibility requires that facilities performing online convective therapies establish a quality management system for fluid preparation that encompasses the design of the systems used to prepare dialysis water, concentrates and dialysis fluid, validation and ongoing verification of the operation of those systems, and training of staff involved in all aspects of fluid preparation.

## References


1 Cheung AK, Levin NW, Greene T, Agodoa L, Bailey J, Beck G, Clark W, Levey AS, Leypoldt JK, Ornt DB, Rocco MV, Schulman G, Schwab S, Teehan B, Eknoyan G: Effects of high-flux hemodialysis on clinical outcomes: results of the HEMO study. J Am Soc Nephrol 2003;14:3251–3263.

2 Locatelli F, Martin-Malo A, Hannedouche T, Loureiro A, Papadimitriou M, Wizemann V, Jacobson SH, Czekalski S, Ronco C, Vanholder R: Effect of membrane permeability on survival of hemodialysis patients. J Am Soc Nephrol 2009;20:645–654

3 Ledebo I: On-line hemodiafiltration: technique and therapy. Adv Ren Replace Ther 1999;6:195–208

4 Polaschegg H-D, Roy T: Technical aspects of online hemodiafiltration; in Ronco C, Canaud B, Aljama P (eds): Hemodiafiltration. Contrib Nephrol. Basel, Karger, 2007, vol 158, pp 68–79.

5 Canaud B, Bragg-Gresham JL, Marshall MR, Desmeules S, Gillespie BW, Depner T, Klassen P, Port FK: Mortality risk for patients receiving hemodiafiltration versus hemodialysis: European results from the DOPPS. Kidney Int 2006;69:2087–2093.

6 Vilar E, Fry A, Wellsted D, Tattersall JE, Greenwood RN, Farrington K: Long-term outcomes in online hemodiafiltration and high-flux hemodialysis: a comparative analysis. Clin J Am Soc Nephrol 2009;4:1944–1953.

7 Santoro A, Mancini E, Bolzani R, Boggi R, Cagnoli L, Francioso A, Fusaroli M, Piazza V, Rapanà R, Strippoli GFM: The effect of online high-flux hemofiltration versus low-flux hemodialysis on mortality in chronic kidney failure: a small randomized controlled trial. Am J Kidney Dis 2008;52:507–518.

8 Blankestijn PJ, Ledebo I, Canaud B: Hemodiafiltration: clinical evidence and remaining questions. Kidney Int 2010;77:581–587

9 Henderson LW, Sanfelippo ML, Beans E: 'On line' preparation of sterile pyrogen-free electrolyte solution. Trans Am Soc Artif Int Organs 1978;24:465–467.

10 Ledebo I: On-line preparation of solutions for dialysis: practical aspects versus safety and regulations. J Am Soc Nephrol 2002;13:S78–S83.

11 International Organization for Standardization: Water for haemodialysis and related therapies (ISO 13959:2009). Geneva, International Organization for Standardization, 2009.

12 Martin K, Laydet E, Canaud B: Design and technical adjustment of a water treatment system: 15 years of experience. Adv Ren Replace Ther 2003;10:122–132.

13 Penne EL, Visser L, van den Dorpel MA, van der Weerd NC, Mazairac AHA, van Jaarsveld BC, Koopman MG, Vos P, Feith GW, Hovinga TKK, van Hamersvelt HW, Wauters IM, Bots ML, Nubé MJ, ter Wee PM, Blankestijn PJ, Grooteman MPC: Microbiological quality and quality control of purified water and ultrapure dialysis fluids for online hemodiafiltration in routine clinical practice. Kidney Int 2009;76:665–672.

14 Kawanishi H, Moriisha M, Sato T, Taoka M: Fully automated dialysis system based on the central dialysis fluid delivery system. Blood Purif 2009;27(suppl 1):56–63.

15 Man NK, Degremont A, Darbord J-C, Collet M, Vaillant P: Evidence of bacterial biofilm in tubing from hydraulic pathway of hemodialysis system. Artif Organs 1998;22:596–600.

16 Stewart PS, Roe F, Rayner J, Elkins JG, Lewandowski Z, Ochsner UA, Hassett DJ: Effect of catalase on hydrogen peroxide penetration into *Pseudomonas aeruginosa* biofilms. Appl Environ Microbiol 2000;66:836–838.
17 Stewart PS, Rayner J, Roe F, Rees WM: Biofilm penetration and disinfection efficacy of alkaline hypochlorite and chlorosulfamates. J Appl Microbiol 2001;91:525–532.
18 Marion-Ferey K, Pasmore M, Stoodley P, Wilson S, Husson GP, Costerton JW: Biofilm removal from silicone tubing: an assessment of the efficacy of dialysis machine decontamination procedures using an in vitro model. J Hosp Infect 2003;53:64–71
19 Ledebo I, Nystrand R: Defining the microbiological quality of dialysis fluid. Artif Organs 1999;23:37–43.
20 Yamaguchi N, Baba T, Nakagawa S, Saito A, Nasu M: Rapid monitoring of bacteria in dialysis fluids by fluorescent vital staining and microcolony methods. Nephrol Dial Transplant 2007;22:612–616.

Richard A. Ward, PhD
Kidney Disease Program, University of Louisville
615 S. Preston Street, Louisville, KY 40202-1718 (USA)
Tel. +1 502 852 5757, Fax +1 502 852 7643, E-Mail richard.ward@louisville.edu

Kawanishi H, Yamashita AC (eds): Hemodiafiltration – A New Era.
Contrib Nephrol. Basel, Karger, 2011, vol 168, pp 89–98

# Biocompatibility of Dialysis Fluid for Online HDF

Tadashi Tomo[a] · Toshio Shinoda[b]

[a]Department of Nephrology (Department of Internal Medicine II, Faculty of Medicine), Oita University Hospital, Oita, and [b]Dialysis Center, Kawakita General Hospital, Tokyo, Japan

## Abstract

We investigated the effects of online hemodiafiltration (HDF) using acetate-free bicarbonate dialysis (AFD) fluid on bioincompatibility as represented by inflammatory markers in patients undergoing maintenance hemodialysis therapy and compared it with conventional acetate-containing bicarbonate dialysis (ACD) fluid. A total of 24 maintenance hemodialysis patients were registered for cross-over design during the 6-month study period (13 males and 11 females, aged 58.2 ± 14.5 years, mean duration of dialysis 10.0 ± 8.0 years, chronic glomerular nephritis in 20 patients, diabetic nephropathy in 2 patients, polycystic kidney in 1 patient, and nephrosclerosis in 1 patient). These patients were subjected to ACD for the first 3 months followed by AFD fluid for the latter 3 months. Blood variables of C-reactive protein and interleukin-6 were determined after each of the first and latter 3-month periods. The filters (membrane surface area, raw material), the conditions of HDF (blood flow rate, dialysate flow rate, dialysis time, dry weight, pre-dilution mode and convective volume) and drug regimen including erythrocyte-simulating agent (drug type, dosage) were unchanged throughout the cross-over study. There appeared to be significantly higher levels of predialysis blood pH and bicarbonate in the AFD phase than in the ACD phase. Blood C-reactive protein and interleukin-6 levels were significantly decreased in AFD group as compared with those seen in ACD group. From these results, it can be suggested that online HDF using AFD fluid contributes to alleviating microinflammation, a prognostic factor for bioincompatible events in hemodialysis patients.



Hemodiafiltration (HDF) has become established as blood purification therapy with the most advanced technologies, which enables both diffusive and enhanced convective removals of uremic solutes by dialysis and ultrafiltration, respectively. Dialysis fluids for dialysis and substitution fluids for filtration were required for HDF therapy. Of HDF therapies, online HDF can be characterized by using highly purified dialysis fluids as a substitution fluid prepared for online provision into the blood. The therapeutic benefits of the online HDF can feed large volumes of substitution fluids which are 20 l/session for post-dilution and 50 l/session for pre-dilution. The large convective volumes are directly injected into blood and therefore not only the composition of substitution fluids in addition to dialysis fluids but also their biocompatibility is of considerable importance. Thus, the purification and composition of substitution fluids can be key factors for its biocompatibility in online HDF therapy.

## Purification of Online Preparation

Purification of dialysis fluids is important when high-flux membranes are given because backfiltration can occur. Also, purification of substitution fluids is a more contributing factor because they are directly injected into blood. In Japan, the purity and quality of online preparation of substitution fluids through dialysis fluids are defined by the following acceptable criteria [1]: (a) sterile and non-pyrogenic; (b) bacterial counts; not more than $10^{-6}$ CFU/ml, and (c) endotoxin level; not more than 0.001 EU/ml (not more than the detectable limit).

## Composition of Dialysis and Substitution Fluids

*Electrolytes*
The composition of substitution fluids is fundamentally based on that of extracellular fluid, however individual electrolyte contained in dialysis fluids is somewhat unbalanced and is therefore required to be adjusted to a standard balance. Sodium concentration is set at 138–140 mEq/l equivalent to that of extracellular fluid. Potassium in dialysis and substitution fluids is allowed to be set at a lower concentration of 2.0 mEq/l than that of extracellular fluid to correct hyperkalemia observed in hemodialysis patients with renal failure. Meanwhile, for patients with hypokalemia, blood potassium level should be compensated by oral intake, drip infusion, or medication during blood purification therapy. Higher calcium concentration in substitution fluids is set at 3.5–3.8 mEq/l because hypocalcemia occurs in most of the hemodialysis patients with renal failure.

*Glucose*
Since a fasting blood glucose levels is approximately 100 mg/dl in human blood, the use of a glucose-free substitution fluid can incidentally cause hypoglycemia, aside from developing symptoms or not. Glucose in substitution fluids is therefore contained so as to reach the final concentration of 100 mg/dl in the blood.

It should be noted that hypoglycemia infrequently occurs even though such a glucose concentration is prepared because glucose is presumably metabolized in the body.

*Buffer*

Many of the dialysis fluids currently used in Japan contain sodium bicarbonate as a buffer source. In the past, sodium acetate had been used as a buffer source because it was useful in avoiding precipitation of calcium carbonate from the dialysis fluid (likely to emerge if sodium bicarbonate is used) [2]. However, the adverse effects of acetate in hemodialysis patients have been known for the past several years and can be associated with intradialytic hypotension and cardiovascular instability; therefore, the primary buffer comprises bicarbonate in standard hemodialysis [3]. The bicarbonate-buffered dialysis fluids currently used in Japan contain small amounts of acetate as an additive to prevent crystallization of calcium and magnesium. Problems arising from such small amounts of acetate contained in the dialysis fluid have also been reported.

Higuchi et al. [4] reported that cytokine production was minimal during acetate-free biofiltration (an acetate-free method of blood purification) and was maximal during bicarbonate dialysis with a dialysis fluid containing small amounts of acetate. This tendency is true for superoxide production by neutrophils as evidenced by a significant elevation in the production during the bicarbonate dialysis as compared with during acetate-free biofiltration [5]. These findings suggest that even small amounts of acetate in dialysis fluid in bicarbonate dialysis can induce microinflammation during blood purification therapy.

The present study was undertaken to examine whether removal of acetate (contained at a concentration of 8–10 mEq/l in the conventional dialysis fluids) from the dialysis fluid would lead to alleviation of bioincompatible events as characterized by microinflammation observed during blood purification therapy in stable patients undergoing maintenance hemodialysis. To this end, online HDF was carried out in these patients and thereby the effects of acetate-free bicarbonate dialysis (AFD) fluid were investigated and compared with conventional acetate-containing bicarbonate dialysis (ACD) fluid.

## Methods

*Patients*

The study involved 24 hemodialysis patients who were receiving online HDF (13 males and 11 females, aged 58.2 ± 14.5 years, mean duration of dialysis 10.0 ± 8.0 years) in a stable clinical condition. Causes of renal failure were chronic glomerular nephritis in 20 patients, diabetic nephropathy in 2 patients, polycystic kidney in 1 patient, and nephro-

**Table 1.** Composition of dialysis fluids tested in the present study

| | Na mEq/l | K mEq/l | Ca mEq/l | Mg mEq/l | Cl mEq/l | $HCO_3^-$ mEq/l | Acetate mEq/l | Glucose g/l |
|---|---|---|---|---|---|---|---|---|
| Acetate (–) dialysate[1] | 140 | 2.0 | 3.0 | 1.0 | 111 | 35 | – | 1.5 |
| Acetate (+) dialysate | 140 | 2.0 | 2.5 | 1.0 | 111 | 30 | 8 | 1.0 |

[1] Citrate 2 mEq/l is added.

sclerosis in 1 patient. Informed consent was obtained from each patient prior to the study.

*Conditions and Procedure for Online HDF*

Online HDF was carried out 3 times weekly for 4–5 h/session with pre-dilution mode (12–18 l/h) at a blood flow rate of 200–300 ml/min and a dialysate flow rate of 500–700 ml/min. The compositions of ACD and AFD fluids tested in this study are presented in table 1. The purity and quality of the dialysis fluids was not more than $10^{-6}$ CFU/ml in terms of bacterial counts and not more than the detectable limit for the endotoxin level at the terminal of dialysis circuit.

The patients enrolled in this study, specified in the 'Patients' section, received treatment with ACD during the first 3 months of the study followed by with AFD during the latter 3 months. During the 6-month study period, comprising the first 3 months, *ACD phase* (June 1 through August 31, 2007) and the latter 3 months, *AFD phase* (September 1 through November 30, 2007), only the dialysis fluid was changed, and the following conditions were kept unchanged: (1) filters (membrane surface area, raw material), (2) settings for HDF, i.e. blood flow rate, dialysate flow rate, dialysis time, dry weight, pre-dilution mode and convective volume, and (3) drug regimen including erythrocyte-simulating agent (drug type, dosage). On the last Monday (for the Monday, Wednesday, and Friday dialysis group) or the last Tuesday (for the Tuesday, Thursday, and Saturday dialysis group) of each of the first and latter 3-month periods, blood was sampled from each patient.

Each blood sample was analyzed as follows: (1) C-reactive protein (CRP; SRL Co., Ltd) and interleukin-6 (IL-6; R&D Systems, USA) as markers related to inflammation. pH and $HCO_3^-$ before hemodialysis session were also analyzed.

*In vitro Study*

The test sample containing neutrophils, which were separated from each blood sample collected from 24 hemodialysis patients from whom informed consent was obtained prior to the study, was exposed to AFD and ACD fluids. Free radical generation was measured using LBP-953 (Berthold) according to the methods reported by Prasad [6] and Takayama et al. [7].

The test sample containing neutrophils was prepared as follows: the whole blood sample (4 ml) was mixed with 1 ml of dextran solution. The mixture was incubated at 30°C for 15 min, and the supernatant was centrifuged at 270 *g* for 6 min at 4°C. The supernatant was removed, and the precipitate was suspended. To remove erythrocytes, cooled hemolytic reagent (3 ml) was added to the suspended precipitate and then the mixture was left standing on ice for 5 min, followed by adding 3 ml of ice-cooled wash solution for peripheral blood lymphocytes (PBL) separation. The supernatant was removed after centrifugation at 270 *g* for 6 min at 4°C and the precipitate was suspended. To this suspension 5 ml of ice-cooled wash solution for PBL separation was added and the mixture was recentrifuged at 270 *g* for 6 min at 4°C. The supernatant was then removed and the precipitate was suspended. The suspension was mixed with 1 ml of ice-cooled wash solution for PBL separation and resuspended. This suspension (10 μl) was mixed with 90 μl of Turk's solution. Following blood cell counting, the cell density of the mixture was adjusted to $1.5 \times 10^6$/ml. Thus, 100 μl of the prepared suspension (neutrophil count, $1.5 \times 10^6$/ml) was used as a test sample.

*Statistical Analysis*
Data are expressed as mean ± SD. Paired t test was used for comparing different dialysis fluids. $p < 0.05$ was regarded as statistically significant.

## Results

*Online HDF Study*
None of the 24 patients enrolled in this study developed any adverse event throughout the 6-month evaluation period (first and latter 3-month periods). This study was well tolerated for all patients with the following conditions to be kept unchanged: (1) settings for dialysis, i.e. the filter (membrane surface area, raw material), blood flow rate, dialysate flow rate, and dry weight; (2) drug regimen (drug type, dosage), and (3) erythrocyte-simulating agent (drug type, dosage).

Predialysis blood pH and bicarbonate levels were found to be significantly higher in the AFD phase than in the ACD phase ($p < 0.05$ and $p < 0.01$, respectively; data not shown). AFD resulted in significant decreases in blood CRP levels as compared with the ACD fluid ($p < 0.05$; data not shown). Such significantly lowered levels were also observed for IL-6 when the dialysis with AFD fluid was performed ($p < 0.05$; fig. 1).

*In vitro Study*
AFD exhibited better biocompatibility as indicated by an evidently smaller amount of free radicals generated from neutrophils when compared with during ACD ($p < 0.05$; fig. 2).

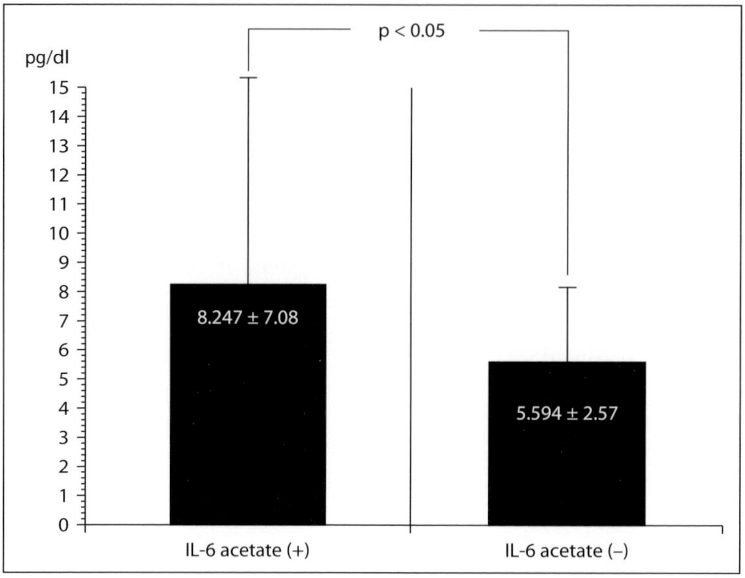


**Fig. 1.** Comparison of IL-6 between ACD and AFD fluids. Data were expressed as mean ± SD of 24 patients.

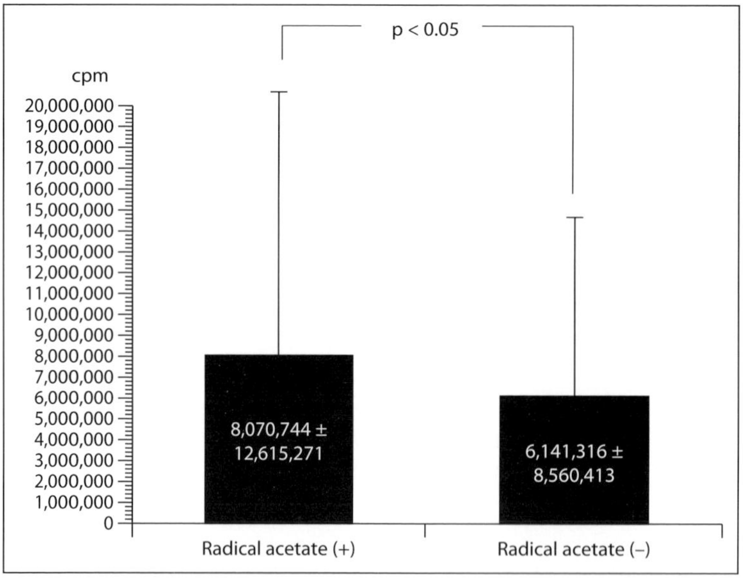


**Fig. 2.** Comparison of free-radical generation between ACD and AFD fluids. Data are expressed as mean ± SD of 24 patients.

## Discussion

Adverse effects of acetate-buffered dialysis fluids due to acetate intolerance have been reported to be associated with higher cardiovascular risks, thus leading to the widespread use of bicarbonate-buffered dialysis fluids [2]. Many of the commercially available dialysis fluids in Japan are bicarbonate-buffered, which somewhat contain acetate (8–10 mEq/l) to prevent salt precipitation. The present study was designed to explore the effects of online HDF therapy with AFD fluid on the prognostic factors for bioincompatible events including inflammation and free radicals in hemodialysis patients, when compared with those with ACD fluid.

Both CRP and IL-6, indicators of inflammatory reactions seen during ACD, decreased significantly after being replaced by AFD. In the present study, the purity and quality of the dialysis fluids at the terminal of dialysis circuit was consistently maintained below $10^{-6}$ CFU/ml in terms of bacterial count and below detectable limits for endotoxin throughout the 6-month evaluation period. Furthermore, the conditional background for online HDF therapy including filter (membrane material, surface area), oral medication and erythrocyte-simulating agent (drug type, dosage) and settings for HDF was kept unchanged, indicating that such situations are unlikely to affect CRP and IL-6 levels. Higuchi et al. [4] reported that cytokine production was significantly reduced during acetate-free biofiltration therapy as compared with during dialysis with ACD, suggesting that the decreases in CRP and IL-6 observed in this study seems to reflect the influence of the absence of acetate in dialysis fluid. IL-6 can induce CRP [8], while the converse is also true, that is, that in response to the reduction in IL-6, CRP production was downregulated in the present study. Both CRP and IL-6 have been reported to serve as predictors of the survival rates in maintenance hemodialysis patients, and lowered CRP and IL-6 levels can contribute to better prognosis including survival advantage, improved clinical status [9].

Also in the neutrophil stimulation test conducted in the present study, the formation of free radicals was considerably limited in the AFD phase as compared with in the ACD phase, suggesting that AFD fluid is more biocompatible. Previous studies done by our group [10] have shown that plasma radicals are decreased in the online HDF therapy, and it seems possible that the decrease in free radical formation is associated with less inflammatory responses in the AFD.

In predialysis analysis of blood pH and bicarbonate level, effective correction of metabolic acidosis was observed in the AFD phase evidenced by a significantly higher pH and bicarbonate level. It can be suggested that the effects depends on the relatively high concentrations of bicarbonate (35 mEq/l) contained in the AFD fluid. Lower predialysis blood levels of bicarbonate have been acknowledged to be associated with a higher risk of mortality for hemodialysis patients, and therefore it is recommended that the predialysis or stabilized serum should be maintained over 22 mEq/l by K/DOQI guidelines [11]. In the present study, the predialysis blood bicarbonate level was 21.3 ± 1.6 mEq/l in the AFD phase, which seems to fail to achieve K/DOQI guidelines. However, the values obtained in this study are the data collected on Monday or Tuesday, after an interdialytic interval of 2 days, whereas the criteria given in the K/DOQI guidelines pertain to the predialysis level obtained after an interdialytic interval of 1 day. Therefore, one would conceive that if blood samples in our study were drawn after an interdialytic interval of 1 day, the values would satisfy the criteria specified in the K/DOQI guidelines.

Limitations in the present study are the small number of subjects (24 patients) and inability to design a complete cross-over study (ACD→AFD→ACD). Sample size in our study had to be limited because it was relatively difficult to keep steady conditions such as dialysis settings and drug regimen for 6 months. The inability to execute a complete cross-over study is accounted for by the aspect that a central dialysis fluid delivery system is introduced in many Japanese medical facilities; namely, if the dialysis fluid were changed for cross-over study, patients other than the subjects of this study would be also involved. It should be considered that 8 of the 24 patients enrolled in our study strongly refused to resume ACD after AFD. Furthermore, our data stem from patients receiving online HDF; however, the studies in hemodialysis patients remain to be investigated.

Our evaluation is based on the comparison between data after 3 months of online HDF with ACD and AFD fluids. When the data at the start of the study (at the start of online HDF with ACD) was added to the evaluation, no significant difference in CRP levels was observed between before and after online HDF with ACD fluid. In contrast, CRP level was significantly decreased 3 months after online HDF with AFD fluid (data not shown). On the basis of these results, it can be suggested that the changes in CRP observed 3 months after online HDF with AFD fluid represent specific effects of the AFD fluid but not reflect the effects of long-term online HDF therapy per se.

## Conclusion

The results obtained in the present study indicate that the online HDF therapy with AFD fluid can significantly alleviate microinflammatory responses as compared with that with ACD fluid. It seems likely that inflammation serves as a trigger for dialysis-related complications in hemodialysis patients and bioincompatible factors associated with dialysis and renal failure play an important role in the generation of the microinflammation (fig. 3). Our data also suggest that even minimal amounts of acetate contained in the dialysis fluid can be bioincompatible for blood purification. Acetate-free dialysis therapy including approach from online supply side of substitution fluid would be expected to

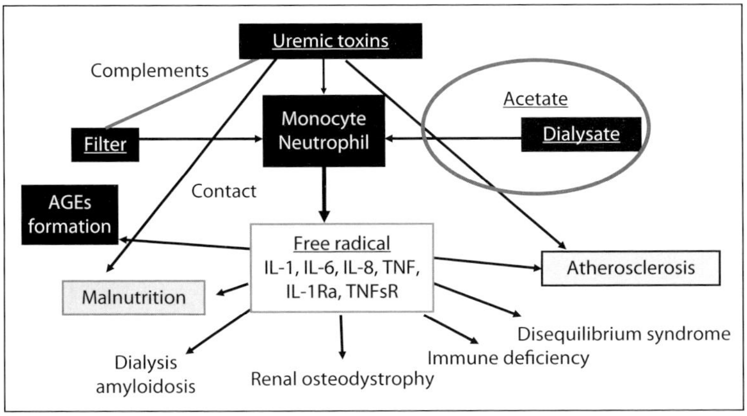


**Fig. 3.** Bioincompatibilities and dialysis-related complications.

open a promising therapeutic avenue for improving biocompatibility for blood purification over conventional acetate-containing bicarbonate blood purification, thus leading to prevention of the onset and progression of dialysis-related complications in dialysis patients.

## References


1 Kawanishi H, Akiba T, Masakane I, Tomo T, Mineshima M, Kawasaki T, Hirakata H, Akizawa T: Standard on microbiological management of fluids for hemodialysis and related therapies by the Japanese Society for Dialysis Therapy 2008. Ther Apher Dial 2009;13:161–166.

2 Mion CM, Hegstrom RM, Boen ST, Scribner BH: Substitution of sodium acetate for sodium bicarbonate in the bath fluid for hemodialysis. Trans Am Soc Artif Intern Organs 1964;10:110–115.

3 Graefe U, Follette WC, Vizzo JE, Goodisman LD, Scribner BH: Reduction in dialysis-induced morbidity and vascular instability with the use of bicarbonate in dialysate. Proc Clin Dial Transplant Forum 1976;6:203–209.

4 Higuchi T, Yamamoto C, Kuno T, Okada K, Soma M, Fukuda N, Nagura Y, Takahashi S, Matsumoto K: A comparison of bicarbonate hemodialysis, hemodiafiltration, and acetate-free biofiltration on cytokine production. Ther Apher Dial 2004;8:460–467.

5 Todeschini M, Macconi D, Fernández NG, Ghilardi M, Anabaya A, Binda E, Morigi M, Cattaneo D, Perticucci E, Remuzzi G, Noris M: Effect of acetate-free biofiltration and bicarbonate hemodialysis on neutrophil activation. Am J Kidney Dis 2002;40:783–793.

6 Prasad K: C-reactive protein increases oxygen radical generation by neutrophils. J Cardiovasc Pharmacol Ther 2004;9:203–209.

7 Takayama F, Egashira T, Yamanaka Y: Assay for oxidative stress injury by detection of luminol-enhanced chemiluminescence in a freshly obtained blood sample: a study to follow the time course of oxidative injury (in Japanese). Nippon Yakurigaku Zasshi 1998;111:177–186.

8 Weinhold B, Bader A, Poli V, Rüther U: Interleukin-6 is necessary, but not sufficient, for induction of the human C-reactive protein gene in vivo. Biochem J 1997;325:617–621.

9 Stenvinkel P, Lindholm B: C-reactive protein in end-stage renal disease: are there reasons to measure it? Blood Purif 2005;23:72–78.
10 Tomo T, Matsuyama K, Nasu M: Effect of hemodiafiltration against radical stress in the course of blood purification. Blood Purif 2006;22(suppl 2):72–77.
11 National Kidney Foundation: K/DOQI clinical practice guidelines for nutrition in chronic renal failure. Am J Kidney Dis 2000;35(suppl 2):S1–S140.

Tadashi Tomo, MD, PhD
Department of Nephrology (Department of Internal Medicine II, Faculty of Medicine)
Oita University Hospital
1-1 Hasama-Machi, Yufu-shi, Oita 879-5593 (Japan)
Tel. +81 97 586 5804, Fax +81 97 549 4245, E-Mail tomo@med.oita-u.ac.jp

Kawanishi H, Yamashita AC (eds): Hemodiafiltration – A New Era.
Contrib Nephrol. Basel, Karger, 2011, vol 168, pp 99–106

# Characteristics of Central Dialysis Fluid Delivery System and Single Patient Dialysis Machine for HDF

Ikuo Aoike

Koyo Medical Clinic, Kamedakoyo, Niigata, Japan

**Abstract**

The central dialysis fluid delivery system (CDDS), with which dialysis fluid is prepared at a single location and sent to each patient station, was developed as a unique system of dialysis in Japan and has been widely used. Maintenance hemodialysis using the single patient dialysis machine (SPDM), with which reverse osmosis water is first sent to each dialysis unit, and the dialysis fluid is prepared and used at each patient station, is used in many areas worldwide other than Japan and some Asian regions. Purification of dialysis fluid is essential for online hemodiafiltration, and it is possible to achieve the target purification level with both CDDS and SPDM by keeping the appropriate procedure. It is therefore desirable to understand the characteristics of both systems and make a selection based on the scale of the facility and the concept of treatment.



## Central Dialysis Fluid Delivery System in Japan

The components of the central dialysis fluid delivery system (CDDS) and flow of dialysis water are shown in figure 1 [2]. Liquid dialysis concentrate is diluted with reverse osmosis (RO) water from the RO apparatus to prepare a solution of the appropriate concentration. This solution is sent to each patient station via the piping system from the central dialysis fluid proportioning unit. Both acid (A) and bicarbonate (B) liquid dialysis concentrates are available in the form of powder as well as liquid concentrate. The powder is first dissolved in RO water in the powder-mixing unit followed by dilution and preparation in the same manner as the liquid concentrates.

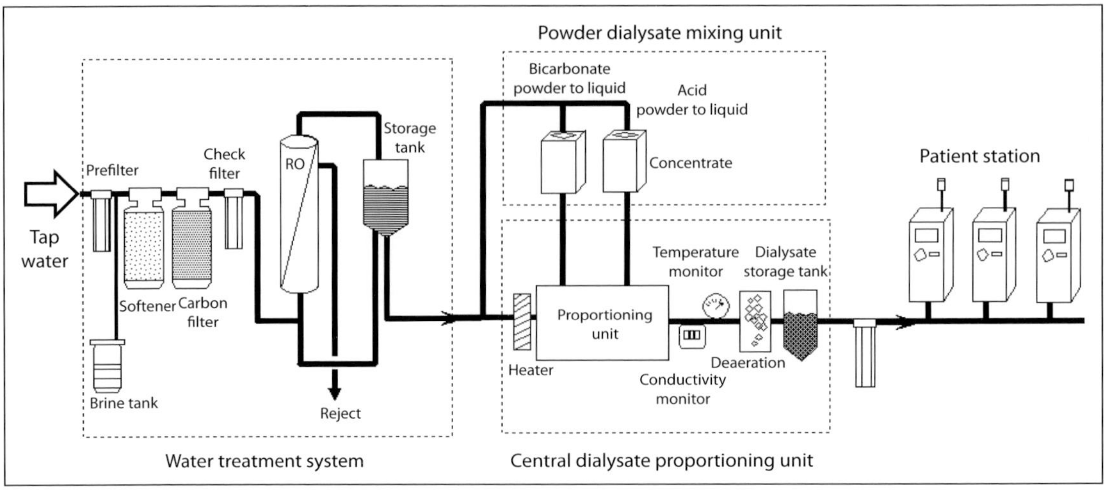


**Fig. 1.** Basic design of CDDS.

The reasons for the wide acceptance of CDDS and the increase in market share in Japan are as follows: (1) Laborsaving: with single patient dialysis machine (SPDM), it is necessary to carry the liquid dialysis concentrate to each apparatus. With CDDS, the dialysis fluid is sent to each patient station via the piping system; therefore, it can save on the work of preparation. (2) Simplified patient station maintenance: with SPDM, every apparatus is equipped with a highly elaborate mechanism for mixing and diluting the dialysis concentrate with RO water to prepare the dialysis fluid. With CDDS, the mechanism is much simpler, can be easily downsized, and maintenance is much easier than that of SPDM. Failure probability is low, and the price is lower. (3) CDDS is laborsaving because there is only one checkpoint for the composition of dialysis fluid. (4) The economic advantage can be obtained easily because of the low cost achieved by points 1–3 above.

These advantages facilitated the prevalence of the dialysis therapy and significantly contributed to the establishment of therapy with stable quality. In Japan, CDDS has a history of safe use for over 40 years. The Japanese Society for Dialysis Therapy (JSDT) conducts a questionnaire survey at dialysis facilities throughout the country every year in order to grasp the current status of dialysis in Japan. The results of the survey are reported in the Registry of the JSDT. According to the Registry of JSDT 2008, 111,690 patient stations at 4,072 facilities were in operation as of December 31, 2008 [1]. Koda and Mineshima [2] reported that SPDM accounts for 12.3% of all dialysis systems in Japan. It is therefore estimated that approximately 98,000 stations are performing hemodialysis by CDDS. As regards the purification of the dialysis fluid, the importance

**Table 1.** Microbiological quality standard for dialysis fluids – attainment level

| | |
|---|---|
| • | Dialysis water (RO water) |
| | Bacteria: <100 CFU/ml |
| | Endotoxin: <0.050 EU/ml |
| • | Standard dialysis fluid |
| | Bacteria: <100 CFU/ml |
| | Endotoxin: <0.050 EU/ml |
| • | Ultrapure dialysis fluid |
| | Bacteria: <0.1 CFU/ml |
| | Endotoxin: <0.001 EU/ml (less than the detection limit) |
| • | Online prepared substitution fluid |
| | Sterile and non-pyrogenic |
| | Bacteria: $<10^{-6}$ CFU/ml |
| | Endotoxin: <0.001 EU/ml (less than the detection limit) |

of which has been fully recognized in recent years, the level is increasing through the efforts of improving the purification method and use of endotoxin retentive filters (ETRFs). It is now possible to fulfill not only the ISO standard (CD), but also the Microbiological Quality Standard for Dialysis Fluids [3] (table 1) in the report of the meeting of JSDT.

Although the patient station of CDDS is a simpler structure than that of SPDM, CDDS still has many system components and it must be noted that CDDS has certain disadvantages, including the following: (1) The mixing unit and central dialysis fluid proportioning unit must be installed and maintained. (2) The RO water line from the RO apparatus to the mixing unit or the central dialysis fluid proportioning unit are not cleaned and disinfected in most systems. (3) No measures are implemented to prevent contamination of the powder-mixing unit except for the cartridge type system DAD model (Nikkiso Co. Ltd). (4) In the event of a problem with the mixing unit or the central dialysis fluid proportioning unit, the whole dialysis unit cannot be used, and dialysis therapy cannot be provided. (5) Since only one composition of dialysis fluid can be selected with CDDS, it is not possible to choose a dialysis fluid suitable for each case.

## SPDM in Japan

Of the underlying diseases at the start of dialysis, chronic renal failure due to diabetic nephropathy was most common after 1998, reaching 43.2% in 2008 and still increasing. Before 1998, however, the largest number of patients who were introduced to dialysis had chronic glomerulonephritis as the underlying disease, and many of them were relatively stable dialysis cases. In Japan, dialysis therapy became widespread, and the number of dialysis facilities increased rapidly from the late 1980s. The number of patient stations is still increasing by more than 3,300 on average every year. The advantages of CDDS seem to play an important role in the increase.

As described above, the rate of the SPDM used in Japan is 12.3%, and the purposes for its use include blood purification in critical care for multiple organ dysfunction syndrome or acute renal failure in the ICU, home dialysis, hemofiltration- or hemodiafiltration (HDF)-specific apparatus, and acetate-free biofiltration. It is estimated that only a few dialysis units use SPDM for maintenance dialysis.

Unlike dialysis patients in the past, current patients represent a group of various clinical states as a result of such factors as patient aging or an increase in hemodynamically unstable diabetic patients with serious complications. In addition, 7.3% of the patients have more than 20 years of dialysis history, the longest of which is 40 years and 8 months [1]. Therefore, the increase in the number of long-term dialysis cases that present with dialysis intolerance symptoms is a major issue now. In the current situation where cases with different clinical states coexist in one dialysis unit, it is becoming increasingly important to choose the mode of dialysis and kind of dialysis fluid appropriate for each patient's clinical state. From this viewpoint, the choice of SPDM is likely to gain in importance in the near future.

A summary of the advantages of SPDM is as follows: (1) It is possible to choose the composition of dialysis fluid. Recently, acetate-free dialysis fluid has become available, so it is now possible to use the fluid composition to suit each case better. (2) The structure of the dialysis unit is simple, so maintenance of the system is easy. (3) It is possible to operate each patient station separately. (4) Maintenance of the piping system is simple because only RO water is sent to each patient station through the pipes and not dialysis fluids, which contain electrolytes or glucose, etc.

The disadvantages of SPDM in comparison with CDDS are as follows: (1) The unit price of the patient station is higher because it includes a mechanism to prepare the dialysis fluid. (2) The interior structure of the patient station is complicated, therefore a drug solution alone may not sufficiently clean and disinfect the station. (3) The RO water branch pipes may not be sufficiently cleaned and disinfected. (4) There is more work to be done for preparation because it is necessary to check the electrolytes and osmotic pressure of the dialysis fluid at each patient station.

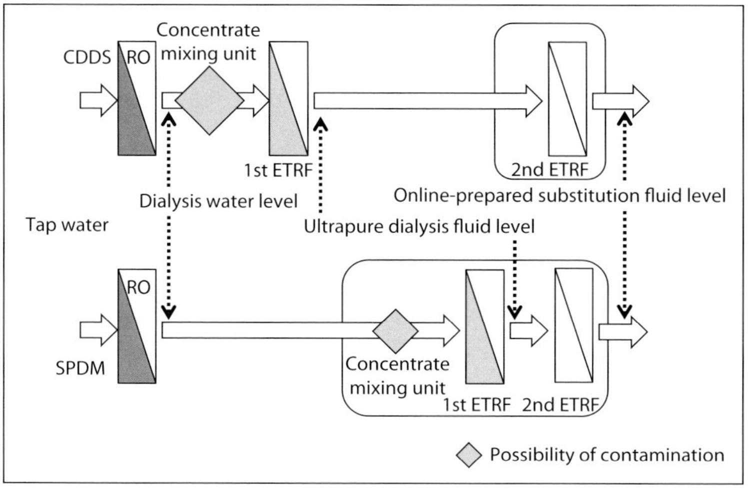


**Fig. 2.** Comparison of the water purification process with CDDS and SPDM.

## Substitution Fluid for Online HDF with CDDS and SPDM

According to the JSDT 2008 standard [3], the purity levels required for dialysis water, from the outlet of RO apparatus to the mixing unit and the central dialysis fluid proportioning unit in CDDS, is the 'dialysis water level' shown in table 1, and that for dialysis fluid, after the central dialysis fluid proportioning unit, is 'dialysis fluid level'. Those requirements are much more strict comparing with ISO standard, especially in required endotoxin level. However, as described above, these segments are often the area where purification management may be insufficient or new contamination is feared; therefore, the first ETRF is mounted after the central dialysis fluid proportioning unit. After the first ETRF, ultrapure dialysis fluid level is applicable. After that, online-prepared substitution fluid level is applied at the second ETRF of the patient machine and used for HDF. In the case of the CDDS mounted with the first ETRF, online HDF therapy can be offered easily in many cases by mounting the second ETRF on each patient machine (fig. 2).

With SPDM, RO water at the dialysis water level is sent to each patient machine. Although asepsis is guaranteed for liquid dialysis concentrates used in the SPDM, the possibility of contamination during the process of suction of the concentrate to the patient machine cannot be ruled out. The prepared dialysis fluid is cleaned by the first ETRF mounted in each patient machine to the ultrapure dialysis fluid level and by the second ETRF to the online-prepared substitution fluid level. The guarantee of water quality by using the second ETRF is significant in both CDDS and SPDM (fig. 2).

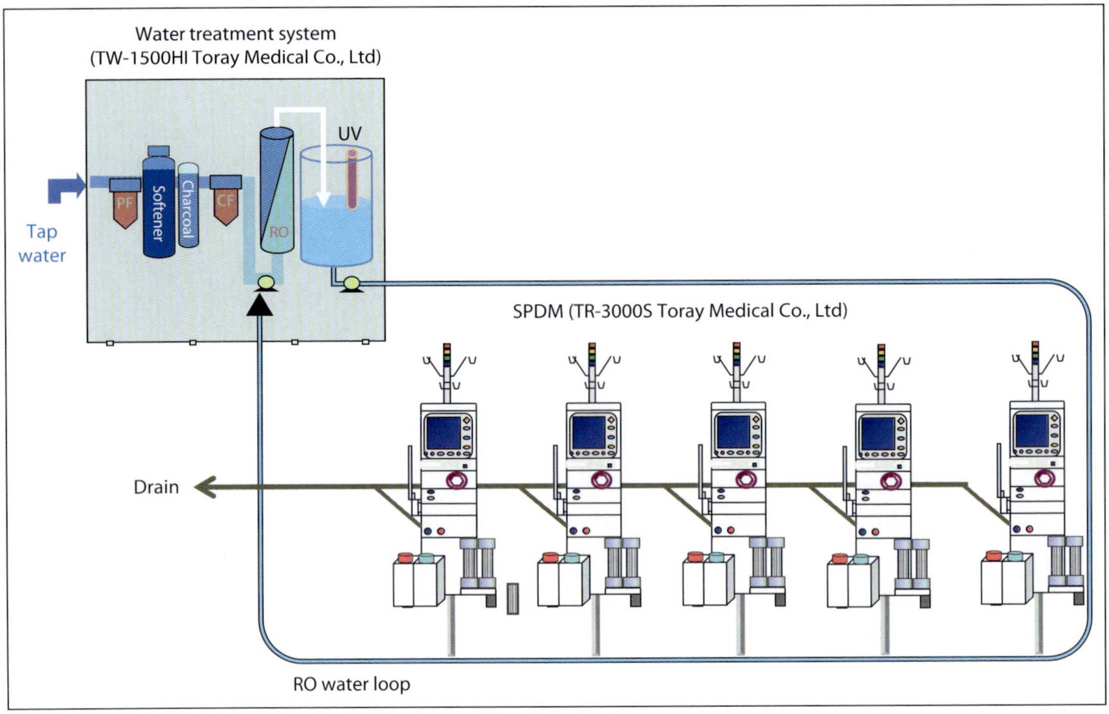


**Fig. 3.** Scheme of SPDM. PF = Pre-filter; CF = check filter; RO = reverse osmosis membrane; UV = ultraviolet lamp; CCF= carbon cartridge filter.

## Maintenance of Purification of Dialysis Fluid

The purity level of CDDS is mainly managed by washing with water and sodium hypochlorite or peracetic acid-based agent, together with washing with acetic acid once to several times weekly in order to remove adhered mineral substances to the pipes. SPDM is managed in a similar manner. However, SPDM is often not used daily, so in some cases the equipment itself and the pipes have not been cleaned sufficiently. Hot water disinfection is not common in Japan, and the hot water function is provided as an option with both CDDS and SPDM. It is speculated that the pipes for dialysis fluid and RO water are disinfected with hot water on an experimental basis at several facilities only. In recent years, an RO apparatus with a function to wash the RO membranes using RO water or hot water has been commercially available in order to achieve a higher level of purification. However, the RO apparatus, recommended piping, and patient stations of CDDS and SPDM of the dialysis units used in Japan are composed of products from different manufacturers mainly for economic reasons. In such cases, it is difficult to ask a single manufacturer for validation,

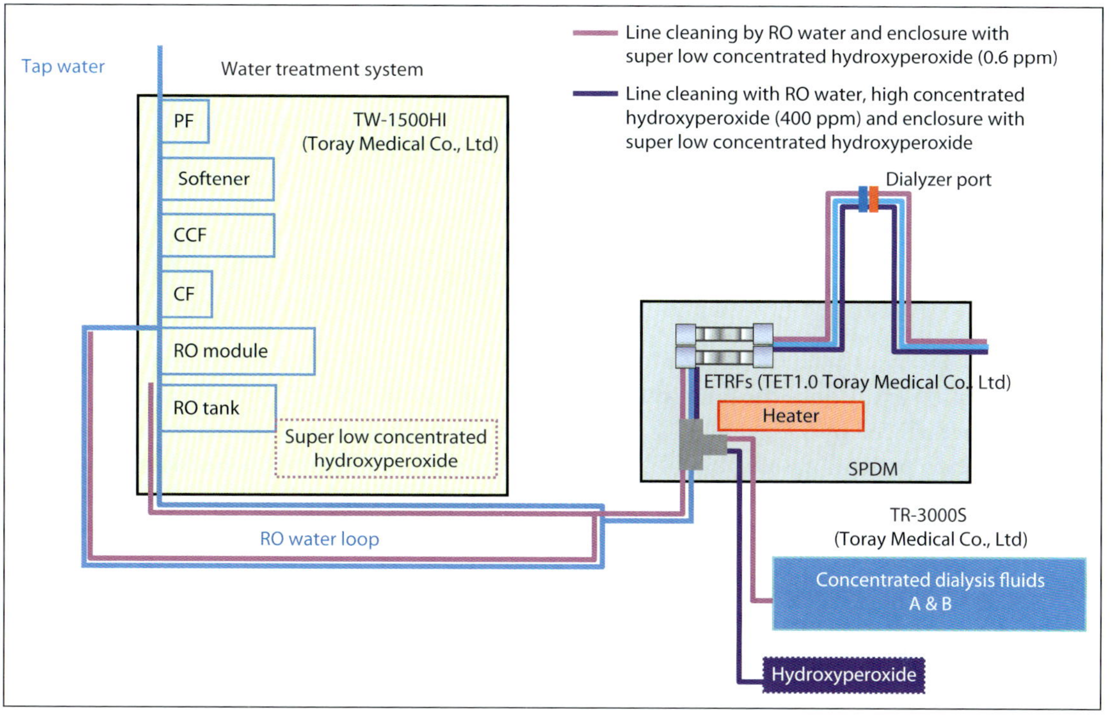


**Fig. 4.** Flow diagram of disinfection of water system and SPDM.

therefore the validation should be done for the whole system on each facility's own responsibility.

## HD and/or Online HDF Using SPDM by Comprehensive Management

As stated above, the structure of CDDS and HD and online HDF using CDDS has been described extensively in other articles. Here, we give a practical example of SPDM with which a high level of purification has been maintained (fig. 3). The system consists of an RO apparatus with the function for washing RO membranes using RO water, a loop piping system for RO water, and a patient station mounted with two ETRFs with a hot water disinfection function.

Peracetic acid-based agent is used to clean the RO water pipes and patient machine, and the equipment is cleaned and disinfected with a concentration of 400 ppm as well as filling with very low concentration agent (0.6 ppm) during the night. A computer program controls cleaning, and branches from the RO water pipes can also be disinfected (fig. 4).

Cleaning with disinfectant is carried out daily and hot water disinfection three times a week. Using these structures and programs, biological inspections (1-week culture on R2A medium) of the RO water just behind the RO apparatus showed a result of 0 CFU/ml. Endotoxins were also measured at a level below the detection limit (<0.001 EU/ml), thus the online-prepared substitution fluid level is achieved and maintained.

## Conclusion

CDDS has been used safely for over 40 years. Online HDF can be put into operation easily once the purification of dialysis fluid is achieved. With SPDM, individualized operation and the choice of dialysis fluid or treatment method to suit each patient's case is possible. The choice between CDDS and SPDEM should be made considering the advantages and disadvantages of both systems based on the scale of the facility and the concept of treatment.

## References


1 Registry of Japanese Society for Dialysis Therapy, 2008.

2 Koda Y, Mineshima M: Advances and advantages in recent central dialysis fluid delivery system. Blood Purif 2009;27(suppl 1):23–37.

3 Kawanishi H, Akiba T, Masakane I, Tomo T, Mineshima M, Kawasaki T, Hirakata H, Akizawa T: The standard on microbiological management of fluids in Japanese Society for Dialysis therapy, 2008. Ther Apher Dial 2009;3:161–166.



Ikuo Aoike
Koyo Medical Clinic, 3-9-25 Kamedakoyo
Konan-ku, Niigata 950-0121 (Japan)
E-Mail kmc8686@an.wakwak.com

Kawanishi H, Yamashita AC (eds): Hemodiafiltration – A New Era.
Contrib Nephrol. Basel, Karger, 2011, vol 168, pp 107–116

# Fully Automated Dialysis System for Online Hemodiafiltration Built into the Central Dialysis Fluid Delivery System

Hideki Kawanishi · Misaki Moriishi

Tsuchiya General Hospital, Hiroshima, Japan

**Abstract**

The fully automated dialysis system was developed as an improvement over a previous patient monitor used in the treatment of hemodialysis, with the aim of standardizing and promoting labor-saving in such treatment. This system uses backfiltration dialysis fluid to perform priming, blood rinse back and rapid fluid replenishment, and causes guiding of blood into the dialyzer by the drainage pump for ultrafiltration. This requires that the dialysis fluid used be purified to a high level. This paper is a report on the author's experience using dialysis fluid maintained at such a high level of purification for the fully automated dialysis system with an online hemodiafiltration function built into the central dialysis fluid delivery system.


Priming, guiding of blood into the dialyzer and blood rinse back for hemodialysis treatment require a certain level of expertise and have proved a stumbling block to the development of automation. A system utilizing backfiltrated dialysis fluid as a means of standardizing and reducing the labor involved in these processes has thus been developed. This system makes active use of backfiltrated dialysis fluid and thus requires strict control of water quality for each patient monitor and the central dialysis fluid delivery system (CDDS), as well as purification of the dialysis fluid used [1, 2].

Against the above background the GC-110N (JMS Co. Ltd, Japan) was developed as a fully automated dialysis system (FADS) able to actively use purified dialysis fluid through backfiltration to automate the priming, blood rinse back and rapid fluid replenishment processes, with each process segueing to the next through the touch of a single button [3, 4]. The GC-110N has been widely used throughout Japan since its introduction in March 2005. Further, an

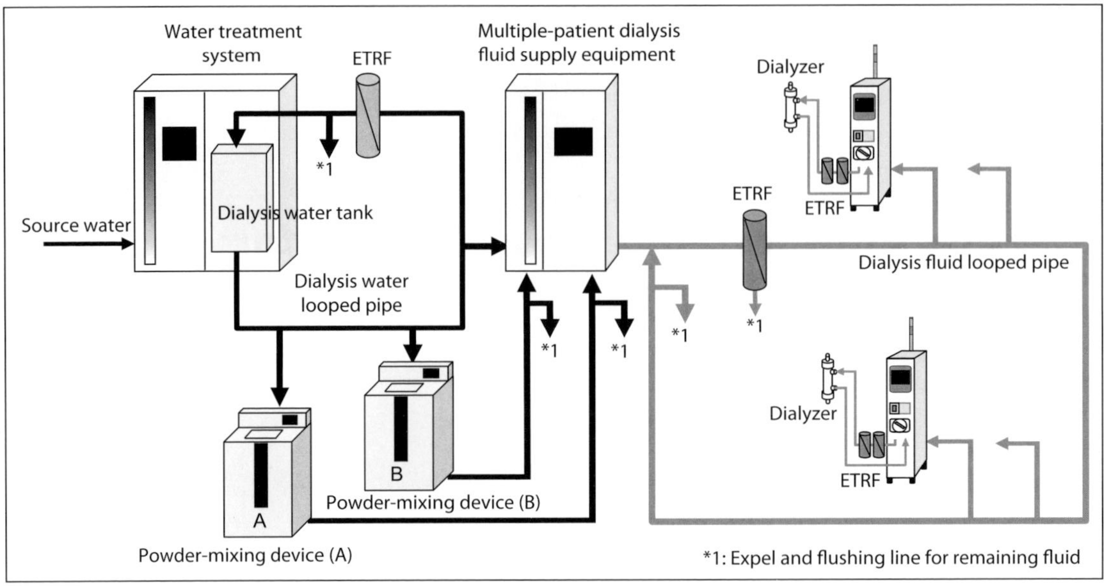


**Fig. 1.** Flowchart of the central dialysis delivery system used to achieve dialysis fluid purification.

online hemodiafiltration (HDF) function using purified dialysis fluid has been used since March 2010. This report intends to investigate the safety and results gained through the long-term use of the FADS with an online HDF function to carry out priming, blood rinse back and rapid fluid replenishment using back-filtrated dialysis fluid.

## Outline of the Central Dialysis Delivery System

Figure 1 shows in flowchart form the processes used by the CDDS to achieve dialysis fluid purification. The source water is then purified into dialysis water using a reverse osmosis (RO) module almost completely free of leaks with a sodium chloride blocking rate of over 99.5%. The dialysis water then accumulates in the dialysis water tank. In order to prevent cross-contamination of the dialysis water, initial water is removed from each line at the startup of the RO equipment, and expels the remaining water when the equipment is stopped. Dialysis water is cycled to the RO module while the equipment is in operation, even when purification is not occurring, to prevent water from pooling inside the equipment. With regard to the dialysis water supply lines, an endotoxin retentive filter (ETRF) is placed at the re-entry mouth of the dialysis water tank as a looped pipe to provide circulation to the dialysis water tank, countering the presence of contaminants inside the pipes and preventing cross-contamination.

The dialysis fluid supply equipment (Multiple-Patient Dialysis Fluid Supply Equipment (MPDFSE)) (BC-Purela01™) mixed A, B solution and dialysis water, and supplied as dialysis fluid to each patient monitor. The pipe connecting the MPDFSE to each patient monitor also has a looped circulation pump in place. This prevents cross-contamination by eliminating dead-end pipes and causing dialysis fluid to circulate back if the flow rate goes above a set level, preventing water accumulation.

## FADS with Online HDF

This FADS uses a sealed capacity control method with constant capacity receptacles (double-chamber method using two diaphragms). This control method uses a dilution pump to pump dialysis fluid from the dialysis fluid supply line to the dialyzer, dilute it into the blood circuit, and then filtrate through the dialyzer an amount of dialysis fluid equal to the volume of dialysis fluid that has been diluted.

At this time, the quality of the dialysis fluid must satisfy the standards for 'online prepared substitution fluid'. Although conventionally a complete filtration system with a single ETRF has been used immediately before the dialyzer to check and control the quality of the filtration fluid, this has been changed to two ETRF units operating in series, with each performing automated integrity testing, to ensure that fluid quality is maintained even if one unit breaks down (fig. 2).

In addition, since the dilution pump is not located inside the unit, a JMS pump that satisfies the required standards for peripheral equipment is used.

## Fully Automated Dialysis System

The FADS is based on the currently available patient monitor, the GC-110 (manufactured by JMS Co. Ltd, Japan), primary improvements including the positive/reverse functions for the drainage and blood pumps and computer controls.

Furthermore, dialysis fluid is used for priming, rapid fluid replenishment and blood rinse back in place of the standard normal saline solution, though normal saline may still be used for these processes as before. Details of this system have been described elsewhere [4].

*Automatic Priming.* Priming is automatically performed with dialysis fluid extracted from the blood circuit through backfiltration from the dialyzer. Two ETRF must be placed in series immediately before the dialyzer of each patient monitor. The operator brings out the dialyzer, blood circuit, and dilution

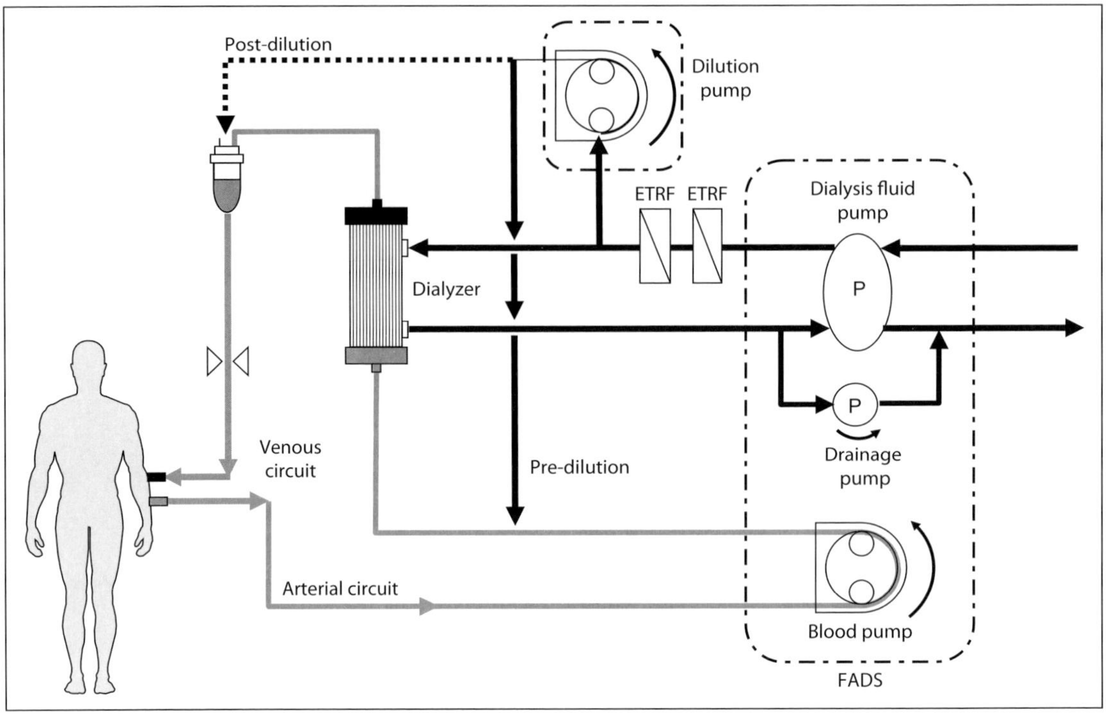


**Fig. 2.** Flowchart of online HDF with fully automated GC-110N console.

circuit for online HDF and attaches them to the FADS, then turns the automatic priming switch on. The FADS allows adjustment of relative speed of the drainage and blood pumps, and enables priming with backfiltrated dialysis fluid to the arterial or venous circuit, or both circuits and the dilution circuit for online HDF, through changing the orientation of the blood pump. Unlike normal saline solution, priming with backfiltration dialysis fluid is unlimited in terms of volume, allowing cleaning of the dialyzer with a large volume of dialysis fluid to fully remove any remaining substances inside the dialyzer or blood circuit.

*Automatic Guiding of Blood into the Dialyzer.* After the completion of the automatic priming process, the operator places the arteriovenous dialysis needles in the patient, connecting up the venous blood circuit to the venous needle and the arterial blood circuit to the arterial needle. The operator then turns the automatic blood removal switch on. The FADS drainage pump begins positive (draining) cycle, and the dialysis fluid inside the blood circuit is discharged from the dialyzer while blood is guided into it. During this process the patient's blood passes through both the arterial and venous blood circuits to the dialyzer, though the flow rate of either circuit can be adjusted by changing the relative speed of the drainage and blood pumps. When insufficient venous blood guiding occurs, the blood guiding can be set to 100% arterial and 0% venous.

The FADS contains functions to detect problems in blood guiding, monitoring lowering of dialysis fluid pressure (indicating defective blood removal) as a safety mechanism.

*Rapid Fluid Replenishment.* When steps are necessary to reinfuse the patient due to a loss of blood pressure or other problem during dialysis, the operator turns the fluid replenishment switch on. The drainage pump changes to a reverse cycle, while the blood pump can simultaneously be reduced in speed or stopped entirely. This causes the backfiltrated dialysis fluid from the dialyzer to be replenished without the normally required need to prepare saline solution and perform complex operations with the patient monitor and blood circuit. The volume of replenishment can also be preset as necessary.

*Automatic Blood Rinse Back.* Once the dialysis is finished and the drainage completed as planned, previous settings automatically cause the blood rinse back process to begin, or switch on a light to show that the machine is stopped in blood rinse back standby mode. In blood rinse back standby mode, the operator can turn the automatic blood rinse back switch on to begin the said process. The FADS drainage pump will then cycle in reverse and rinse back the blood inside the blood circuit and the backfiltrated dialysis fluid from the dialyzer to the patient.

The dialysis fluid will move along both the arterial and venous circuits to push blood back into the patient, while the arteriovenous ratio can be adjusted through changing the relative speed of the drainage and blood pumps.

## Dialysis Fluid Quality Control Standards

The manufacturer's fluid quality standards and control standards for using the FADS (GC-110N) are shown table 1.

The fluid quality standards of the Japanese Society for Dialysis Therapy (JSDT) require an endotoxin concentration <0.05 EU/ml and a bacterial count <100 CFU/ml for both dialysis water and dialysis fluid. For ultrapure dialysis fluid, the standards are no more than 0.001 EU/ml for endotoxin concentration and 0.1 CFU/ml for bacterial count [5].

The fluid quality standards for GC-110N require for dialysis water an endotoxin concentration <0.05 EU/ml and a bacterial count <100 CFU/ml, measured once every 3 months. When online HDF is used, the dialysis fluid supplied to patient monitor must have an endotoxin concentration <0.05 EU/ml and a bacterial count <100 CFU/ml, with at least two patient monitor units measured each month and all patient monitor units measured at least once each year. Backfiltration dialysis fluid must have an endotoxin concentration <0.001 EU/ml and a bacterial count <0.1 CFU/ml, with the system validated by a dialysis

**Table 1.** Comparison of fluid quality standards for GC-110N and the JSDT 2008

| Item | | JSDT (2008) | |
|---|---|---|---|
| fluid | measurement | standard value | frequency |
| Dialysis water | endotoxin EU/ml | <0.050 | every 3 months |
| | bacteria CFU/ml | <100 | |
| Dialysis fluid delivery line | endotoxin EU/ml | – | – |
| | bacteria CFU/ml | – | – |
| Dialysis fluid | endotoxin EU/ml | <0.050 | min. 2 units/month (all units/year) |
| | bacteria CFU/ml | <100 | |
| Backfiltrate dialysis fluid/ ultrapure dialysis fluid | endotoxin EU/ml | <0.001 | all units every 2 weeks until the system stabilizes; min. 2 units/month (all units/ year) |
| | bacteria CFU/ml | <0.1 | |
| Online prepared substitution fluid | endotoxin EU/ml | <0.001 non-pyrogenic | all units every 2 weeks until the system stabilizes; all units/month |
| | bacteria CFU/ml | $<10^{-6}$ sterile | all units every 2 weeks until the system stabilizes; min. 2 units/month (all units/ year) |

Note: Sterility of $10^{-6}$ CFU/ml of online prepared substitution fluid is impossible to detect. Dialysis fluid used for preparation of substitution fluid should be maintained to the quality of ultrapure dialysis fluid.

| GC-110N fluid quality standards | | | |
|---|---|---|---|
| when automated functions are used, but online HDF is not used | | when online HDF is used | |
| standard value | frequency | standard value | frequency |
| <0.050 | every 3 months | <0.050 | every 3 months |
| <100 | | <100 | |
| – | – | <0.050 | min. 2 units/ month (all units/ year) |
| – | – | <100 | |
| – | – | – | – |
| – | – | – | – |
| <0.001 | all units every 2 weeks until the system stabilizes; min. 2 units/month (all units/ year) | – | – |
| <0.1 | | – | – |
| – | – | <0.001 | all units every 2 weeks until the system stabilizes; all units/ month |
| – | – | $<10^{-6}$ (standard at time of measurement <0.1) | all units every 2 weeks until the system stabilizes; min. 2 units/ month (all units/ year) |

fluid manufacturer every 2 weeks until it has stabilized, followed by measurements of at least two patient monitor units every month and all patient monitor units measured at least once each year. Online prepared substitution fluid must have an endotoxin concentration <0.001 EU/ml and a bacterial count of $10^{-6}$ CFU/ml; however, it is not possible to measure a bacterial count of $10^{-6}$ CFU/ml. This standard is maintained by the ETRF at a standard value for ultrapure dialysis fluid <0.1 CFU/ml. Endotoxin concentration is validated by a dialysis fluid manufacturer every 2 weeks until the system has stabilized, and then all patient monitor units are measured each month. Bacterial count is validated by a dialysis fluid manufacturer every 2 weeks until the system has stabilized, followed by measurements of at least two patient monitor units every month and all patient monitor units are measured at least once each year.

Here we will discuss the reasons for the differences in fluid quality standards between the FADS and JSDT.

The recommendation from JSDT for online HDF includes a requirement to maintain $10^{-6}$ CFU/ml of online prepared substitution fluid even if one ETRF leaks. It also indicates that it is possible to validate the quality of online prepared substitution fluid with the ETRF inhibition functionality.

Based on this recommendation, two ETRF units are mounted in series on this FADS after the patient monitor (immediately before the dialyzer).

In addition, we believed that it would be possible to maintain the quality of online prepared substitution fluid with the ETRF inhibition functionality if the standard for bacteria in the dialysis fluid at the entrance to the unit was no more than 100 CFU/ml, based on test results that indicate an LRV (logarithmic reduction value) of the specified ETRF endotoxin inhibition function of 4 or greater and an LRV of the bacteria inhibition function of 8 or greater. Therefore, we decided to not use ultrapure dialysis fluid for controlling dialysis fluid (immediately before the final ETRF) that creates online prepared substitution fluid, and instead controlled the entrance to the unit at 100 CFU/ml. (The same method was applied for endotoxin.)

In comparison with the JSDT fluid quality standards, this standard of no more than 100 CFU/ml is the same value as for standard dialysis fluid, and therefore the values for 'standard dialysis fluid' are applicable as the control standard.

Further, when using this FADS to perform online HDF, the sample sites for testing backfiltrate dialysis fluid and online prepared substitution fluid are the same, and therefore controlling online prepared substitution fluid will also maintain the quality of backfiltrate dialysis fluid.

## Fluid Quality Control Method

The control method involves the establishment of a Dialysis Equipment Safety Control Committee headed by a Medical Equipment Safety Control Supervisor to perform maintenance and maintain records according to the control plan. It is necessary to provide training for committee members, after which they can use online prepared substitution fluid that has been validated by a medical agency [5].

This type of control requires maintenance by the medical agency that uses GC-110N. If it is discovered that values are not in compliance with fluid quality standards, automated functions (priming, blood rinse back, and rapid fluid replenishment processes with backfiltration dialysis fluid, and blood removal through drainage) and online HDF must be shut down immediately. In addition, when online HDF is used, it is necessary to replace ETRF at least once every 6 months.

## Discussion

The FADS GC-110N (JMS Co. Ltd.) acquired approval to manufacture and sell in Japan in March 2005 as a dialysis monitoring equipment with systems allowing the priming, blood rinse back and rapid fluid replenishment processes to be carried out one after another at the touch of a single button, working through the active use of backfiltration for purified dialysis fluid [3, 4]. This dialysis equipment has been in clinical use for 5 years, with dialysis fluid used for backfiltration produced at a constant level of purity equivalent to ultrapure dialysis fluid. This ultrapure dialysis fluid is passed through the dialyzer for backfiltration (gaining results equivalent to single-use ETRF) to be used in priming, blood rinse back and rapid fluid replenishment, while the backfiltrated dialysis fluid used is in a sterile and non-pyrogenic state, equivalent to online prepared substitution fluid [6, 7]. Further, changes made in 2010 allow the use of online HDF. The main changes involve the installation and control methods for ETRF. Although conventionally a complete filtration system has been used with a single ETRF unit immediately before the dialyzer to check and control the quality of the filtration fluid, this has been changed to two ETRF units operating in series, with each performing automated integrity testing, to ensure that fluid quality is maintained even if one unit breaks down.

The control standards for this system are based on the fluid quality standards of the JSDT [5]. Accordingly, membrane filter methods are essential for the scheduled bacteria measurement. Bacterial sampling is made once a month for dialysis water and dialysis fluid using a 37-mm membrane filter (0.45 μm) (sample: 100 ml, Japan PALL Co. Ltd, Tokyo, Japan, and ADVANTEC Co. Ltd, Tokyo, Japan; culture medium: m-TGE broth ampules). Neither endotoxin concentrations nor bacteria have yet been found in any of these tests since the system was introduced in July 2005.

The benefit of FADS is improved work efficiency through the reduction of the time required for starting and blood rinse back, and the simplification of rapid fluid replenishment in emergencies. In addition, since the dialysis treatment from cannulation to the end is a completely closed circuit, risk due to hazards such as aeration and blood contamination has been reduced. Further, the simplification of operations for hemodialysis treatment has reduced the possibility for various types of human errors. These are just a few examples of the increased efficiency in dialysis provided by the online HDF function. This equipment is the world's first online HDF unit built into CDDS to provide online HDF to multiple patients simultaneously.

## References


1 Baurmeister U, Travers M, Vienken J, Harding G, Million C, Klein E, Pass T, Wright R: Dialysate contamination and backfiltration may limit the use of high-flux dialysis membranes. ASAIO Trans 1989;35:519–522.

2 Leypoldt JK, Schmidt B, Gurland HJ: Measurement of backfiltration rates during hemodialysis with highly permeable membranes. Blood Purif 1991;9:74–78.

3 Tsuchiya S, Moriishi M, Takahashi N, Watanabe H, Kawanishi H, Kim ST, Masaoka K: Experience with the JMS fully automated dialysis machine. ASAIO J 2003;49:547–553.

4 Kawanishi H, Moriishi M, Sato T, Taoka M: Fully automated dialysis system based on the central dialysis fluid delivery system. Blood Purif 2009;27(suppl 1):56–63.

5 Kawanishi H, Akiba T, Masakane I, Tomo T, Mineshima M, Kawasaki T, Hirakata H, Akizawa T: The standard on microbiological management of fluids for hemodialysis and related therapies in Japanese Society for Dialysis Therapy, 2008. Ther Apher Dial 2009;13:161–166.

6 Ledebo I, Nystrand R: Defining the microbiological quality of dialysis fluid. Artif Organs 1999;23:37–43.

7 ISO11663, Quality of dialysis fluid for haemodialysis and related therapies, 2009.



Hideki Kawanishi, MD
Tsuchiya General Hospital, 3-30 Nakajima-cho
Naka-ku, Hiroshima 730-8655 (Japan)
Tel. +81 82 243 9191, Fax +81 82 241 1865, E-Mail h-kawanishi@tsuchiya-hp.jp

Kawanishi H, Yamashita AC (eds): Hemodiafiltration – A New Era.
Contrib Nephrol. Basel, Karger, 2011, vol 168, pp 117–128

# New Uremic Toxins – Which Solutes Should Be Removed?

Griet Glorieux · Raymond Vanholder

Renal Division, University Hospital Gent, Gent, Belgium

**Abstract**

Chronic kidney disease (CKD) is characterized by the progressive retention of a myriad of compounds, several of which play a role in cardiovascular damage, a major cause of mortality in CKD. Over the past years, especially protein-bound compounds (e.g. indoxylsulfate and *p*-cresylsulfate) and/or middle molecules (e.g. AGEs, cytokines and dinucleoside polyphosphates) have been identified as some of the main toxins involved in vascular lesions affecting endothelial cell, leukocyte, platelet and/or vascular smooth muscle cell function in CKD. Many of these solutes, however, are difficult to remove by standard dialysis strategies. The removal of protein-bound solutes remains limited because only the free fraction of the solute is available for, mostly diffusive, removal, while removal of the larger middle molecules (mostly larger peptidic compounds) can be obtained by increasing dialyzer pore size and by applying convective strategies. In addition, new therapeutic strategies pursuing specific removal (e.g. by adsorption) and/or pharmacological neutralization of the molecular impact of the responsible compounds are explored, aiming at an improved outcome in CKD patients.



Retention of uremic solutes starts from the moment kidney function declines. The kinetics of this process are, however, far from clear. Although during the last few years an immense progress has been made in the identification and quantification of uremic solutes [1], a large number of retention solutes remain unidentified [2]. The presence of an indefinite number of posttranscriptional modifications of retention solutes, as a result of oxidation, glycation, cysteination, as well as of several other chemical processes, with each of these structural variants possibly exerting a pathophysiologic impact that differs from the mother compound, hampers the process of mapping the uremic retention solutes even more. Although many compounds and/or their functional role remain unknown further identification and classification is compulsory before a targeted and possibly also tailored treatment will be possible. For the time being, uremic solutes are preferentially classified according to the physicochemical characteristics affecting their clearance during dialysis which, as of today, is still the main therapeutic option for their removal. Traditionally, this subdivision focuses on three types of molecules: the small water-soluble compounds (molecular weight (MW <500 Da), the larger 'middle molecules' (MW >500 Da) and the protein-bound compounds [1].

Recent reviews point out that removal of small water-soluble compounds is important for 'acute mortality' (e.g. related to hyperkalemia, sodium removal), but that for the chronic cardiovascular problems of the uremic syndrome, the protein-bound solutes and the middle molecules seem to play a more essential role [3]. Whereas the small water-soluble compounds, of which urea is the prototype, are easily removed by whatever dialysis strategy, the protein-bound toxins and middle molecules require more sophisticated strategies.

In this review we will focus on those compounds with convincing biological effects, especially affecting the major cell types involved in cardiovascular disease. Next, their removal and the related obstacles will be discussed with a reflection on how this knowledge can be translated into therapeutic measures improving outcome in chronic kidney disease (CKD) patients. The flowchart of the suggested approach is illustrated in figure 1.

## Toxicity of Specific Uremic Retention Solutes

### *Protein-Bound Solutes*

Several protein-bound molecules have been linked to cardiovascular problems, either through a proinflammatory impact or by causing endothelial or other vascular dysfunction. A few important ones are discussed more in detail below. Extended information on the pathophysiological role of specific protein-bound molecules as well as to protein-bound solutes in general can be found in a recent monography reviewing on the current status in uremic toxicity [4].

#### p-*Cresylsulfate*

The amino acids tyrosine and phenylalanine, generated from nutritional proteins, are metabolized by the intestinal flora into 4-hydroxyphenylacetic acid which is decarboxylated to *p*-cresol. However, unconjugated *p*-cresol is not detectable in normal and uremic plasma while during its passage through the intestinal mucosa, a cytosolic sulfotransferase metabolizes *p*-cresol into *p*-cresylsulfate, its main conjugate. Nevertheless, most of the pioneering research on the phenolic uremic retention compounds focused on the concentration and the toxicity of the mother compound *p*-cresol. This was caused by the fact that

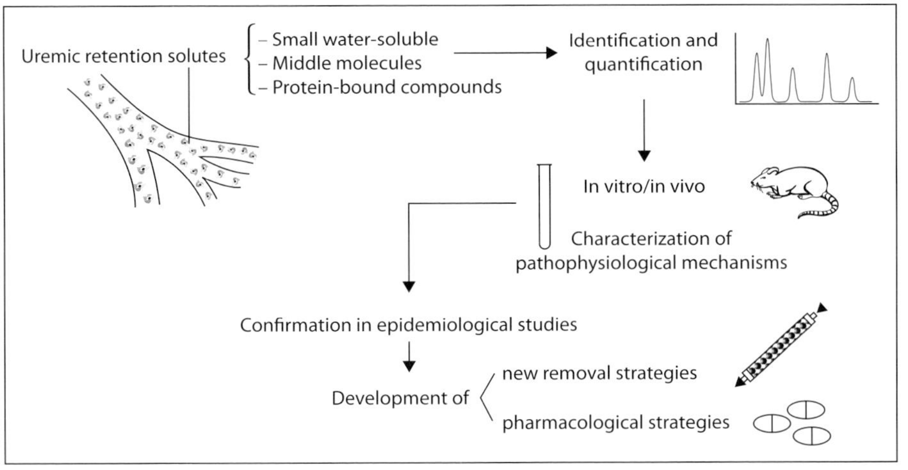


**Fig. 1.** Flowchart of suggested approach in evaluating the effect of uremic retention solutes, aiming at improved outcome in CKD patients.

previously measured *p*-cresol values were the resultant of the hydrolysis of *p*-cresylsulfate as a consequence of sample deproteinization by acidification. In this way, serum levels of *p*-cresol, in uremic patients, were shown to be increased about tenfold, and those of the free non-protein-bound *p*-cresol were even more substantially increased. *p*-Cresol, per se, was demonstrated to affect the inflammatory response by decreasing the reaction of activated polymorphonuclears and decreasing the endothelial cell response to inflammatory cytokines in vitro. Recently, the biological effects of *p*-cresylsulfate were evaluated in vitro, revealing a proinflammatory effect on unstimulated leukocytes [5] and induction of shedding of endothelial microparticles [6], suggesting its contribution to the propensity to vascular damage in renal patients.

Nevertheless, previously held conclusions about protein binding and relationship to overall and cardiovascular mortality in dialysis patients as well as to the development of infection probably are still valid, since there is very likely a correlation between former *p*-cresol estimations and current *p*-cresylsulfate measurements [7]. Moreover, a recent cohort study showed that free of *p*-cresylsulfate is a predictor of survival in CKD [8].

*Homocysteine (Hcy)*

Hcy, a sulfur-containing amino acid, is produced by the demethylation of dietary methionine. Moderate hyperhomocysteinemia is an independent risk factor for cardiovascular disease in the general population. Patients with chronic kidney failure have serum Hcy levels two- to fourfold above normal. Hcy increases the proliferation of vascular smooth muscle cells, one of the most prominent hallmarks of atherosclerosis [9]. Moderate hyperhomocysteinemia may induce endothelial dysfunction and generate oxidative oxygen species. Hcy-induced superoxide anion generation is responsible for NF-κB activation and subsequent monocyte chemoattractant protein-1 expression in macrophages inducing inflammatory responses [10]. The administration of excessive quantities of the Hcy precursor methionine to rats induces atherosclerosis-like alterations in the aorta. Hcy also disrupts several anticoagulant functions in the vessel wall, which results in enhanced thrombogenicity. Studies evaluating the potential of folic acid or 5-methyltetrahydrophosphate to decrease Hcy levels in chronic kidney disease emanated in contradictory results being, on the one hand, not able to reduce levels and on the other hand, if so, without affecting outcome parameters.

*Indoxylsulfate (IS)*

Indole, an aromatic heterocyclic structure, can be produced by bacteria as a degradation product of tryptophan which is subsequently sulfated by hepatic enzymes to produce IS. IS is the most abundant indolic compound in the body of uremic patients. The evidence of its biological, toxic effects has extended over the past years. IS has been linked to endothelial damage, inhibition of endothelial regeneration and repair, and endothelial and human aortic smooth muscle cell free radical production [11]. Induction of oxidative stress by IS promotes proliferation of human aortic smooth muscle cells. Recent data suggest a pro-fibrotic and pro-hypertrophic effect of IS on cardiac fibroblasts and a proinflammatory effect on monocytic cells [12]. Furthermore, IS is a potent endogenous agonist for the human aryl hydrocarbon receptor, a ligand-activated transcription factor involved in the regulation of multiple cellular pathways. Its prolonged activation by IS may contribute to the cellular toxicity observed in dialysis patients. IS has also been related to renal fibrosis and progression of renal failure. In the rat, IS induces aortic calcification, with aortic wall thickening and expression of osteoblast-specific proteins. In hemodialysis patients, IS is associated with markers related to atherosclerosis [13]. A recent cohort study showed that IS is associated with cardiovascular disease and mortality in CKD [14].

*Phenylacetic Acid (PAA)*

PAA is a degradation product of the amino acid, phenylalanine. Plasma concentrations of PAA in patients with CKD stage 5 strongly exceed those in healthy controls. PAA was shown to inhibit inducible nitric oxide synthase expression and consequently, NO production [15], and subsequently was identified as an inhibitor of $Ca^{2+}$ ATPase activity in CKD stage 5. PAA was recently shown to increase formation of ROS in VSMCs and to have inhibitory effects on macrophage-killing function.

In a study by Scholze et al. [16], an association between plasma PAA levels and arterial vascular properties in patients with CKD stage 5 was demonstrated.

*Guanidines*

The guanidines are small water-soluble protein breakdown products; although their protein binding is not cleared out yet, their pathophysiological effects are convincing. In addition, their kinetic behavior diverges from that of urea, which makes them, like the protein-bound solutes, 'difficult to remove' by dialysis. Guanidines are structural metabolites of arginine and are retained in uremia. Among them are well-known uremic retention solutes such as creatinine and guanidine, and more recently detected moieties such as asymmetric and symmetric dimethylarginine (ADMA and SDMA). Guanidine levels have been determined in serum, urine, cerebrospinal fluid and brain of uremic patients.

Guanidino compounds have mainly been implicated in neurotoxicity [17]. Potential cardiovascular impact was, until recently, mainly attributed to ADMA, which inhibits inducible nitric oxide synthase, an endothelial protective enzyme [18]. However, in addition, a mixture of guanidino compounds was shown to suppress the natural killer cell response to interleukin-2 and free radical production by neutrophils. In more recent studies, guanidino compounds have been shown to enhance baseline immune function, related to vascular damage, and methylguanidine and guanidino acetic acid were shown to significantly enhancing the LPS-stimulated production of TNF-α by normal monocytes. In addition, they also have been related to a decreased protein binding of Hcy, another compound with vessel-damaging potential (see above).

Schepers et al. [19] demonstrated that SDMA, considered the inert counterpart of ADMA, stimulates free radical production by monocytes by acting on $Ca^{2+}$ entry via store-operated channels. This proinflammatory effect may trigger vascular pathology and may be involved in altering the prevalence of cardiovascular disease in CKD.

*Middle Molecules*

Apart from these protein-bound molecules, also middle molecules have a toxic impact on the cardiovascular system, although it is of note that several of the middle molecules are protein-bound as well.

Up till now, at least 40 middle molecules or groups of middle molecules have been identified [20]; a quantity far outnumbered, however, by the amount of as yet unidentified solutes [2]. Many of these middle molecules have been linked to cardiovascular problems, either by being proinflammatory, by generating endothelial dysfunction or smooth muscle cell proliferation or by enhancing coagulation. New compounds are discovered regularly, such as recently uridine adenosine tetraphosphate, a very strong vasoconstrictive agent. Below, the biological effect of some specific middle molecules is discussed more in detail. Extended information on the pathophysiological role of middle molecules, such as $\beta_2$-microglobulin, resistin, adiponectin, the cytokines, leptin, immunoglobulin light chains, parathyroid hormone, the dinucleoside polyphosphates and the advanced glycation end-products can also be found in recent reviews on the current status in uremic toxicity [4].

*Advanced Glycation End-Products (AGEs)*

AGEs are glycation adducts formed in the later stages of protein glycation reactions. Protein glycation was originally considered as a posttranslational modification that was situated mostly on extracellular proteins. It is now known that AGE residues are also formed on short-lived cellular and extracellular proteins. Cellular proteolysis forms AGE-free adducts from these proteins, which normally have high renal clearance, but this declines markedly in CKD, leading to profound increases in plasma AGE-free adducts [21] inducing an increase in leukocyte oxidative stress. For many years, the biologic effect of AGE had been studied mainly with artificially prepared compounds, which might not be representative of AGE really present in uremia, such as fructoselysine, N-ε-carboxymethyllysine, pyrraline, or pentosidine. Glorieux et al. [22] demonstrated the proinflammatory effect of several AGE compounds that are retained in uremia, Arg I (arginine modified with glyoxal), carboxyethyllysine, and carboxymethyllysine, demonstrating increased production of free radicals by monocytic cells. It is interesting that one of the studied AGE (Arg II) had no effect at all on leukocytes, showing that the behavior of a number of compounds belonging to a specific group cannot automatically be extrapolated to all solutes of this group.

The binding of the AGE compounds to their receptor RAGE, extracting them from the circulation and/or inducing biological responses has recently been questioned. Other RAGE ligands have been reported such as the extracellular newly identified RAGE-binding protein (EN-RAGE), S100A12. Recently, mean plasma S100A12 levels were shown to be twice as high in HD patients compared to healthy controls; they correlated with the carotid intimal media thickness in HD patients [23]. The link AGE/RAGE might be found in the following: activation of RAGE by S100A12 was shown to decrease the expression of glyoxalase 1 (Glo1). Downregulation of Glo1 is known to increase local concentrations of methylglyoxal and glyoxal and related AGE residue formation. Recently, methylglyoxal modifications of vascular type IV collagen were shown to cause endothelial detachment, anoikis and inhibition of angiogensis. Increased numbers of circulating endothelial cells are indicative for endothelial damage and prognostic for cardiovascular disease in renal failure [24].

*Dinucleoside Polyphosphates*

Dinucleoside polyphosphates are a group of substances involved in the regulation of vascular tone as well as in the proliferation of vascular smooth muscle cells and mesangial cells. Specific members of this group, the diadenosine polyphosphates, were detected in hepatocytes, human plasma and platelets. In addition, concentrations of diadenosine polyphosphates are increased in platelets from hemodialysis patients. Recently, uridine adenosine tetraphosphate (Up4A) was identified as a novel endothelium-derived vasoconstrictive factor. It was also shown to be released from renal tubular cells upon stimulation, whereby it acted as a strong vasoconstrictive mediator on afferent arterioles, suggesting a functional role of Up4A as an autocrine hormone for glomerular perfusion. Plasma Up4A concentrations were increased in juvenile hypertensive patients compared with juvenile normotensive subjects; it also correlated with left ventricular mass and intima media wall thickness which could be attributed to its proliferative effect on vascular smooth muscle cells. Its vasoconstrictive effects, its plasma concentration and its release upon stimulation strongly suggest that Up4A has a functional vasoregulatory role [25]. Dinucleoside polyphosphates were also shown to activate leukocytes as defined by their capacity to induce free radical production which in its turn might contribute to the chronic inflammatory status of the uremic patients [26].

*Resistin*
Resistin is a 12.5-kDa protein. In humans, resistin is mainly produced by macrophages and is released predominantly by human visceral white adipose tissue macrophages. Serum concentrations of resistin are markedly increased in CKD patients with both advanced or mild to moderate renal function impairment, as compared to controls [27]. In patients with CKD, resistin levels correlate with CRP and TNF-α and even with BMI as a covariate suggesting it may play a role in the subclinical inflammation associated with CKD.

Resistin was shown to significantly attenuate neutrophil chemotaxis in response to the chemotactic peptide fMLP, at concentrations corresponding to those measured in serum samples of uremic patients. In addition, resistin decreases the *Escherichia coli-* and PMA-activated oxidative burst by neutrophils. From this point of view, resistin can contribute to the disturbed immune response in uremic patients, playing a role in uremic inflammation. Furthermore, resistin was shown to be present in human atherosclerotic lesions and therefore has a potential role in atherogenesis. Pathophysiologically relevant concentrations of resistin increase endothelial cell adhesion molecule expression, possibly contributing to increased atherosclerosis risk. Plasma resistin positively correlates with leukocyte counts, high-sensitivity CRP, and endothelin-1 after adjustment for age, sex and BMI [28]. Therefore, resistin may be involved in the development of coronary artery disease by influencing systemic inflammation and endothelial activation.

## Removal of Protein-Bound Uremic Solutes and Middle Molecules

To protect patients against the cardiovascular as well as other side effects of the uremic syndrome, it seems in accordance with our current pathophysiological concepts to pursue the removal of protein-bound and middle molecules as much as possible.

Application of high-flux hemodialysis has no considerable impact on the removal of the protein-bound solutes [29]. Convective strategies, on the other hand, increased removal compared to diffusive removal, with postdilution hemodiafiltration (HDF) being superior to both predilution HDF and predilution hemofiltration [30]. In contrast, Krieter et al. [31] could not detect a difference in removal of the protein-bound solutes, *p*-cresylsulfate and IS, between post-HDF and high-flux HD. Daily hemodialysis was shown to decrease the predialysis concentration of protein-bound solutes, as compared to a classical alternate-day dialysis regime. Peritoneal dialysis (PD), however, seemed to be inferior to high-flux hemodialysis in removing protein-bound molecules, in spite of a better preserved residual renal function and considerable transperitoneal albumin loss. In spite of this lower removal with PD, plasma concentrations of protein-bound solutes were also lower in PD patients, pointing to possible differences in intestinal generation and/or metabolism [32]. Whatever the mechanisms, since free plasma concentration determines toxicity, the latter finding seems to be pathophysiologically more relevant than the lower clearance with PD.

Much is expected from adsorptive strategies to enhance removal of the protein-bound solutes. One option is fractionated plasma separation and adsorption (Prometheus®). Indeed, a pilot study showed effective removal of protein-bound solutes but was hampered by troublesome coagulation problems. Removal of protein-bound solutes was also enhanced by adding sorbent to the dialysate. Since the intestine is a major source of uremic toxin generation and/or uptake, administration of pre- and probiotics could contribute to the decrease in plasma levels as was recently suggested by reduced generation rates of *p*-cresylsulfate after administration of the prebiotic oligofructose-inulin to HD patients [33].

In contrast to what was observed for the protein-bound solutes, removal of middle molecules can be accomplished by applying dialysis membranes with a large enough pore size (so-called high-flux membranes). Removal through large pores can be enhanced by applying convection, especially if used in a HDF setting [34]; the amount of cleared middle molecules is correlated to the quantity of plasma water removed and replaced in an equivoluminous manner [34]. The relative improvement in adequacy due to convection becomes more pronounced as the MW of the compounds to be removed increases, since the amount of convective clearance is independent of MW as long as membrane pore size is large enough to allow transfer.

Among convective strategies, both postdilution HDF and predilution hemofiltration are superior to predilution HDF for removal of middle molecules [30]. Of note, partial removal via the kidneys, as long as residual renal function is preserved, becomes relatively more important as the MW of the compounds to be removed increases and/or the molecules in question are difficult to remove by dialysis for other reasons (e.g. protein binding). As a consequence, dialytic strategies which preserve renal function, such as PD or high-flux hemodialysis, are preferable in this context. A recent evaluation in the ongoing CONTRAST study confirmed an effective lowering of $\beta_2$-microglobulin levels by HDF but especially in patients without residual kidney function. It was demonstrated that removal of the middle molecules can be further enhanced by increasing dialysis frequency together with prolonging the dialysis session. In a setting applying the Genius® dialysis system, $\beta_2$-microglobulin removal increased almost twofold, only by increasing dialysis time from 4 to 8 h, in spite of an unaltered Kt/V urea [35]. The reason for this observation is that more time is allowed for $\beta_2$-microglobulin, with its multicompartmental behavior, to move from the extravascular to the intravascular compartment, from where it can be removed by the dialysis procedure.

## Interventional Outcome Studies Based on Removal

The question arises in how far improving the removal of protein-bound solutes and the middle molecules could have an impact on the outcome of patients treated by hemodialysis or related strategies.

As the removal of the protein-bound molecules is poor, no interventional trials with extracorporeal strategies focusing on these compounds have been undertaken so far. AST-120 (Kremezin®) is an intestinal sorbent with the capacity to decrease plasma concentration of IS [36] and maybe other protein-bound uremic solutes such as the cresols as well. A short-term prospective clinical study in humans with AST-120 demonstrated a decrease of plasma concentration of IS, but showed, next to significant improvements in malaise, no other clinical benefit [36]. However, recently, AST-120 (Kremezin®) has been associated with postponement of the start of dialysis, a better presentation of estimated glomerular filtration rate and, if applied before the start of dialysis, with better outcomes once dialysis was undertaken [37].

As removal of middle molecules can easily be achieved by large-pore high-flux dialysis, much more outcome data on this topic are available. A number of retrospective trials and secondary analyses of randomized controlled trials have shown survival superiority for the high-flux membranes in a hemodialysis setting, as compared to low-flux membranes. A subanalysis of the HEMO study focusing on cardiovascular outcome demonstrated a significance in favor of high-flux membranes for patients enrolled in the study after several years of preceding dialysis [38]. The Membrane Permeability Outcome (MPO) study demonstrated survival outcome superiority of high-flux dialysis in dialysis patients with a serum albumin $\leq$4 g/dl at inclusion and at a secondary analysis in diabetics [38].

Interventional outcome studies using convective strategies are still ongoing. One small trial, comparing online hemofiltration to low-flux dialysis illustrated a survival superiority for hemofiltration [39].

In brief, a number of recent data suggest an improvement of outcomes when increasing membrane pore size in a hemodialysis setting; the differences were each time found in subgroups of the studied populations. Whether adding convection results in a supplementary benefit has still not entirely been proven in well-conceived randomized controlled trials, although indirect arguments, such as the relation between $\beta_2$-microglobulin concentration and outcome [40], as well as pathophysiological evidence accumulated over time plead in favor of this strategy.

## Conclusions

Retention of protein-bound and middle molecules to a large extent mediates uremic toxicity and especially cardiovascular complications in CKD. Dialytic removal of middle molecules can be increased by the use of high-flux membranes and further enhanced by adding convection. The data for protein-bound solutes remain less convincing, with postdilution HDF being the most efficient of the available convective strategies. Only a few studies suggest that outcome improves with dialysis on high-flux membranes. Inclusion of new removal methods (e.g. adsorption) and pharmaceutical strategies blocking responsible pathways could contribute to the aim of improving outcome of CKD patients.

## References


1 Vanholder R, De Smet R, Glorieux G, Argiles A, Baurmeister U, Brunet P, Clark W, Cohen G, De Deyn PP, Deppisch R, Descamps-Latscha B, Henle T, Jorres A, Lemke HD, Massy ZA, Passlick-Deetjen J, Rodriguez M, Stegmayr B, Stenvinkel P, Tetta C, Wanner C, Zidek W: Review on uremic toxins: classification, concentration, and interindividual variability. Kidney Int 2003;63:1934–1943.

2 Weissinger EM, Kaiser T, Meert N, de Smet R, Walden M, Mischak H, Vanholder RC: Proteomics: a novel tool to unravel the pathophysiology of uraemia. Nephrol Dial Transplant 2004;19:3068–3077.

3 Vanholder R, Van Laecke S, Glorieux G: What is new in uremic toxicity? Pediatr Nephrol 2008;23:1211–1221.

4 Vanholder R: Progress in uremic toxin research. Semin Dial 2009;22:321–468. 2009.

5 Schepers E, Meert N, Glorieux G, Goeman J, Van der Eycken J, Vanholder R: *p*-Cresylsulphate, the main in vivo metabolite of *p*-cresol, activates leucocyte free radical production. Nephrol Dial Transplant 2007;22:592–596.

6 Meijers BK, Van Kerckhoven S, Verbeke K, Dehaen W, Vanrenterghem Y, Hoylaerts MF, Evenepoel P: The uremic retention solute *p*-cresyl sulfate and markers of endothelial damage. Am J Kidney Dis 2009;54:891–901.

7 Meijers BK, Bammens B, De Moor B, Verbeke K, Vanrenterghem Y, Evenepoel P: Free *p*-cresol is associated with cardiovascular disease in hemodialysis patients. Kidney Int 2008;73:1174–1180.

8 Liabeuf S, Barreto DV, Barreto FC, Meert N, Glorieux G, Schepers E, Temmar M, Choukroun G, Vanholder R, Massy ZA: Free *p*-cresylsulphate is a predictor of mortality in patients at different stages of chronic kidney disease. Nephrol Dial Transplant 2010;25:1183–1191.
9 Kielstein JT, Salpeter SR, Buckley NS, Cooke JP, Fliser D: Two cardiovascular risk factors in one? Homocysteine and its relation to glomerular filtration rate. A meta-analysis of 41 studies with 27,000 participants. Kidney Blood Press Res 2008;31:259–267.
10 Au-Yeung KK, Yip JC, Siow YL, O K: Folic acid inhibits homocysteine-induced superoxide anion production and nuclear factor-κB activation in macrophages. Can J Physiol Pharmacol 2006;84:141–147.
11 Dou L, Jourde-Chiche N, Faure V, Cerini C, Berland Y, Dignat-George F, Brunet P: The uremic solute indoxyl sulfate induces oxidative stress in endothelial cells. J Thromb Haemost 2007;5:1302–1308.
12 Lekawanvijit S, Adrahtas A, Kelly DJ, Kompa AR, Wang BH, Krum H: Does indoxyl sulfate, a uraemic toxin, have direct effects on cardiac fibroblasts and myocytes? Eur Heart J 2010 (in press).
13 Raff AC, Meyer TW, Hostetter TH: New insights into uremic toxicity. Curr Opin Nephrol Hypertens 2008;17:560–565.
14 Barreto FC, Barreto DV, Liabeuf S, Meert N, Glorieux G, Temmar M, Choukroun G, Vanholder R, Massy ZA: Serum indoxyl sulfate is associated with vascular disease and mortality in chronic kidney disease patients. Clin J Am Soc Nephrol 2009;4:1551–1558.
15 Jankowski J, van der Giet M, Jankowski V, Schmidt S, Hemeier M, Mahn B, Giebing G, Tolle M, Luftmann H, Schluter H, Zidek W, Tepel M: Increased plasma phenylacetic acid in patients with end-stage renal failure inhibits iNOS expression. J Clin Invest 2003;112:256–264.
16 Scholze A, Jankowski V, Henning L, Haass W, Wittstock A, Suvd-Erdene S, Zidek W, Tepel M, Jankowski J: Phenylacetic acid and arterial vascular properties in patients with chronic kidney disease stage 5 on hemodialysis therapy. Nephron Clin Pract 2007;107:c1–c6.
17 D'Hooge R, Van de Vijver G, Van Bogaert PP, Marescau B, Vanholder R, De Deyn PP: Involvement of voltage- and ligand-gated $Ca^{2+}$ channels in the neuroexcitatory and synergistic effects of putative uremic neurotoxins. Kidney Int 2003;63:1764–1775.
18 Kielstein JT, Impraim B, Simmel S, Bode-Boger SM, Tsikas D, Frolich JC, Hoeper MM, Haller H, Fliser D: Cardiovascular effects of systemic nitric oxide synthase inhibition with asymmetrical dimethylarginine in humans. Circulation 2004;109:172–177.
19 Schepers E, Glorieux G, Dhondt A, Leybaert L, Vanholder R: Role of symmetric dimethylarginine in vascular damage by increasing ROS via store-operated calcium influx in monocytes. Nephrol Dial Transplant 2009;24:1429–1435.
20 Vanholder R, Van Laecke S, Glorieux G: The middle-molecule hypothesis 30 years after: lost and rediscovered in the universe of uremic toxicity? J Nephrol 2008;21:146–160.
21 Thornalley PJ: Glycation free adduct accumulation in renal disease: the new AGE. Pediatr Nephrol 2005;20:1515–1522.
22 Glorieux G, Helling R, Henle T, Brunet P, Deppisch R, Lameire N, Vanholder R: In vitro evidence for immune activating effect of specific AGE structures retained in uremia. Kidney Int 2004;66:1873–1880.
23 Mori Y, Kosaki A, Kishimoto N, Kimura T, Iida K, Fukui M, Nakajima F, Nagahara M, Urakami M, Iwasaka T, Matsubara H: Increased plasma S100A12 (EN-RAGE) levels in hemodialysis patients with atherosclerosis. Am J Nephrol 2009;29:18–24.
24 Segal MS, Bihorac A, Koc M: Circulating endothelial cells: tea leaves for renal disease. Am J Physiol Renal Physiol 2002;283:F11–F19.
25 Jankowski V, Tolle M, Vanholder R, Schonfelder G, van der Giet M, Henning L, Schluter H, Paul M, Zidek W, Jankowski J: Uridine adenosine tetraphosphate: a novel endothelium-derived vasoconstrictive factor. Nat Med 2005;11:223–227.
26 Schepers E, Glorieux G, Jankowski V, Dhondt A, Jankowski J, Vanholder R: Dinucleoside polyphosphates: newly detected uraemic compounds with an impact on leucocyte oxidative burst. Nephrol Dial Transplant 2010 (in press).

27 Axelsson J, Bergsten A, Qureshi AR, Heimburger O, Barany P, Lonnqvist F, Lindholm B, Nordfors L, Alvestrand A, Stenvinkel P: Elevated resistin levels in chronic kidney disease are associated with decreased glomerular filtration rate and inflammation, but not with insulin resistance. Kidney Int 2006;69:596–604.

28 Hu WL, Qian SB, Li JJ: Decreased C-reactive protein-induced resistin production in human monocytes by simvastatin. Cytokine 2007;40:201–206.

29 Lesaffer G, De Smet R, Lameire N, Dhondt A, Duym P, Vanholder R: Intradialytic removal of protein-bound uraemic toxins: role of solute characteristics and of dialyser membrane. Nephrol Dial Transplant 2000;15:50–57.

30 Meert N, Eloot S, Waterloos MA, Van Landschoot M, Dhondt A, Glorieux G, Ledebo I, Vanholder R: Effective removal of protein-bound uraemic solutes by different convective strategies: a prospective trial. Nephrol Dial Transplant 2009;24:562–570.

31 Krieter DH, Hackl A, Rodriguez A, Chenine L, Moragues HL, Lemke HD, Wanner C, Canaud B: Protein-bound uraemic toxin removal in haemodialysis and post-dilution haemodiafiltration. Nephrol Dial Transplant 2010;25:212–218.

32 Vanholder R, Meert N, Van Biesen W, Meyer T, Hostetter T, Dhondt A, Eloot S: Why do patients on peritoneal dialysis have low blood levels of protein-bound solutes? Nat Clin Pract Nephrol 2009;5:130–131.

33 Meijers BK, De Preter V, Verbeke K, Vanrenterghem Y, Evenepoel P: *p*-Cresyl sulfate serum concentrations in haemodialysis patients are reduced by the prebiotic oligofructose-enriched inulin. Nephrol Dial Transplant 2010;25:219–224.

34 Lornoy W, Becaus I, Billiouw JM, Sierens L, Van Malderen P, D'Haenens P: On-line haemodiafiltration. Remarkable removal of $\beta_2$-microglobulin. Long-term clinical observations. Nephrol Dial Transplant 2000;15(suppl 1):49–54.

35 Eloot S, Van Biesen W, Dhondt A, Van de WH, Glorieux G, Verdonck P, Vanholder R: Impact of hemodialysis duration on the removal of uremic retention solutes. Kidney Int 2008;73:765–770.

36 Schulman G, Agarwal R, Acharya M, Berl T, Blumenthal S, Kopyt N: A multicenter, randomized, double-blind, placebo-controlled, dose-ranging study of AST-120 (Kremezin®) in patients with moderate to severe CKD. Am J Kidney Dis 2006;47:565–577.

37 Ueda H, Shibahara N, Takagi S, Inoue T, Katsuoka Y: AST-120 treatment in pre-dialysis period affects the prognosis in patients on hemodialysis. Ren Fail 2008;30:856–860.

38 Locatelli F, Martin-Malo A, Hannedouche T, Loureiro A, Papadimitriou M, Wizemann V, Jacobson SH, Czekalski S, Ronco C, Vanholder R: Effect of membrane permeability on survival of hemodialysis patients. J Am Soc Nephrol 2009;20:645–654.

39 Penne EL, Blankestijn PJ, Bots ML, van den Dorpel MA, Grooteman MP, Nube MJ, van der Tweel I, ter Wee PM: Effect of increased convective clearance by on-line hemodiafiltration on all cause and cardiovascular mortality in chronic hemodialysis patients – the Dutch CONvective TRAnsport STudy (CONTRAST): rationale and design of a randomised controlled trial [ISRCTN38365125]. Curr Control Trials Cardiovasc Med 2005;6:8.

40 Cheung AK, Greene T, Leypoldt JK, Yan G, Allon M, Delmez J, Levey AS, Levin NW, Rocco MV, Schulman G, Eknoyan G: Association between serum $\beta_2$-microglobulin level and infectious mortality in hemodialysis patients. Clin J Am Soc Nephrol 2008;3:69–77.



Griet Glorieux
Nephrology Section, 0K12IA, University Hospital
De Pintelaan, 185, BE–9000 Gent (Belgium)
Tel. +32 9 3324511, Fax +32 9 3324599, E-Mail griet.glorieux@UGent.be

Kawanishi H, Yamashita AC (eds): Hemodiafiltration – A New Era.
Contrib Nephrol. Basel, Karger, 2011, vol 168, pp 129–133

# Beta-2-Microglobulin as a Uremic Toxin: the Japanese Experience

Akira Fujimori

Blood Purification and Kidney Center, Konan Hospital, Kobe, Japan

**Abstract**

Gejyo and coworkers identified $\beta_2$-microglobulin ($\beta_2$-MG) as the major constitutional protein of dialysis-related amyloidosis (DRA) a quarter of a century ago. Since then, $\beta_2$-MG has been the most extensively studied low molecular weight protein in end-stage renal disease. The onset of DRA may be prevented by the use of high-flux dialysis membranes, especially when high-volume hemodiafiltration is used in the treatment of uremic patients. Adsorption therapy is another choice to improve the removal of $\beta_2$-MG. There seems to be a relative risk reduction in mortality when patients are treated with dialysis membranes that have a higher clearance of $\beta_2$-MG. 

## $\beta_2$-Microglobulin and Dialysis-Related Amyloidosis

$\beta_2$-Microglobulin ($\beta_2$-MG) is a polypeptide with a molecular weight of 11,800 daltons. Gejyo et al. [1, 2] first identified $\beta_2$-MG as the constitutive protein of dialysis-related amyloidosis (DRA). DRA is characterized by peripheral joint osteoarthropathy manifested by joint stiffness, pain, and swelling. Unlike other types of amyloidosis, $\beta_2$-MG amyloid is confined largely to osteoarticular sites. However, amyloid deposition is found in the internal organs like stomach and heart, and in some cases results in gastrointestinal and cardiac disorders. Clinical manifestations almost never appear before 5 years of dialysis therapy. Incidence correlates with increased age of the individual and elapsed time on dialysis.

$\beta_2$-MG is mainly produced by lymphocytes but all nuclear cells generate the substance. When urinary clearance of $\beta_2$-MG is impaired, $\beta_2$-MG starts to accumulate in the body. The essential factor of DRA is thought to be long-term exposure to systemic accumulation of $\beta_2$-MG. However, serum concentrations of native $\beta_2$-MG were found not to correlate with the risk of development of

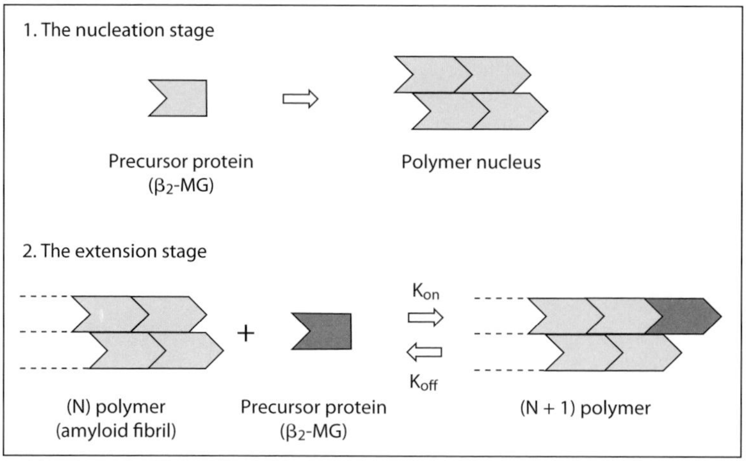


**Fig. 1.** Polymer nucleus-dependent polymerization model. The model for amyloid fibril formation is comprised of two processes: (1) the nucleation stage covers the polymer nucleus formation process from precursor proteins such as $\beta_2$-MG, and (2) the extension stage, in which the fibrils elongation process takes place, following the tenets of the first order kinetic model.

DRA [2], but rather the isoforms, glycated $\beta_2$-MG or polymers of $\beta_2$-MG in tissue were found to be amyloidogenic [3, 4]. Naiki et al. [5] developed a model in which an in vitro reaction of amyloid fibril formation was possible. They called it the polymer nucleus-dependent polymerization model (fig. 1). This model is comprised of two processes, the nucleation stage, which covers the polymer nucleus formation process from precursor protein, and the extension stage, in which the elongation process of the fibrils takes place. In the latter process, the precursor protein molecules bind one after another, resulting in elongation of the fibrils.

## Therapeutic Approaches

Although fundamental treatment for DRA has not been established, elimination of $\beta_2$-MG accumulation is thought to be effective to prevent DRA. Here, the influence of high-flux dialysis, hemodiafiltration (HDF), and hemoadsorption on the removal of $\beta_2$-MG is reviewed.

### *High-Flux Dialysis*

Today, high-flux (high-performance) dialyzers are widely used and accumulating evidence indicates that high-flux membranes are superior to cuprophane (or unmodified cellulose membranes) in removing $\beta_2$-MG. This can be achieved by direct flux across the membrane, adsorption to the membrane, or a combination of both.

The Niigata Research Program [6] revealed that in patients previously dialyzed with cellulosic membranes, serum $\beta_2$-MG concentrations fell from around 40 mg/l to around 30 mg/l after switching to PMMA membranes (Toray Industries, Japan), which was associated with reduction of joint pain scores. In a group of patients exclusively treated with PMMA, joint pain scores were kept at a low level and onset of DRA was not observed.

To study the impact of the dialysis membranes on surgery for carpal tunnel syndrome (CTS) as well as mortality, a multivariate Cox regression analysis with time-dependent covariates was conducted on 819 patients from March 1968 to November 1994 at a single center [7]. 248 of the patients were either switched from the conventional (cuprophane) to high-flux dialysis or treated only with high-flux membranes. Of the 819 patients at the beginning of the study, 51 underwent CTS surgery and 206 died. The relative risk of CTS surgery was reduced to 0.503 ($p<0.05$) and mortality to 0.613 ($p<0.05$) by dialysis on high-flux membranes, compared with the conventional membranes. Serial measurements of $\beta_2$-MG were persistently and significantly lower in patients on high-flux dialysis. Thus, high-flux dialysis substantially improved morbidity and mortality through elimination of $\beta_2$-MG and other low molecular weight proteins.

*Hemodiafiltration*

HDF is the process in which standard high-flux membrane efficiency is improved by using a high degree of ultrafiltration to use the process of convection in removing $\beta_2$-MG. According to the Japanese Society for Dialysis Therapy Statistical Survey, the relative risk of the onset of DRA associated with the high-flux dialysis was 0.424, offline HDF was 0.104, online HDF was 0.039, push/pull HDF was 0.009, and adsorption column combined with hemodialysis was 0.039 when the deterioration risk of DRA in low-flux dialysis was the reference [8]. In HDF, convection is combined with diffusion, and as a consequence, maximal clearance over a large molecular weight spectrum is achieved. Because of the high ultrafiltration, large quantities of substitution fluid are required to replace the volumes lost by the patient. Since the use of large volume of bottled (or bagged) substitution fluid is cost-consuming, online HDF, where purified dialysate is used, has drawn attention. Unlike European countries, where individual preparation system is used, Kim [9] made every effort to establish the online system with centrally delivered dialysate solution. The central dialysate delivery system (CDDS) requires three consecutive endotoxin (ET) removal filters to keep the infusion solution sterile and ET-free. Sato and Koga [10] reported the efficacy of online HDF operated on CDDS. Low molecular weight proteins ($\beta_2$-MG, prolactin, $\alpha_1$-microglobulin, and $\alpha_1$-acid glycoprotein) were more effectively removed in this online HDF than hemodialysis using the same dialyzers. Removal of low molecular weight protein was enhanced as the molecular weight increased. They also reported the recovery from joint pain and restricted joint motion.

*Hemoadsorption*

Gejyo et al. [11] using the Lixelle-300 device (Kaneka Corp., Osaka, Japan) (a cellulose-beaded sorbent with ligands covalently binding $\beta_2$-MG) combined with dialysis removed >200–300 mg of $\beta_2$-MG per session. The same group subsequently reported improvement in clinical symptoms and prevention of additional bone cysts [12]. In another study, ET removal was shown in vitro [13]. It was also shown that the use of the hemoadsorption device is associated with reductions in IL-1β, IL-1-receptor-α, IL-6, 1L-8, and TNF-α of 31.4, 39.3, 36.4, 76.2, and 71.6%, respectively [14]. Lysozyme (5%) and retinol-binding protein, markers of small molecular weight proteins, are also reduced in concentration. Increases in blood pressure and recovery from shock have also been reported. The same device is capable of removing digoxin [15]. Hypotension was the most frequent adverse event observed. A smaller device has been associated with less hypotension [16]. In one patient, using the Lixelle adsorption column together with high-flux membrane, $\beta_2$-MG was maintained at under 20 mg/dl; within 6 months, DRA symptoms in the right hand of a patient, refractory to other DRA therapy, had completely disappeared and the motor nerve latency almost normalized [17].

## Conclusion

$\beta_2$-MG is major constitutional protein of DRA. Aggressive removal of $\beta_2$-MG by HFD, HDF, and adsorption column leads to reduction of the risk of DRA and, possibly, to improvement of patient morbidity and mortality.

## References


1 Gejyo F, Yamada T, Odani S, Nakagawa Y, Arakawa M, Kunitomo T, Kataoka H, Suzuki M, Hirasawa Y, Shirahama T, et al: A new form of amyloid protein associated with chronic hemodialysis was identified as $\beta_2$-microglobulin. Biochem Biophys Res Commun 1985;129:701–706.

2 Gejyo F, Homma N, Suzuki Y, Arakawa M: Serum levels of $\beta_2$-microglobulin as a new form of amyloid protein in patients undergoing long-term hemodialysis. N Engl J Med 1986;314:585–586.

3 Miyata T, Inagi R, Wada Y, Ueda Y, Iida Y, Takahashi M, Taniguchi N, Maeda K: Glycation of human $\beta_2$-microglobulin in patients with hemodialysis-associated amyloidosis: identification of the glycated sites. Biochemistry 1994;33:12215–12221.

4 Gorevic PD, Munoz PC, Casey TT, DiRaimondo CR, Stone WJ, Prelli FC, Rodrigues MM, Poulik MD, Frangione B: Polymerization of intact $\beta_2$-microglobulin in tissue causes amyloidosis in patients on chronic hemodialysis. Proc Natl Acad Sci USA 1986;83:7908–7912.

5 Naiki H, Higuchi K, Nakakuki K, Takeda T: Kinetic analysis of amyloid fibril polymerization in vitro. Lab Invest 1991;65:104–110.
6 Aoike I, Gejyo F, Arakawa M: Learning from the Japanese Registry: how will we prevent long-term complications? Niigata Research Programme for $\beta_2$-Microglobulin Removal Membrane. Nephrol Dial Transplant 1995;10(suppl 7):7–15.
7 Koda Y, Nishi S, Miyazaki S, Haginoshita S, Sakurabayashi T, Suzuki M, Sakai S, Yuasa Y, Hirasawa Y, Nishi T: Switch from conventional to high-flux membrane reduces the risk of carpal tunnel syndrome and mortality of hemodialysis patients. Kidney Int 1997;52:1096–1101.
8 Nakai S, Iseki K, Tabei K, Kubo K, Masakane I, Fushimi K, Kikuchi K, Shinzato T, Sanaka T, Akiba T: Outcomes of hemodiafiltration based on Japanese dialysis patient registry. Am J Kidney Dis 2001;38:S212–S216.
9 Kim ST: Characteristics of protein removal in hemodiafiltration. Contrib Nephrol. Basel, Karger, 1994, vol 108, pp 23–37.
10 Sato T, Koga N: Centralized on-line hemodiafiltration system utilizing purified dialysate as substitution fluid. Artif Organs 1998;22:285–290.
11 Gejyo F, Homma N, Hasegawa S, Arakawa M: A new therapeutic approach to dialysis amyloidosis: intensive removal of $\beta_2$-microglobulin with adsorbent column. Artif Organs 1993;17:240–243.
12 Gejyo F, Kawaguchi Y, Hara S, Nakazawa R, Azuma N, Ogawa H, Koda Y, Suzuki M, Kaneda H, Kishimoto H, Oda M, Ei K, Miyazaki R, Maruyama H, Arakawa M, Hara M: Arresting dialysis-related amyloidosis: a prospective multicenter controlled trial of direct hemoperfusion with a $\beta_2$-microglobulin adsorption column. Artif Organs 2004;28:371–380.
13 Tsuchida K, Takemoto Y, Sugimura K, Yoshimura R, Yamamoto K, Nakatani T: Adsorption of endotoxin by $\beta_2$-microglobulin adsorbent column (Lixelle): the new approach for endotoxinemia. Ther Apher 2002;6:116–118.
14 Tsuchida K, Takemoto Y, Sugimura K, Yoshimura R, Nakatani T: Direct hemoperfusion by using Lixelle column for the treatment of systemic inflammatory response syndrome. Int J Mol Med 2002;10:485–488.
15 Kaneko T, Kudo M, Okumura T, Kasiwagi T, Turuoka S, Simizu M, Iino Y, Katayama Y: Successful treatment of digoxin intoxication by haemoperfusion with specific columns for $\beta_2$-microgloblin adsorption (Lixelle) in a maintenance haemodialysis patient. Nephrol Dial Transplant 2001;16:195–196.
16 Hiyama E, Hyodo T, Kondo M, Otsuka K, Honma T, Taira T, Yoshida K, Uchida T, Endo T, Sakai T, Baba S, Hidai H: Performance of the newer type (Lixelle type S-15) on direct hemoperfusion $\beta_2$-microglobulin adsorption column for dialysis-related amyloidosis. Nephron 2002;92:501–502.
17 Shiota E, Fujinaga M: Remission of a recurrent carpal tunnel syndrome by a new device of the hemodialysis method in a long-term hemodialysis patient. Clin Nephrol 2000;53:230–234.



Akira Fujimori, MD
Blood Purification and Kidney Center, Konan Hospital
1-5-16 Kamokogahara, Higashinada-ku
Kobe 658-0064 (Japan)
E-Mail louie@kcc.zaq.ne.jp

Kawanishi H, Yamashita AC (eds): Hemodiafiltration – A New Era.
Contrib Nephrol. Basel, Karger, 2011, vol 168, pp 134–138

# Markers and Possible Uremic Toxins: Japanese Experiences

Eriko Kinugasa

Department of Internal Medicine, Showa University Northern Yokohama Hospital, Yokohama, Japan

## Abstract

Oxidative stress and resultant accumulation of advanced glycation end products (AGEs) are closely related to the development of cardiovascular disease, which is the major cause of death among end-stage renal disease patients. Several markers of oxidative stress, such as malondialdehyde, oxidized low-density lipoprotein, AGEs and 8-hydroxydeoxyguanosine, are significantly elevated in circulating blood and/or tissue levels. Vitamin E is one of the scavengers opposed to oxidative stress and has been bonded to the dialyzer membrane surface to suppress oxidative stress related to hemodialysis itself. Vitamin E-coated dialyzers are widely used in Japan and several favorable clinical effects have been reported. Improved biocompatibility leads to decreased activation of circulating blood cells and these are related to reduced doses of heparin, improvement of anemia, and dose reduction in erythropoiesis-stimulating agents. Improvement of the cytokine network and immunological system is also suggested. It is expected that regression of atherosclerosis and slowed vascular calcification might occur parallel with reduction of oxidative stress by vitamin E-coated dialyzer. An improvement of endothelial function and dialysis hypotension during dialysis has also been reported. In small studies in Japan, improvement of nutritional state, insulin resistance and quality of life have been suggested. Although a larger scale control study will be needed, hemodialysis with vitamin E-coated membrane might become another powerful treatment modality other than hemodiafiltration.


It has been reported that the population of dialysis patients in Japan at the end of 2008 was 283,421, and the number of dialysis patients per million people was about 2,220 [1]. The dialysis patient population is increasing every year, although about 27,000 patients die annually. The main cause of death in these patients is cardiovascular disease (CVD), which accounts for about 35% of all causes of death in Japan. It is well known that the risk for CVD in end-stage renal disease (ESRD) patients is substantially higher than that in the general population. Some of the traditional cardiovascular risk factors are applicable to ESRD patients and non-traditional risk factors, such as oxidative stress and advanced glycation end products (AGEs), are also associated with the prevalence of CVD and the development of long-term complications of ESRD such as dialysis-related amyloidosis (dialysis-related amyloidosis and $\beta_2$-microglobulin are reviewed in the following chapter).

Although hemodiafiltration (HDF) may achieve a better reduction in AGE levels compared with conventional hemodialysis treatment, the incidence of HDF in Japan is only 7–8%. Therefore, the effects of hemodialysis with vitamin E-coated membrane on oxidative stress and AGEs are briefly reviewed.

## Oxidative Stress and AGEs in ESRD

Oxidative stress is defined as a perturbation in the pro- and antioxidant balance. In the presence of oxidative stress, oxidation of carbohydrates and lipids may lead to the formation of reactive carbonyl compounds and advanced glycosidation and lipoxidation end products. Formation of AGEs is initiated by the non-enzymatic reaction between glucose and proteins. In this reaction, a labile Schiff's base is produced and followed by its rearrangement into the Amadori compound, finally into a wide range of AGEs, such as carboxymethyllysine, pyrraline, pentosidine, imidazolone, glyoxal dimer and methylglyoxal dimer. AGEs accumulate in accordance with the progression of chronic kidney disease stage. A marked elevation of serum AGEs is noted in ESRD, but with no difference between patients with and without diabetes mellitus, indicating that renal excretion has an important role in AGE metabolism.

Although chronic kidney disease per se is a pro-oxidant state, extracorporeal circulation with less biocompatible membrane may accelerate the oxidative state. There are several papers regarding the relationship between atherosclerosis and oxidative stress and/or AGE accumulation. Increased AGE levels are associated with extensive coronary artery calcification in ESRD patients [2], furthermore, AGE levels increased in concert with carotid artery intima-media thickness in patients starting hemodialysis treatment [3].

AGEs accumulate in the extracellular matrix, such as protein-protein cross-linking, which may induce arterial or cardiac stiffness. Furthermore, lipoprotein undergoes glycation and AGE modification of lipoprotein may increase vascular deposition of low-density lipoprotein (LDL), which induces vascular inflammation and the development of atherosclerosis. Inflammation is enhanced by the interaction between AGEs and AGE-specific receptor (RAGE). RAGE has been identified on various cells, such as monocytes, mesangial cells and endothelial cells. AGEs induce the production of interleukin-1, insulin-like growth factor-1, and tumor necrosis factor-α by binding RAGE. AGEs accumulate within endothelial cells via RAGE and cause endothelial dysfunction.

AGE-modified $\beta_2$-microglobulin interacts with monocytes, then mediates monocyte chemotaxis and induces production of proinflammatory cytokines [4]. AGEs are also suspected as being the cause of peritoneal sclerosis in peritoneal dialysis patients [5].

## Vitamin E-Coated Dialysis Membrane

Vitamin E (α-tocopherol) is a powerful scavenger that protects plasma molecules and cell membranes from oxidative damage. Vitamin E-coated dialysis membrane has been developed in Japan (Asahi Kasei Kuraray Medical Co. Ltd), and many favorable clinical effects have been reported. Originally, vitamin E was bonded to regenerated cellulosic membrane, but now vitamin E-coated polysulfone dialyzer is available.

## Clinical Effects of Vitamin E-Coated Dialyzer

Firstly, better biocompatibility has been observed with vitamin E-coated dialysis membrane, such as reduced platelet activation, decreases in the frequency of dialyzer clotting and reduction of heparin dose. Decreased leukocyte activation and the release of interleukin-6 from stimulated monocytes during hemodialysis have also been noted [6–8]. Improvement of the cytokine network and immunological reaction was also suggested in an in vitro peripheral blood mononuclear cell study [9]. In some patients with severe eosinophilia, dialysis with vitamin-E coated membrane resulted in a significant improvement of eosinophilia [10]. As an antioxidative effect, serum levels of malondialdehyde, AGEs and 8-hydroxydeoxyguanosine significantly decreased 6 months after changing dialysis membrane from polysulfone to vitamin E-coated cellulosic membrane [11]. Improvement of anemia and reduced doses of erythropoiesis-stimulating agents have also noted using vitamin E-coated dialyzer, probably due to antioxidative effects, lessened erythrocyte membrane damage and improvement of erythrocyte survival [10, 11].

Surprisingly, regression of atherosclerosis was suggested by a randomized prospective control study lasting 1 year [11]. It was reported that decreases in intima-media thickness were noted in patients using vitamin E-coated cellulosic membrane with simultaneous improvement of the rheological changes in circulating erythrocytes and blood viscosity. There is another report regarding the antiatherosclerotic effects of vitamin E-coated membrane [12]. Concurrent therapy with LDL apheresis and hemodialysis using vitamin E-coated dialyzer resulted in the improvement of intima-media thickness, pulse wave velocity, serum level of interleukin-6 and C-reactive protein among ESRD patients suffering from peripheral artery disease, compared to the treatment with LDL apheresis and usual dialysis membrane. Similarly, an improvement of the superficial skin pressure and ankle-brachial index was noted among patients with diabetic hemodialysis patients treated with vitamin E-coated dialyzer [13]. It might delay the development of aortic calcification with the treatment of vitamin E-coated dialyzer for a 2-year observation period [14].

The effects on improvement of endothelial dysfunction by vitamin E-coated membrane are also reported in several studies [15]. During hemodialysis, the plasma nitric oxide level significantly increased at the end of dialysis with cellulosic membrane compared to the predialysis level, while it decreased at the end of dialysis with vitamin E-coated cellulosic membrane [7]. Another study demonstrates that dialysis-related endothelial dysfunction was improved with the use of a vitamin E-coated dialyzer [16]. Endothelial function was evaluated by flow-mediated dilation during reactive hyperemia using high-resolution ultrasound Doppler echocardiography before and after a single dialysis session. After hemodialysis by non-coated membrane, flow-mediated dilation was impaired with an increment of plasma levels of oxidized LDL. On the contrary, dialysis with vitamin E-coated membrane prevented dialysis-induced flow-mediated dilation. Although dialysis hypotension is frequently associated with diabetic patients, improvement of blood pressure fall was demonstrated by switching dialyzers, that is from a conventional one to a vitamin E-coated dialyzer. Other favorable clinical effects on nutritional state, insulin resistance and quality of life have been evaluated in small studies in Japan.

## Conclusion

Vitamin E-coated hemodialyzers work effectively from the point of antioxidative stress. Reduction of several makers, showing oxidative stress and carbonyl stress, is closely related to the improvement of cell function and indicator of atherosclerosis. Although a larger scale control study will be needed, hemodialysis with vitamin E-coated membrane might become another powerful treatment modality other than HDF. A multicenter randomized prospective control study (the VEESA study) is currently in progress in Japan.

## References


1 Patient Registration Committee, Japanese Society for Dialysis Therapy: An overview of regular dialysis treatment in Japan as of 31 December 2008. Jpn J Dial Ther 2010;43:1–35.

2 Taki K, Takayama F, Tsuruta Y, Niwa T: Oxidative stress, advanced glycation end product, and coronary artery calcification in hemodialysis patients. Kidney Int 2006;70;218–224.

3 Suilman ME, Stenvinkel P, Jogestrand T, Maruyama Y, Qureshi AR, Barany P, Heinburger O, Lindholm B: Plasma pentosidine and total homocysteine levels in relation to change in common carotid intima-media area in the first year of dialysis therapy. Clin Nephrol 2006;66:418–425.
4 Miyata T, Hori O, Zhang J, Yan SD, Ferran L, Iida Y, Schmidt AM: The receptor for advanced glycation end products (RAGE) is a central mediator of the interaction of AGE-$\beta_2$-microglobulin with human mononuclear phagocytes via an oxidant-sensitive pathway. Implication for the pathogenesis of dialysis-related amyloidosis. J Clin Invest 1996;98:1088–1094.
5 Nakamura S, Tachikawa T, Tobita K, Miyazaki S, Sakai S, Morita T, Hirasawa Y, Weigle B, Pischetsrieder, Niwa T: Role of advanced glycation end products and growth factors in peritoneal dialysis. Am J Kidney Dis 2003;41(suppl 1):S61–S67.
6 Girndt M, Lender S, Kaul H, Sester U, Sester M, Kohler H: Prospective crossover trial of the influence of vitamin E-coated dialyzer membranes on T-cell activation and cytokine inducer. Am J Kidney Dis 2000;35:95–104.
7 Libetta C, Zucch M, Gori E, Sepe V, Galli F, Meloni F, Milanesi F, Canton AD: Vitamin E-loaded dialyzer resets PBMC-operated cytokine network in dialysis patients. Kidney Int 2004;65:1473–1481.
8 Kojima K, Oda K, Homma H, Takahashi K, Kanda Y, Inokami T, Uchida S: Effect of vitamin E-bonded dialyzer on eosinophilia in haemodialysis. Nephrol Dial Transplant 2005;20:1932–1935.
9 Satoh M, Yamasaki Y, Nagake Y, Kasahara J, Hashimoto M, Nakanishi N, Makino H: Oxidative stress is reduced by the long-term use of vitamin E-coated dialysis filters. Kidney Int 2001;59:1943–1950.
10 Nakatan T, Takamoto Y, Tsuchida K: The effect of vitamin E-bonded dialyzer membrane on red blood cell survival in hemodialyzed patients. Artif Organs 2003;27:214–217.
11 Kobayashi S, Moriya H, Aso K, Ohtake T: Vitamin E-bonded hemodialyzer improves atherosclerosis associated with a rheological improvement of circulating red blood cells. Kidney Int 2003;63:1881–1887.
12 Nakamura T, Kawagoe Y, Matsuda T, Takahashi Y, Sekizuka K, Ebihara I, Koide H: Effects of LDL apheresis and vitamin E-modified membrane of carotid atherosclerosis in hemodialyzed patients with arteriosclerosis obliterans. Kidney Blood Press Res 2003;26:185–191.
13 Kida N, Kunimitsu M, Kaneda A, Shimatani K, Kiyota M, Wakikata T, Nagahara M, Takeda A, Shiota M, Okajima M: Effect of vitamin-E bonded hemodialyzer on improvement of skin perfusion pressure in hemodialytic patients with end-stage chronic renal failure. Vitamembrane 2009;32–36.
14 Mune M, Yukawa S, Kishino M, Otani H, Kimura K, Nishikawa O, Takahashi T, Kodama N, Saika Y, Yamada Y: Effect of vitamin E on lipid metabolism and atherosclerosis in ESRD patients. Kidney Int 1999:56(suppl 7):S126–S129.
15 Baragetti I, Furiani S, Vetteroretti S, Raselli S, Maggi FM, Galli F, Catapano AL, Buccianti G: Role of vitamin E-coated membrane in reducing advanced glycation end products in hemodialysis patients: a pilot study. Blood Purif 2006;24:369–376.
16 Miyazaki H, Matsuoka H, Itabe H, Usui M, Ueda S, Okuda S, Imaizumi T: Hemodialysis impairs endothelial function via oxidative stress: effects of vitamin E-coated dialyzer. Circulation 2000;101:1002–1006.

Eriko Kinugasa, MD
Department of Internal Medicine, Showa University Northern Yokohama Hospital
35-1 Chigasaki-Chuoh, Tsuzuki-ku, Yokohama 224-8503 (Japan)
E-Mail kinugasa@med.showa-u.ac.jp

Kawanishi H, Yamashita AC (eds): Hemodiafiltration – A New Era.
Contrib Nephrol. Basel, Karger, 2011, vol 168, pp 139–145

# Biocompatibility of the Dialysis Membrane

Yoshiaki Takemoto · Toshihidei Naganuma · Rikio Yoshimura

Department of Urology, Osaka City University, Graduate School of Medicine, Osaka, Japan

**Abstract**

Biocompatibility of dialysis membranes can be defined as the sum of specific interactions between blood and the dialysis membranes. In the early phase of hemodialysis therapy, acute side effects are the main issues for treatments of ESRD patients and biocompatibility of dialysis membranes are evaluated from aspects of acute reactions. Recently, chronic reactions that are not specifically acutely detrimental to the patients are focused for biocompatibility of dialysis membranes. These reactions include for example complement activation, contact pathway activation, platelet activation, monocyte activation and neutrophil activation during the hemodialysis treatments. In this paper, blood-membrane interactions will be emphasized for evaluating the biocompatibility of dialysis membranes.



Hemodialysis is a therapeutic procedure that is performed to approximate the physiological conditions of the blood by extracorporeal circulation. However, one problem that cannot be avoided while performing extracorporeal circulation is the contact of the blood with foreign materials, namely the dialysis membrane. When blood vessels are damaged and the blood comes in contact with matter other than the vascular endothelial cells, the humoral and cellular pathways mediate certain responses including blood-membrane interactions, which are defined by biocompatibility.

Early studies on biocompatibility in hemodialysis therapy have focused on acute reactions that are specifically detrimental to the patients. Over the years, however, various responses have been elucidated, and recent studies have focused on chronic responses that are not specifically acutely detrimental to the patients. Such blood-membrane interactions have been summarized as shown in figure 1, indicating an extremely intricate tangle of pathways [1].

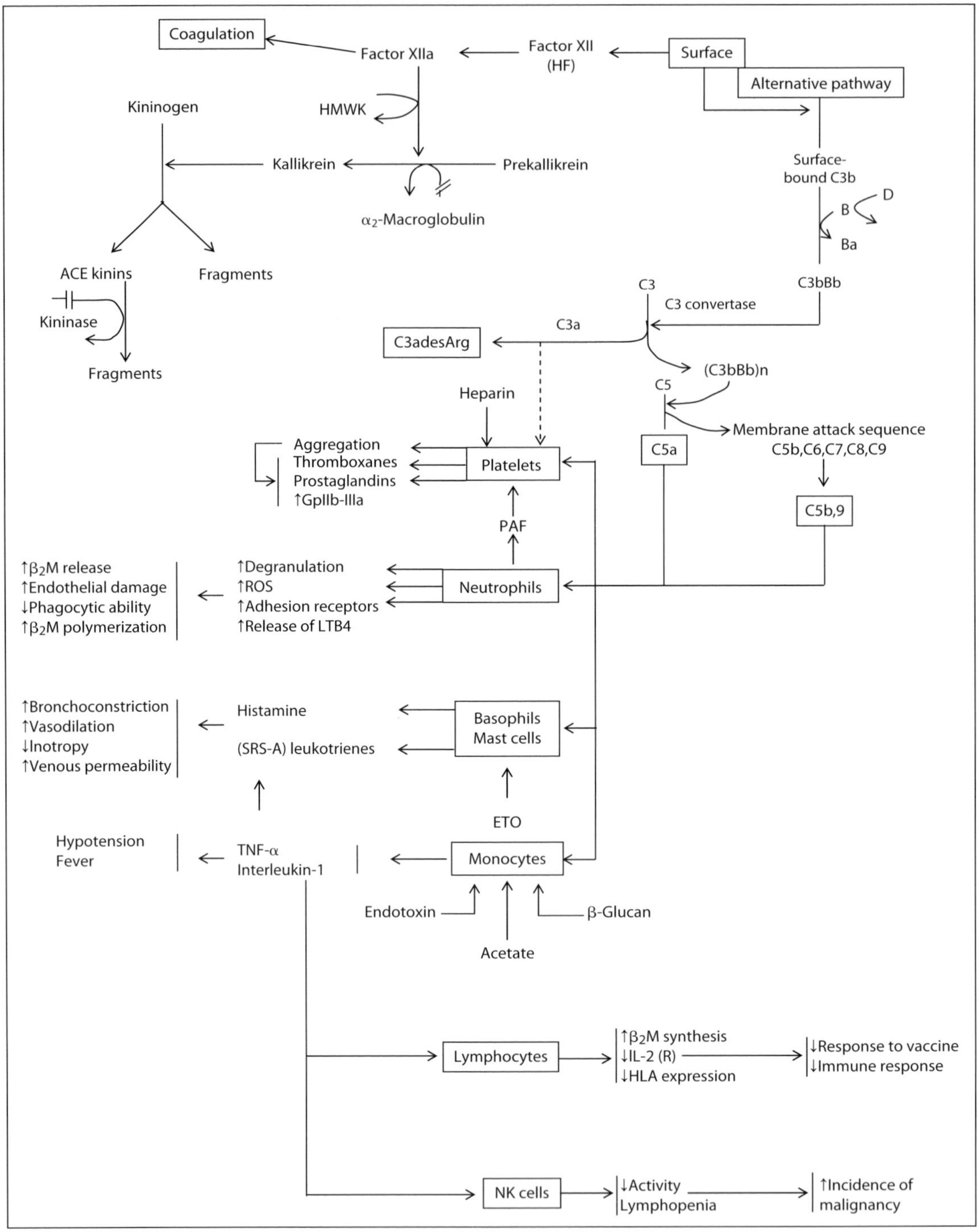


**Fig. 1.** Schematic diagram of multiple pathways involved in blood-membrane interactions [from 1].

## Complement Activation

Ever since transient neutropenia and hypoxemia which occur during dialysis with cellulosic membranes have been attributed to the activation of the alternative complement pathway by Craddock et al. [2] in 1997, complement activation has been extensively studied. Because the activation of complement is maximum at about 15 min following initiation of hemodialysis with cellulosic membranes, it has been used as a classic index of biocompatibility. As the mechanism of complement activation, free OH radicals present on the surfa ce of the cellulosic membranes bind with C3b in the blood, causing the activation of the alterative complement pathway. During this process, blood levels of C3a and C5a known as anaphylatoxins increase, and these substances have also been used as markers of biocompatibility. Because OH radicals that activate complement are not present in synthetic polymeric membranes and because some of these membranes can adsorb C3a and C5a, these markers have often been used as with the changes in neutrophil counts in comparing synthetic polymeric membranes with cellulosic membranes.

## Contact Pathway Activation

When the dialysis membrane comes in contact with blood, the intrinsic coagulation factor XII as well as the coagulation system are activated. At the same time, the kinin-kallikrein system is activated, and bradykinin is generated. If there is little interaction between the dialysis membrane and coagulation factor, the membrane can be considered highly biocompatible with superior antithrombogenicity. Bradykinin has attracted attention because it is a potent vasodilator and induces anaphylactic reactions through heightened vascular permeability, but it has not become a major problem, as it is usually rapidly degraded by a kinase. However, this kinase is the same as angiotensin-converting enzyme (ACE), and if the patient is taking an ACE inhibitor as an antihypertensive drug, the degradation of bradykinin may be delayed, causing low blood pressure, chest symptoms, respiratory problems accompanying mucous membrane edema and other symptoms of shock. In addition, because materials with a strong negative electrical charge can remarkably increase factor XII activation, when using the AN69 dialysis membrane with its strong negative charge or performing LDL apheresis using dextran sulfate column, enhanced bradykinin generation and slowed degradation can occur at the same time, increasing the risk of severe anaphylactic shock [3–5].

## Platelet Activation

Platelets are activated when they come in contact with the dialysis membrane, and their numbers are thought to decrease as they adhere to the membrane

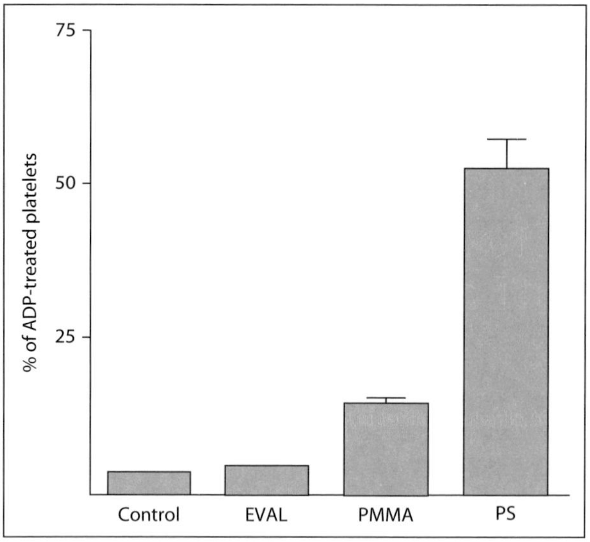


**Fig. 2.** Expression of P-selectin on the surface of platelets after incubation with hemodialysis membrane was measured by cell-based ELISA [from 8].

surface and aggregate. Because activated platelets release various factors, they have been regarded as favorable markers of biocompatibility. The serum level of PF4 which is released from the platelets has been reported to increase immediately after coming into contact with dialysis membranes having strong hydrophobic properties in an ex vivo experiment as shown in figure 2 [6]. Similarly, the levels thromboxane $B_2$ and BTG, which are also released by platelet activation, have been reported to increase in dialysis membranes with strong hydrophobic properties [7]. Recently, it has been reported that the expression of P-selectin on the platelet membrane caused by activated platelets coming into contact with the dialysis membrane can be used as an index of biocompatibility (fig. 3). This study also indicated that P-selectin expression is increased in dialysis membranes having strong platelet adherence [8].

## Monocyte Activation

In the interleukin hypothesis proposed by Henderson et al. [9] in 1983, monocytes activated by coming into contact with regenerated cellulosic membranes were found to produce and secrete IL-1, causing short-term complications such as fever and low blood pressure. Later, it was shown that inflammatory cytokines such as IL-6, IL-8 and tumor necrosis factor are also produced from monocytes, not only through contact with the dialysis membrane, but also by contaminants in the dialysate. Because endotoxins that are present in the contaminated dialysate

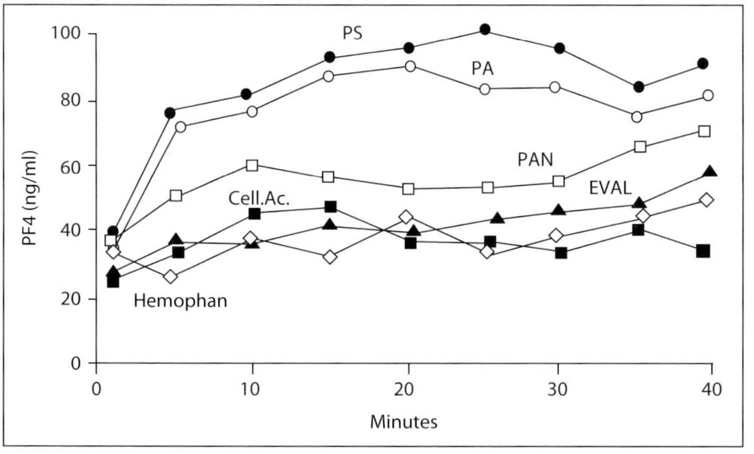


**Fig. 3.** Ex vivo model: release of PF4 from platelets after blood-membrane interaction with different dialyzer membranes [from 6].

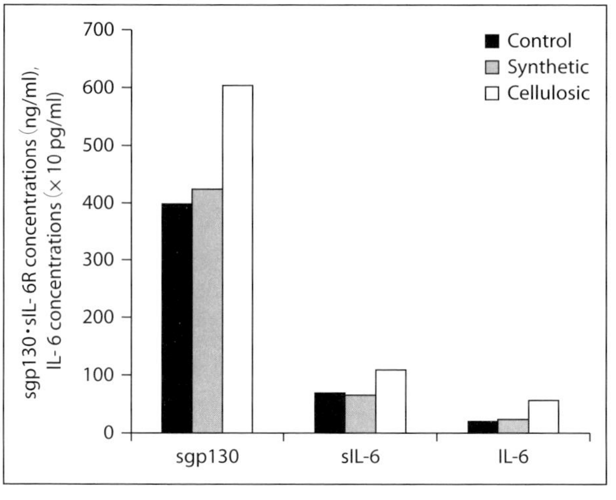


**Fig. 4.** Plasma circulating levels of sgp130, sIL-6R, IL-6 in 10 healthy controls patients, 11 patients who had ESRD and were undergoing dialysis treatment with cellulosic membranes, and 10 ESRD patients who were treated with synthetic membranes [from 10].

can highly produce and stimulate cytokines, the purity of the dialysate has become as important as the material of the membrane when evaluating biocompatibility in hemodialysis. Many studies are currently being made and it has recently been reported that the blood concentrations of IL-6, which is an inflammatory cytokine as well as its soluble receptors sIL-6R and sgp130, are significantly higher in patients using cellulosic membranes compared to normal controls and patients using polymeric membranes (PS, EVAL), which suggests that these substances may also be used as markers of biocompatibility (fig. 4) [10].

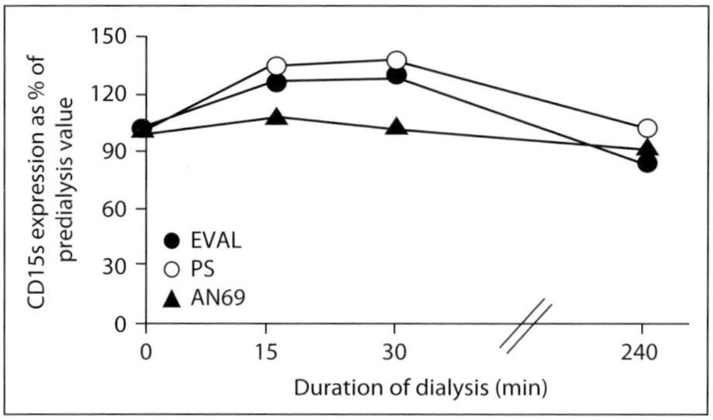


**Fig. 5.** Changes in CD15s expression on neutrophil surface during hemodialysis using ethylene vinyl alcohol (EVAL), polysulfone (PSF) and polyacrylonitrile co-sodium methalyl sulfonate (AN69) membranes. $p < 0.05$ EVAL vs. AN69 [from 11].

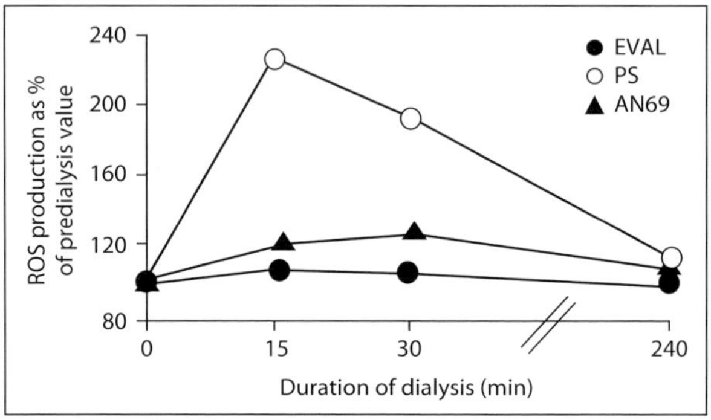


**Fig. 6.** ROS (hydrogen peroxide) production by neutrophil population during hemodialysis using ethylene vinyl alcohol (EVAL), polysulfone (PSF) and polyacrylonitrile co-sodium methalyl sulfonate (AN69) membranes. $p < 0.001$ PSF vs. EVAL and AN69 $p < 0.05$ EVAL vs. AN69 [from 11].

## Neutrophil Activation

Neutrophil activation by the dialysis membrane has been evaluated by the expression of adhesion molecules on the neutrophil membrane. In that report, the expression rate of CD15s, which is an adhesion molecule on leukocytes, was measured during dialysis using different dialysis membranes, and as shown in figure 5, the rate was significantly lower in the AN69 membrane compared to the EVAL membrane, indicating superior biocompatibility [11]. In the same report, the function of neutrophils was studied by the production of reactive oxygen species (ROS). It has also been reported that when activated platelets adhere to neutrophils, the neutrophils are activated, increasing the production of ROS, and ROS production by neutrophils is the mildest using the EVAL membrane which is considered to have superior biocompatibility against platelets (fig. 6).

## Conclusion

Early studies on the biocompatibility of dialysis membranes focused on direct reactions mainly in regenerated cellulosic membranes. With the advent of synthetic polymeric membranes, biocompatibility has been evaluated in comparison to that of regenerated cellulosic membranes. In the future, not only differences in biocompatibility of synthetic polymeric membranes, which are more biocompatible than regenerated cellulosic membranes, but also the biocompatibility of hemodialysis therapy as a system needs to be investigated.

## References


1 Hakim RM: Clinical implications of hemodialysis membrane biocompatibility. Kidney Int 1993;44:484–494.
2 Craddock PR, Hammerschmidt D, White JG, et al: Complement (C5a)-induced granulocyte aggregation in vitro. A possible mechanism of complement-mediated leukostasis and leucopenia. J Clin Invest 1977;60:260–264.
3 Tielemans C, Madhoun P, Lenaers M, et al: Anaphylactoid reactions during hemodialysis on AN69 membranes in patients receiving ACE inhibitors. Kidney Int 1990;38:982–984.
4 Verresen L, Fink E, Lemke HD, et al: Bradykinin is a mediator of anaphylactoid reactions during hemodialysis with AN69 membranes. Kidney Int 1994;45:1497–1503.
5 Olbricht CJ, Schaumann D, Fischer D: Anaphylactoid reaction, LDL apheresis with dextran sulfate and ACE inhibitors. Lancet 1992;340:908–909.
6 Von Sengbush G, Baurmeister U, Vienken J: Adaptability of cellulosic membranes to different biocompatibility parameters. Contrib Nephrol. Basel, Karger, 1987, vol 59, pp 126–133.
7 Horl WH, Riegel W, Steinhaur HB, Wanner C, Schollmeyer P, Scaefer RM, Heidland A: Plasma levels of main granulocyte components during hemodialysis. Contrib Nephrol. Basel, Karger, 1987, vol 59, pp 35–43.
8 Itoh S, Suzuki C, Tsuji T: Platelet activation through interaction with hemodialysis membranes induces neutrophils to produce reactive oxygen species. J Biomed Mater Res 2006;77A:294–303.
9 Henderson LW, Koch KM, Dinarello CA, et al: Hemodialysis hypotension: the interleukin-1 hypothesis. Blood Purif 1983;1:3–8.
10 Memoli B, Grandaliano G, Soccio M, Postiglione L, Guida B, Biesti V, Esposito P, Procino A, Marrone D, Michael A, Andreucci M, Schena FP, Pertosa G: In vitro modulation of soluble antagonistic IL-6 receptor synthesis and release in ESRD. J Am Soc Nephrol 2005;16:1099–1107.
11 Sirolli V, Ballone E, Diliberato L, Dimascio R, Cappelli P, Albertazzi A, Bonomini M: Leukocyte adhesion molecules and leukocyte-platelet interactions during hemodialysis: effects of different synthetic membranes. Int J Artif Organs 1999;22:536–542.



Yoshiaki Takemoto, MD
Department of Urology, Osaka City University, Graduate School of Medicine
1-5-7 Asahi-machi, Abeno-ku, Osaka 545-8586 (Japan)
Tel. +81 6 6645 2394, Fax +81 6 6633 9131, E-Mail ytakemoto@msic.med.osaka-cu.ac.jp

Kawanishi H, Yamashita AC (eds): Hemodiafiltration – A New Era.
Contrib Nephrol. Basel, Karger, 2011, vol 168, pp 146–152

# Choice of Dialyzers for HDF

Akihiro C. Yamashita[a] · Kenji Sakurai[b]

[a]Department of Human and Environmental Science, Shonan Institute of Technology, Fujisawa and [b]Hashimoto Clinic, Sagamihara, Japan


## Abstract

Commercial dialyzers were investigated both in vivo and in vitro for a better selection of dialyzers for hemodiafiltration (HDF) therapy. In in vivo online HDF, since a reduction rate of $\alpha_1$-microglobulin ($\alpha_1$-MG) was determined by the amount of albumin loss regardless of blood flow rate ($Q_B$), ultrafiltration rate ($Q_F$), and the performance of dialyzer, there is no preference for choice of dialyzers to remove $\alpha_1$-MG except for albumin sieving. It was clinically verified that albumin leakage mainly occurred in the first 60 min of treatment even in HD with a polysulfone dialyzer. Ultrafiltration may be more carefully started in order to reduce albumin loss. In an in vitro study, the sieving coefficient for albumin took a peak value at the beginning of the experiment in all polysulfone membrane dialyzers, which corresponded well with the clinical results stated above. Although polymethylmethacrylate membrane dialyzers allowed to penetrate only a limited amount of albumin, they could adsorb a bigger amount of albumin than that penetrated. If dialyzers are used under high $Q_B$, post-dilution may be preferred because pre-dilution should increase the apparent blood flow rate as well as blood pressure at the inlet. If dialyzers are used under relatively low $Q_B$, either one of two dilution methods can be applied; however, with pre-dilution it may be easier to control the loss of albumin than with the post-dilution technique. In other words, it would be recommended to employ less albumin-leakage dialyzers when a post-dilution HDF is performed with a large amount of fluid exchange. 

The concept of removing so-called middle molecules from the blood of patients with end-stage renal disease has been widely accepted since the early 1970s [1]. The concept was later extended to larger solutes such as low molecular weight proteins including $\beta_2$-microglobulin ($\beta_2$-MG, MW 11,800), inflammatory cytokines or even greater ones [2]. For removing low molecular weight proteins, hemodiafiltration (HDF) may be considered a superior tool to conventional hemodialysis (HD) due to the larger amount of ultrafiltration or convective mass transfer across the membrane. Although many high-flux dialyzers

**Table 1.** A list of investigated dialyzers

| | Brand name | Membrane material | Investigation system | Modality | Flow rate [ml/min] | | | Manufacturer |
|---|---|---|---|---|---|---|---|---|
| | | | | | $Q_B$ | $Q_{DTot}$ | $Q_S$ | |
| 1 | TS-2.1UL | PS | in vivo | pre-dilution HDF | 240 | 500 | 208, 238 | Toray Medical Co., Tokyo, Japan |
| 2 | FDY-210GW | PEPA | in vivo | HD | 200 | 500 | – | Nikkiso Co., Tokyo, Japan |
| 3 | | PEPA | in vivo | pre-dilution HDF | 200, 240 | 500 | 208, 238 | |
| 4 | | PEPA | in vivo | post-dilution HDF | 200 | 500 | 42 | |
| 5 | FDY-250GW | PEPA | in vivo | HD | 200, 240 | 500 | – | |
| 6 | | PEPA | in vivo | pre-dilution HDF | 200, 240 | 500 | 167, 208, 250 | |
| 7 | APS-25SA | PS | in vivo | HD | 200 | 500 | – | Asahi Kasei-Kuraray Medical Co., Tokyo, Japan |
| 8 | | PS | in vivo | pre-dilution HDF | 200, 240 | 500 | 208 | |
| 9 | APS-21E | PS | in vivo | HD | 200 | 500 | – | |
| 10 | | PS | in vivo | pre-dilution HDF | 200 | 500 | 208 | |
| 11 | FX-S 140 | PS | in vivo | HD | 200, 250, 300 | 500 | – | Fresenius Medical Care Co., Bad Homburg, Germany |
| 12 | BG-1.6PQ | PMMA | in vitro | ultrafiltration | 200 | – | 10 | Toray Medical Co. |
| 13 | FLX-15GW | PEPA | in vitro | ultrafiltration | 200 | – | 10 | Nikkiso Co. |

$Q_B$ = Blood flow rate; $Q_{DTot}$ = total dialysis fluid flow rate; $Q_S$ = substitution fluid flow rate; PS = polysulfone; PEPA = polyester polymer alloy; PMMA = polymethylmethacrylate.

are commercially available, there are not many analyses on the choice of dialyzers best suited for a particular treatment, especially for HDF. We have investigated the diffusive and convective transport of several commercial dialyzers with a variety of performances in vivo as well as in vitro for the purpose of better selection of commercial models for HDF with a large amount of fluid exchange.

## Materials and Method

Commercial dialyzers were investigated both in vivo and in vitro. The dialyzers tested are listed in table 1.

*In vivo Observations.* HD, pre-dilution online HDF, or post-dilution online HDF were performed, and the loss of albumin was clinically evaluated in each treatment. The reduction rate of $\alpha_1$-microglobulin ($\alpha_1$-MG, MW 33,000), one of the largest target solutes that should be removed [3] by the treatment, was calculated. The blood flow rate ($Q_B$) ranged from 200 to 240 ml/min, the total dialysate flow rate ($Q_{DTot}$), a sum of intrinsic dialysis fluid flow that entered into the dialyzer and substitution fluid flow $Q_S$ that was 0 (HD), 45 (post-dilution HDF) or 215 ml/min (pre-dilution HDF), was fixed to 500 ml/min in all studies, and ultrafiltration rate ($Q_F$) was approximately 15 ml/min larger than $Q_S$. A study was also done for a commercial model in which albumin concentration in the outlet of dialysis fluid was measured frequently during the course of conventional HD varying $Q_B$ from 200 to 300 ml/min to identify when albumin leaked across the membrane.

*In vitro Observations.* A 2,000-ml aqueous test solution that included a solute of interest was prepared and was pumped into a dialyzer with adsorption characteristics at $Q_B$ = 200 ml/min and was returned to the same tank. Ultrafiltration was induced by another roller pump at $Q_F$ = 10 ml/min and was also returned to the tank, expecting to achieve a steady state after starting the experiment with a small time delay due to the dilution by preloaded phosphate buffer solution that controlled the pH at 7.40. Time courses of penetrated as well as adsorbed albumin were measured in order to clarify the mechanism of removal.

## Results and Discussion

*In vivo Observations.* Figure 1 shows the relationship between the $\alpha_1$-MG reduction rate and amount of albumin loss in various modalities of treatment including conventional HD, pre- or post-dilution online HDF with varying $Q_B$, $Q_S$ and with many different dialyzers in 1 patient. A high correlation between $\alpha_1$-MG reduction rate and albumin loss was found, although there was a twofold different molecular weight. One of the reasons why they were well correlated was that the Stokes radii of these two solutes (31.0 Å for $\alpha_1$-MG and 35.5 Å for albumin [4], respectively) do not change much. In other words, although removing such solutes larger than $\beta_2$-MG may be desired in recent clinical HDF therapy,

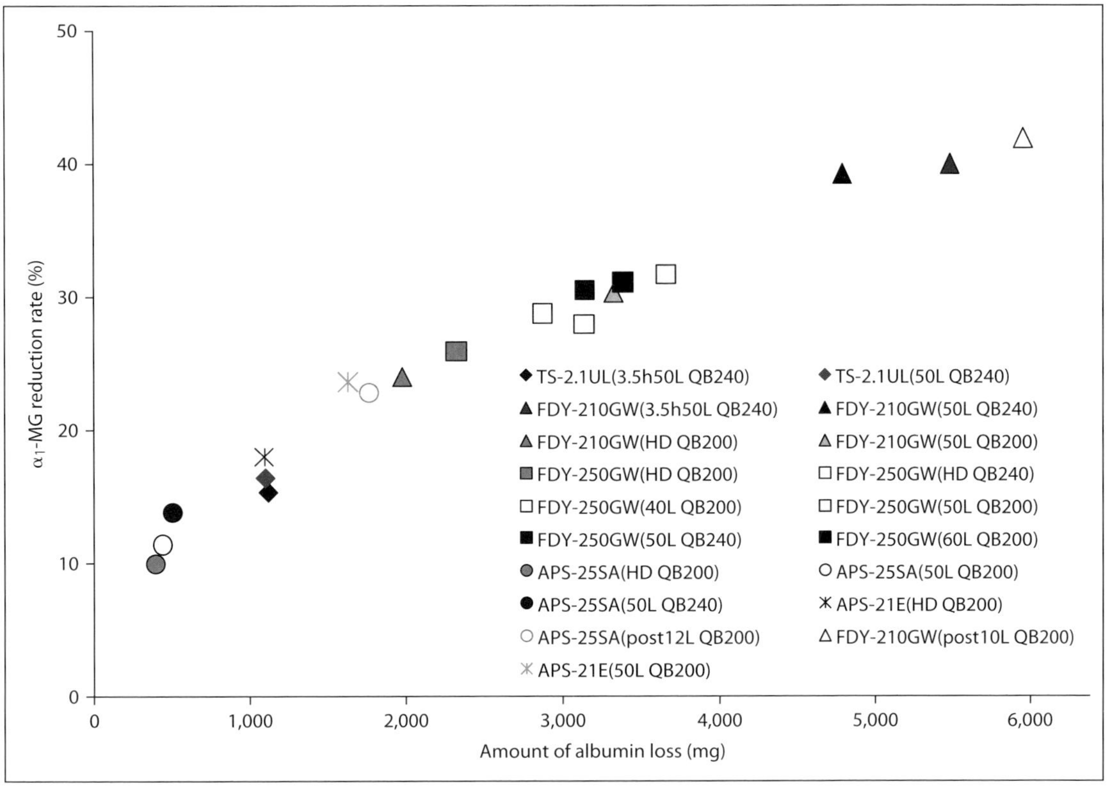


**Fig. 1.** Relationship between $\alpha_1$-MG reduction rate and amount of albumin loss. $Q_{Dtotal} = Q_{Dnet} + Q_S = 500$ ml/min. Volumes in parentheses are the amount of substitution fluid in pre-dilution HDF unless otherwise specified. 'post' indicates post-dilution HDF.

$\alpha_1$-MG may not be very well separated from albumin no matter which membrane is employed. In addition, if the reduction rate of 30% in $\alpha_1$-MG is desired, approximately 3 g of albumin loss may be counted no matter which dialyzer and/or which modality have been chosen. Therefore, it is the albumin loss that determines the choice of dialyzers in terms of removing $\alpha_1$-MG regardless of the modality of treatment.

A study was also done for the FX-S140 dialyzer (polysulfone membrane) in which albumin concentration in the outlet of dialysis fluid was measured, with a varying $Q_B$ from 200 to 300 ml/min (fig. 2). The albumin concentration in the dialysis fluid rapidly decreased from 100 to 20 μg/ml for the first 60 min and was kept almost constant thereafter. These results corresponded well with a previously published report [5]. Moreover, the higher the blood flow rate, the lower the concentration of albumin was found to be. This may be due to the fact that the higher the blood flow rate, the more albumin molecules enter into the

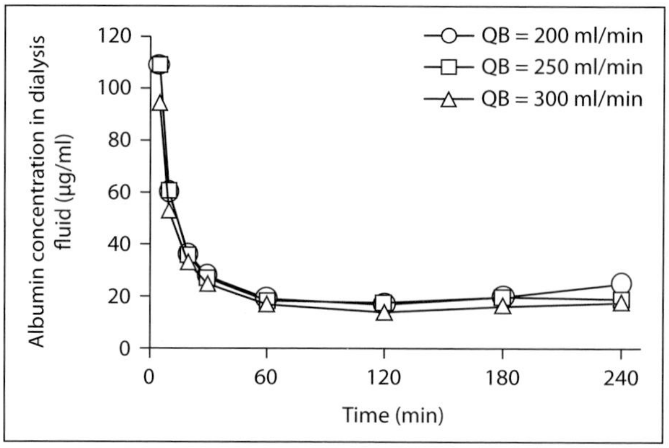


**Fig. 2.** Time course of albumin concentration in dialysis fluid at the outlet of the dialyzer.

dialyzer per unit time. A higher degree of fouling may have occurred, which lowered the albumin loss.

In the series of pre-dilution online HDF studies, $Q_B$ ranged between 200 and 240 ml/min. However, if $Q_B$ was chosen >300 ml/min, pre-dilution with improved removal of middle molecules ($Q_S$ >200 ml/min) may hardly be possible because a much higher pressure at the blood inlet may be expected due to a greater apparent $Q_B$ (>500 ml/min), as well as insufficient hydraulic permeability for performing pre-dilution HDF. Under such circumstances, there would be no choice available other than post-dilution HDF [6].

*In vitro Observations.* Time courses of *sc* for albumin in various dialyzers were measured in aqueous solution in vitro (data not shown). The *sc* took the maximum value immediately after starting the experiment in polysulfone dialyzers, which implied a large amount of initial albumin loss as reported clinically [5]. More attention should be paid to albumin leakage at the beginning of treatment when the membrane pores are still not covered by protein molecules. In order to avoid a large amount of albumin loss, use of blood dilution before ultrafiltration or pre-dilution may be suited although removal of most other solutes may be matched between pre- and post-dilution HDF treatments. In other words, if the membrane with relatively low *sc* for albumin is chosen, use of post-dilution may be preferred in order to remove more middle molecules.

Both PMMA and PEPA are known to have strong adsorption characteristics. Figure 3 compared the amount of penetrated and adsorbed albumin in the aqueous ultrafiltration experiment. Penetrated albumin in PMMA looked much smaller than that in PEPA, however PMMA adsorbed much more albumin than PEPA, and the adsorbed albumin loss could be sevenfold more than that found with permeation, whereas albumin loss due to permeation and adsorption was

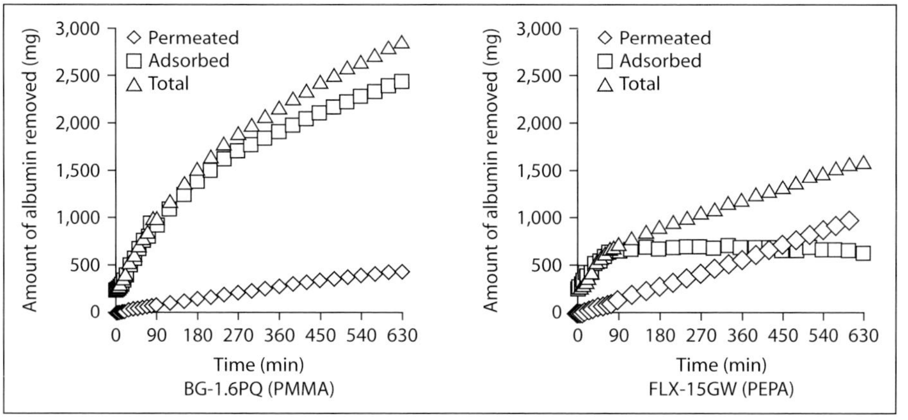


**Fig. 3.** Albumin loss by ultrafiltration (permeated) and by adsorption (adsorbed) in two dialyzers with adsorption characteristics.

comparable in PEPA. Albumin loss in PMMA membrane cannot be easily evaluated just by measuring the concentration of the ultrafiltrate.

## Conclusions

It is the albumin loss that determines the choice of dialyzers in terms of removing $\alpha_1$-MG, one of the largest target solutes to remove, regardless of the modality of the treatment. Under high $Q_B$ (>300 ml/min), post-dilution is preferred to pre-dilution. The dialyzer with a large surface area and relatively low sieving coefficient for albumin may be the first choice to avoid much albumin loss. Under relatively low $Q_B$ (<250 ml/min), both pre- and post-dilution can be clinically utilized. The dialyzer with a relatively low *sc* for albumin may be used in the post-dilution and that with relatively high *sc* for albumin may be selected in the pre-dilution.

## References


1 Babb AL, Popovich RP, Christopher TG, Scribner BH: The genesis of the square-meter hour hypothesis. Trans Am Soc Artif Intern Organs 1971;17:81–91.

2 Vanholder R, De Smet R, Glorieux G, Argiles A, Baurmeister U, Brunet P, Clark W, Cohen G, De Deyn PP, Deppisch R, Descamps-Latscha B, Henle T, Jorres A, Lemke HD, Massy ZA, Passlick-Deetjen J, Rodriguez M, Stegmayr B, Stenvinkel P, Tetta C, Wanner C, Zidek W: Review on uremic toxins: classification, concentration, and interindividual variability. Kidney Int 2003;63:1934–1943.

3 Bernier I, Dautigny A, Glatthaar BE, Lergier W, Jolles J, Gillessen D, Jolles P: Alpha-1-microglobulin from normal and pathological urines. Biochim Biophys Acta 1980;626:188–196.

4 Dawes WA: Quantitative Problems in Biochemistry. New York, Longman, 1980, pp 1–43.

5 Ahrenholz PG, Winker RE, Michelsen A, Lang DA, Bowey SK: Dialysis membrane-dependent removal of middle molecules during hemodiafiltration: the $\beta_2$-microglobulin/albumin relationship. Clin Nephrol 2004;62:21–28.

6 Canaud B, Bragg-Gresham JL, Marshall MR, Desmeules S, Gillespie BW, Depner T, Klassen P, Port FK: Mortality risk for patients receiving hemodiafiltration versus hemodialysis: European results from the DOPPS. Kidney Int 2006;69:2087–2093.



Akihiro C. Yamashita, PhD, Prof.
Department of Human and Environmental Science
Shonan Institute of Technology, 1-1-25 Tsujido-Nishikaigan
Fujisawa, Kanagawa 251-8511 (Japan)
Tel./Fax +81 466 30 0234, E-Mail yama@la.shonan-it.ac.jp

Kawanishi H, Yamashita AC (eds): Hemodiafiltration – A New Era.
Contrib Nephrol. Basel, Karger, 2011, vol 168, pp 153–161

# Estimation of Internal Filtration Flow Rate in High-Flux Dialyzers by Doppler Ultrasonography

Michio Mineshima

Department of Clinical Engineering, Tokyo Women's Medical University, Tokyo, Japan

**Abstract**

Several types of dialyzer with enhanced internal filtration have been introduced for clinical application as a means of improving the efficiency of solute removal, and the enhanced internal filtration in these dialyzers has increased the convective transport of the solute besides the diffusive transport. The internal filtration flow rates ($Q_{IF}$) of the dialyzer, however, have never been evaluated precisely. In this study, blood flow velocity in a cross-sectional plane of a dialyzer was measured by pulse Doppler ultrasonography to evaluate $Q_{IF}$. An in vitro study using bovine blood was carried out to determine the local blood flow velocity profile with a probe slider that enables the probe to move in parallel along a dialyzer. A good correlation between observed blood velocity ($u_B(0)$) and blood flow rate ($Q_B(0)$) at the inlet portion of the dialyzer was obtained during the in vitro study. Blood flow rate profiles along the dialyzer ($Q_B(z)$) could be estimated from the product of blood velocity $u_B(z)$ and the total cross-sectional area of the blood flow path ($S_B$) of the hollow fibers. The maximum internal filtration flow rate value ($Q_{IF\text{-}Max}$) was estimated as $Q_B(0) - [Q_B(z)]_{Min}$, where $[Q_B(z)]_{Min}$ is the minimum value of $Q_B(z)$. The Doppler ultrasonography described in this paper is a useful method for bedside monitoring of $Q_{IF}$ in several dialyzers, because it is noninvasive to the patient and produces reliable data with higher reproducibility.



As shown in figure 1, the pressure drops of blood and dialysate flow in a countercurrent manner induce internal filtration/backfiltration in commercially available dialyzers. When there is less net filtration by the dialyzer, filtration through the membrane from blood to dialysate occurs in the upstream blood flow, and backfiltration from dialysate to blood downstream. Internal filtration/backfiltration depends on membrane permeability and the dialyzer specifications. In 1996, Dellanna et al. [1] reported the clinical application of dialyzers

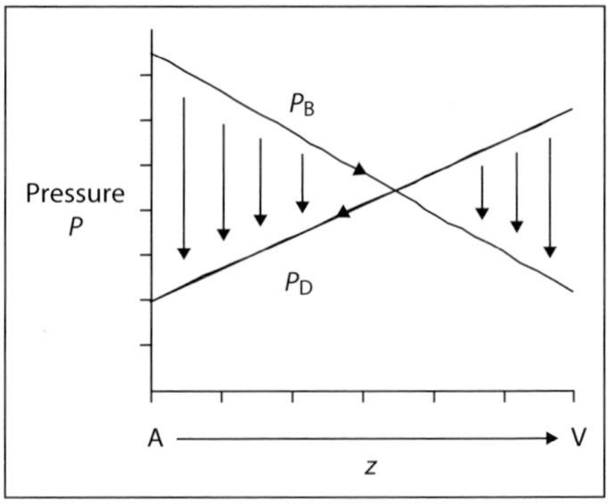


**Fig. 1.** Internal filtration/backfiltration in a dialyzer.

designed for enhanced internal filtration as a means of increasing solute clearance. The enhanced internal filtration in these dialyzers increased convective transport of the solute besides diffusive transport. We examined the effects of internal filtration on the efficiency of solute removal in an analytical and experimental study [2]. The results of the analytical study showed that although internal filtration seemed to be affected by several parameters, namely blood flow rate ($Q_B$), dialysate flow rate ($Q_D$), the patient's hematocrit, plasma total protein level, the effective length ($L_{eff}$), inner diameter ($D$), and density ratio ($DR$) of the hollow fibers, the internal filtration flow rate ($Q_{IF}$) value increased markedly at a smaller $D$, longer $L_{eff}$, and larger $DR$ values. An in vitro evaluation with myoglobin solution showed the same tendencies as in the analytical study. Internal filtration enhanced hemodialysis (IFEHD) seems to be more effective and convenient than hemodiafiltration (HDF) therapy, since IFEHD requires no additional equipment, such as a roller pump.

In this paper, we measured blood flow velocity in a cross-sectional plane of the dialyzer by pulse Doppler ultrasonography in order to evaluate $Q_{IF}$ [3]. An in vitro study with bovine blood was carried out to determine the local blood flow velocity profile with a newly designed probe slider that enables parallel movement of the probe along the dialyzer.

## Materials and Methods

Figure 2 is a photograph of the setup for the in vitro experiment. Part of the bovine blood in the tank was fed to the dialyzer at a preset flow rate and returned to the tank during dialysis at a dialysate flow rate of 500 ml/min. The net filtration rate was set at zero on a commercially available dialysis machine (model NCU-5; Nipro Corp., Osaka, Japan).

Figure 3 is a photograph of the newly designed probe slider used in the in vitro experiment. We positioned the dialyzer horizontally on the slider in a water bath and

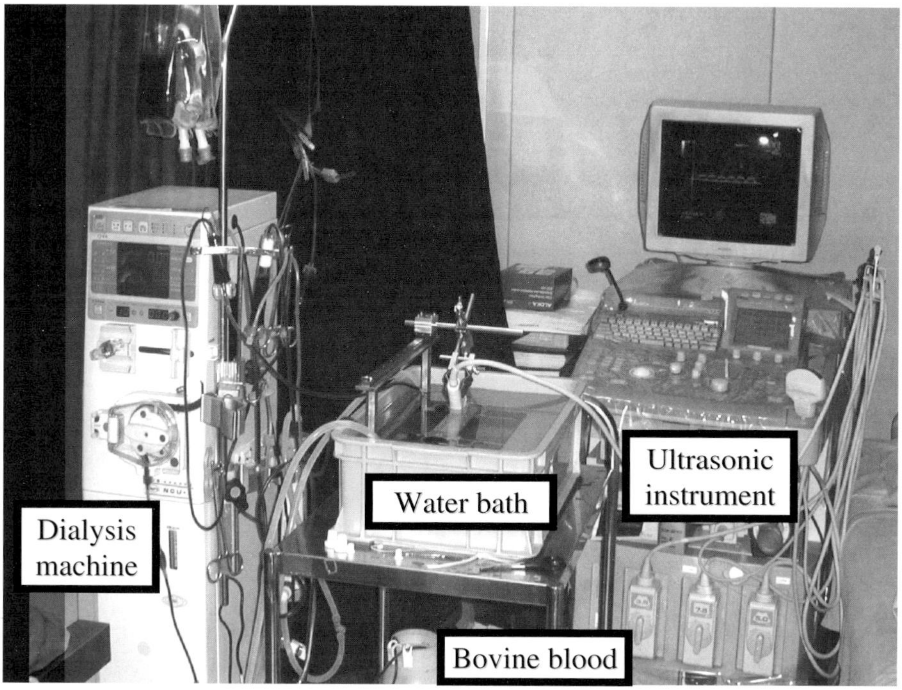


**Fig. 2.** A photograph of the in vitro experiment with bovine blood.

submerged it in the water. The probe holder can slide lengthwise in parallel with the dialyzer, and the slider makes it possible to measure the distribution of blood flow velocity values along the dialyzer.

The Doppler effect is a well-known phenomenon in which the motion of the source of a sound in relation to a receiver causes an apparent change in the frequency of the sound that can be measured. As shown in figure 4, the Doppler shift is defined as the difference between transmitted frequency and observed frequency of the ultrasound beam. The average velocity of blood flow in a cross-sectional plane in the dialyzer could be calculated by the Doppler shift equation:

$$f_D = \frac{2Vf\cos\theta}{c} \quad (1)$$

where $f_D$ = Doppler shift, $f$ = frequency transmitted by the transducer, $V$ = blood flow velocity, $c$ = velocity of the sound beam, and $\theta$ = angle of the insonation.

We used a ProSound 5000 detector (Aloka Co. Ltd, Tokyo, Japan) for ultrasonography and chose a probe having a pulse-wave Doppler $f$ value 7.5 MHz.

As shown in figure 5, the Doppler ultrasonography operating conditions were: (a) sampling rate: 810 Hz; (b) sampling depth ($L_D$): 1 cm from the inner surface of the jacket; (c) sampling gate width ($L_W$): 2 cm, and (d) angle of the beam ($\theta$): 65°. These conditions were selected based on the results of trial and error attempts to achieve reproducible blood flow velocity measurements.

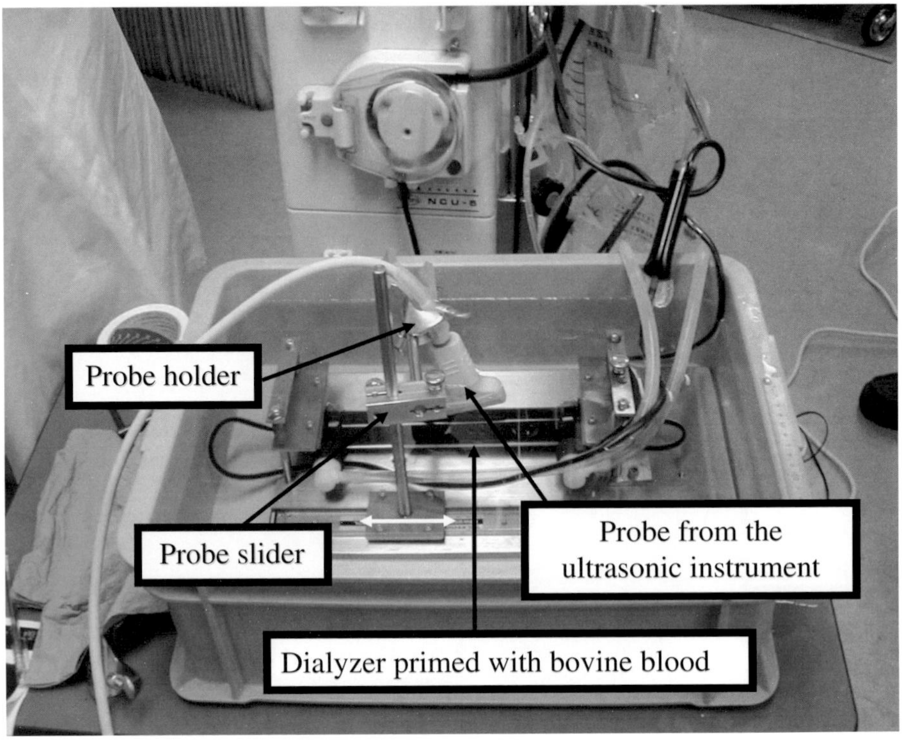


**Fig. 3.** A photograph of the probe slider used in the in vitro experiment.

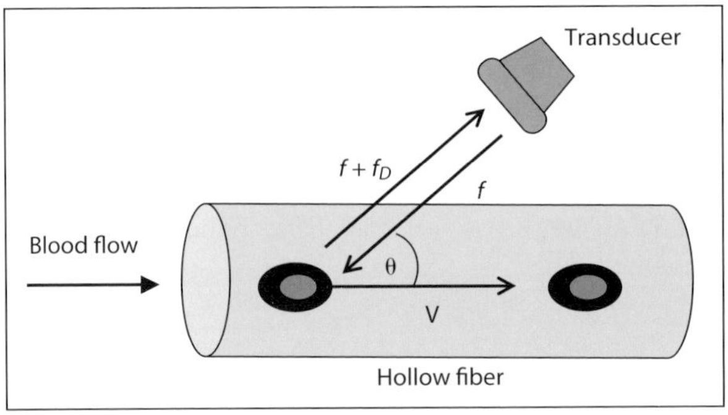


**Fig. 4.** Doppler shift of the ultrasound beam.

Two types of dialyzers containing a CTA membrane (Nipro Corp.) were used in the in vitro experiments with bovine blood. Their specifications are listed in table 1. The FB-150F is a commercially available high-flux dialyzer. The FB-150IF has a smaller inner diameter, 135 μm, and a larger number of hollow fibers for the same surface area. Its

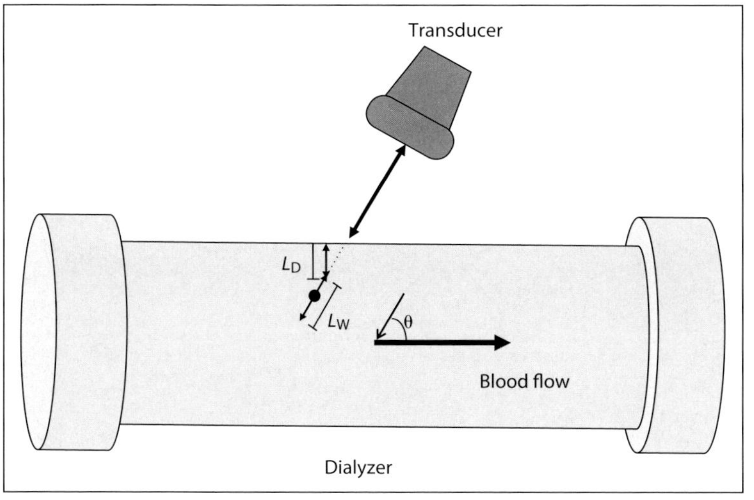


**Fig. 5.** Operating conditions of Doppler ultrasonography.

**Table 1.** Specifications of dialyzers used in the *in vitro* experiments

| | FB-150F | FB-150IF |
|---|---|---|
| Membrane surface area, $m^2$ | 1.5 | 1.5 |
| Inner diameter of the fiber (*D*), μm | 200 | 135 |
| Effective length of the fiber ($L_{eff}$), cm | 22.7 | 21.6 |
| Fiber density ratio (*DR*), % | 52.7 | 47.2 |
| Inner diameter of the jacket, mm | 32.7 | 31.2 |

ultrafiltration coefficient is almost the same as that of the FB-150F. The blood flow rate ($Q_B$), dialysate flow rate ($Q_D$), and net filtration flow rate ($Q_F$) were 100–400, 500, and 0 ml/min, respectively.

## Results

Figure 6 is a photograph of the B mode and the Doppler mode under typical experimental conditions. As shown on the left side of the photograph, we adjusted the sampling point before measurement and then determined the time-blood flow velocity profile on the right side of the photograph. This profile

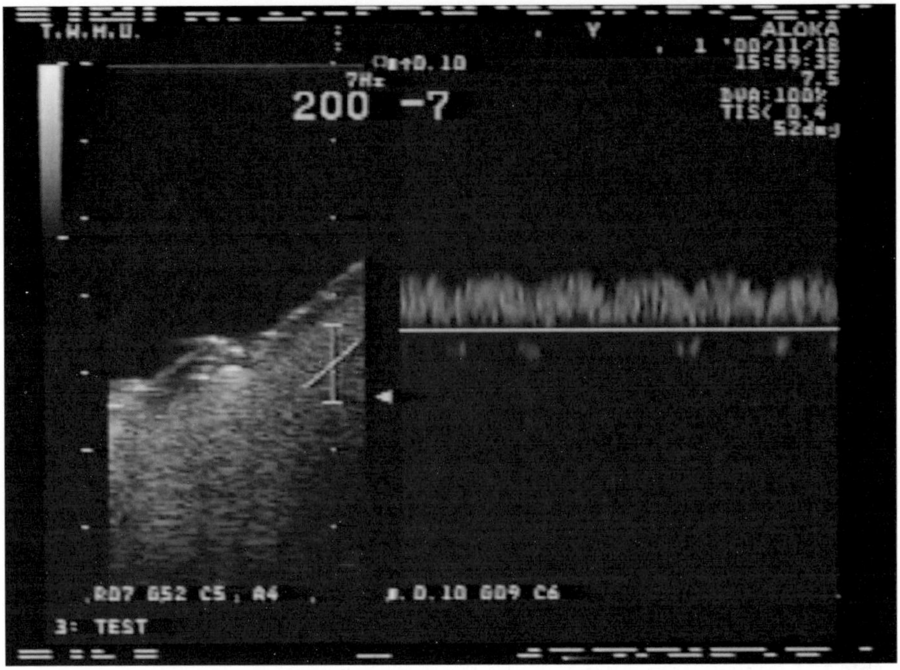


**Fig. 6.** A photograph of the B mode and the Doppler mode of the in vitro experiment.

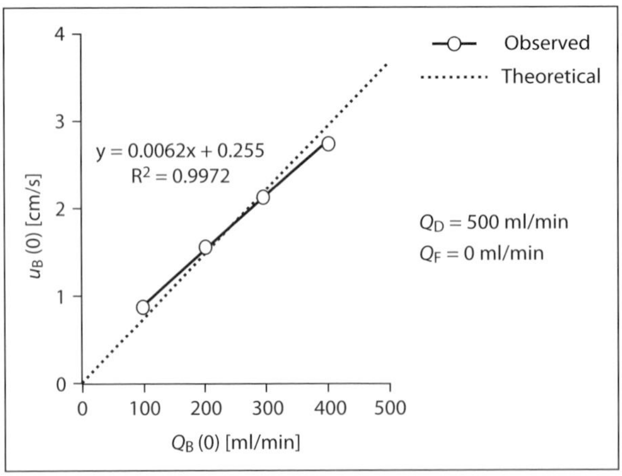


**Fig. 7.** A relationship between the observed blood velocity, $u_B(0)$, and the blood flow rate, $Q_B(0)$, at the inlet potion of the FB-150IF dialyzer.

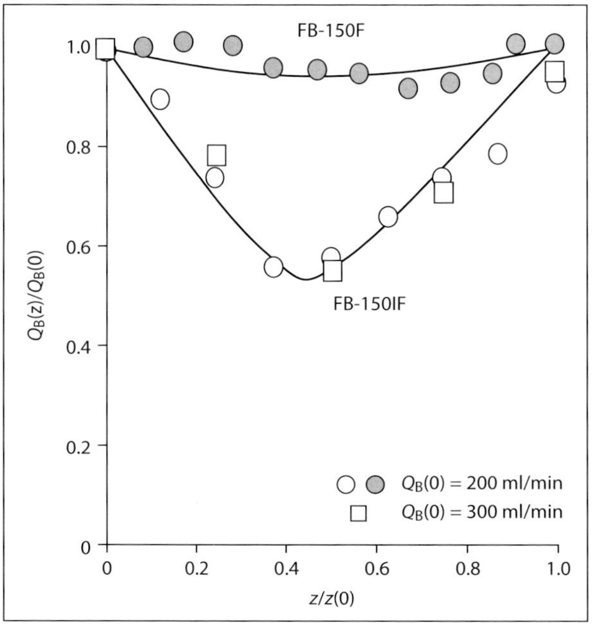


**Fig. 8.** Blood flow rate profiles along the dialyzer.

shows periodic changes caused by the pulsatile blood flow induced by the motion of the roller pump.

Figure 7 shows the relationship between observed blood velocity ($u_B(0)$) and blood flow rate ($Q_B(0)$) at the inlet potion of the FB-150IF dialyzer. A good correlation was obtained during the experiment. The theoretical line was calculated by using the following equation:

$$u_B(0) = Q_B(0)/S_B \tag{2}$$

where $S_B$ is the total cross-sectional area of the blood flow path in the hollow fibers.

Figure 8 shows the $Q_B$ profiles along the dialyzer. The $Q_B(z)$ value was calculated as the product of $u_B(z)$ and $S_B$. The FB-150IF dialyzer showed a greater change in the blood flow rate than the FB-150F dialyzer, meaning that the FB-150IF has larger internal filtration than the FB-150F dialyzer.

Table 2 shows the maximum internal filtration flow rate values ($Q_{IF\text{-}Max}$) obtained in the bovine blood experiments. The $Q_{IF\text{-}Max}$ value was defined as $Q_B(0) - [Q_B(z)]_{Min}$, where $[Q_B(z)]_{Min}$ is the minimum value of $Q_B(z)$. At a $Q_B(0)$ of 200 ml/min, the FB-150IF has a $Q_{IF\text{-}Max}$ of 78.3 ml/min, which is nearly six times higher than that of the FB-150F, despite having the same membrane surface area.

**Table 2.** Maximum internal filtration flow rates, $Q_{IF\text{-}Max}$

| Blood flow rate $Q_B(0)$, ml/min | $Q_{IF\text{-}Max}$, ml/min | |
|---|---|---|
| | FB-150F | FB-150IF |
| 100 | 17.6 | 53.6 |
| 200 | 12.5 | 78.3 |
| 300 | 16.2 | 116.4 |

Flow rates: dialysate flow rate ($Q_D$) = 500 ml/min; net filtration rate ($Q_F$) = 0 ml/min.

## Discussions

IFEHD, defined as HD therapy with a dialyzer designed for enhanced internal filtration, seems more efficient and convenient than HDF therapies, such as conventional HDF using sterile replacement fluid [4], online HDF using purified dialysate as replacement fluid [5], and push & pull HDF by using a reservoir and performing filtration and backfiltration alternately [6], because IFEHD needs no additional equipment, such as a roller pump, reservoir, etc. However, since the $Q_{IF}$ values of the dialyzers had never been evaluated precisely, there were no clear estimates of their solute removal characteristics, and selecting the operating conditions for the IFEHD treatment was difficult.

Since 1992, Ronco's group has performed several studies to estimate internal filtration along dialyzers by using a gamma camera [7, 8] and computerized helical scanning technique [9, 10], while Hardy et al. [11], measured the local ultrafiltration flow rates in dialyzers by magnetic resonance imaging. Although excellent data were obtained for several dialyzers, these methods are somewhat complicated and could not be used in clinical practice. The Doppler ultrasonography method described in this paper, on the other hand, is a useful method for a bedside monitoring of the internal filtration flow rate of dialyzers because it is noninvasive to the patient and produces reliable data with higher reproducibility. This method can be used to measure local blood velocity in several 'black-box' type devices, including hemofilters, direct hemoadsorbers, membrane oxygenators as well as hemodialyzers.

## Conclusions

To estimate the internal filtration flow rate of the dialyzers, pulse Doppler ultrasonography in a cross-sectional plane can measure the blood flow velocity in the hollow fibers of hemodialyzers. A good correlation between the observed blood velocity and the blood flow rate at the inlet portion of the dialyzers was obtained in an in vitro study with bovine blood, and the maximum internal filtration flow rate based on the blood flow rate profiles along the dialyzers could be estimated by this method.

## References


1 Dellanna F, Wuepper A, Baldamus CA: Internal filtration – advantage in haemodialysis? Nephrol Dial Transplant 1996;11(suppl 2):83–86.

2 Mineshima M, Ishimori I, Ishida K, Hoshino T, Kaneko I, Sato Y, Agishi T, Tamamura N, Sakurai H, Masuda T, Hattori H: Effects of internal filtration on the solute removal efficiency of a dialyzer. ASAIO J 2000;46:456–460.

3 Sato Y, Mineshima M, Ishimori I, Kaneko I, Akiba T, Teraoka S: Effect of hollow fiber length on solute removal and quantification of internal filtration rate by Doppler ultrasound. Int J Artif Organs 2003;26:129–134.

4 Leber HW, Wizemann V, Goubeaud G, Rawer P, Schutterle G: Simultaneous hemofiltration/hemodialysis: an effective alternative to hemofiltration and conventional hemodialysis in the treatment of uremic patients. Clin Nephrol 1978;9:115–121.

5 Rindi P, Pilone N, Ricco V, Cioni L: Clinical experience with a new hemodiafiltration system. ASAIO Trans 1988;34:765–768.

6 Usuda M, Shinzato T, Sezaki R, Kawanishi A, Maeda K, Kawaguchi S, Shibata M, Toyoda T, Asakura Y, Ohbayashi S: New simultaneous HF and HD with no infusion fluid. Trans Am Soc Artif Intern Organs 1982;28:24–27.

7 Ronco C, Brendolan A, Feriani M, Milan M, Conz P, Lupi A, Berto P, Bettini M, La Greca G: A new scintigraphic method to characterize ultrafiltration in hollow fiber dialyzers. Kidney Int 1992;41:1383–1393.

8 Ronco C, Brendolan A, Lupi A, Metry G, Levin NW: Effects of a reduced inner diameter of hollow fibers in hemodialyzers. Kidney Int 2000;58:809–817.

9 Ronco C, Brendolan A, Crepaldi C, Rodighiero M, Everard P, Ballestri M, Cappelli G, Spittle M, La Greca G: Dialysate flow distribution in hollow fiber hemodialyzers with different dialysate pathway configurations. Int J Artif Organs 2000;23:601–609.

10 Ronco C, Brendolan A, Crepaldi C, Rodighiero M, Scabardi M: Blood and dialysate flow distributions in hollow-fiber hemodialyzers analyzed by computerized helical scanning technique. J Am Soc Nephrol 2002;13(suppl 1):S53–S61.

11 Hardy PA, Poh CK, Liao Z, Clark WR, Gao D: The use of magnetic resonance imaging to measure the local ultrafiltration rate in hemodialyzers. J Memb Sci 2002;204:195–205.



Dr. Michio Mineshima
Department of Clinical Engineering, Tokyo Women's Medical University
8-1 Kawada-cho, Shinjuku-ku, Tokyo 162-8666 (Japan)
Tel. +81 3 3353 8112, ext. 37203, Fax +81 3 5269 7760, E-Mail mmine@ce.twmu.ac.jp

Kawanishi H, Yamashita AC (eds): Hemodiafiltration – A New Era.
Contrib Nephrol. Basel, Karger, 2011, vol 168, pp 162–172

# Management of Anemia by Convective Treatments

Francesco Locatelli · Celestina Manzoni · Lucia Del Vecchio · Salvatore Di Filippo · Giuseppe Pontoriero · Andrea Cavalli

Department of Nephrology, Dialysis and Renal Transplant, Alessandro Manzoni Hospital, Lecco, Italy

**Abstract**

Anemia secondary to chronic kidney disease is a complex syndrome. Adequate dialysis can contribute to its correction by removing small and possibly medium/large molecules that may inhibit erythropoiesis. A clear relationship among hemoglobin, erythropoiesis-stimulating agent (ESA) dose and increase in dialysis dose has been pointed out by a number of prospective and retrospective studies. Increasing attention has also been paid to the relationship between dialysis, increased inflammatory stimulus and ESA response, as dialysate contamination and low compatible treatments may increase cytokine production and consequently inhibit erythropoiesis. As medium/large molecular weight inhibitors can be removed only by more permeable membranes, convective treatments and, particularly, online treatments, could theoretically improve anemia correction by two mechanisms: higher removal of medium and large solutes (possibly containing bone marrow inhibitors) and reduced microbiological and pyrogenic contamination of the dialysate. Unfortunately, available results are conflicting. Large, prospective, randomized studies on this topic are still needed. 

Anemia is one of the major clinical problems of patients with chronic kidney disease (CKD) on renal replacement therapy (RRT) and, together with hypertension, causes cardiac hypertrophy and subsequent dilation. Given that cardiovascular disease is the major cause of morbidity and mortality in these patients, great effort should be done to prevent, reverse or at least reduce this complication.

Over the last 20 years, the availability of erythropoiesis-stimulating agents (ESA) has led to the almost complete disappearance of the severe anemia of end-stage renal disease requiring repeated blood transfusions; it has also reduced left ventricular hypertrophy [1] and led to a direct improvement in myocardial function. According to the most recent international guidelines, the target hemoglobin in CKD patients receiving ESA should be between 11 and 12 g/dl [2]. Recently, the possibility that excessive ESA dose, together with aiming at higher hemoglobin target, may be harmful has emerged [3–5]. In this perspective, any effort aimed at reducing ESA requirements in order to obtain the desired hemoglobin target has become of extreme importance.

## Pathogenesis of Anemia in Chronic Kidney Disease

The most important trigger of anemia in CKD patients is a reduction in erythropoiesis caused by reduced renal production of erythropoietin (EPO). This is often a relative deficiency: EPO levels may be in the normal range but insufficient for a patient being anemic. In addition, a number of other factors can contribute to the pathogenesis of anemia in CKD patients and influence the response to ESA therapy. Although absolute or relative iron deficiency is probably the most important factor, occult blood loss, infection, inflammation, malnutrition, oxidative stress, and dialysis dose are also important. Less frequent problems are hyperparathyroidism with marrow fibrosis, aluminium toxicity, vitamin $B_{12}$ and folic acid deficiency, hemolysis, bone marrow disorders, hemoglobinopathies, and carnitine deficiency (absolute or dialysis-related). ACE inhibitors and angiotensin II receptor antagonists may also play a role. Moreover, shortened survival of red blood cells is often present.

The observation that the start of dialytic treatment can improve anemia suggests that in CKD patients erythropoiesis is influenced by the retention of uremic toxins. A number of metabolites have been implicated, including various amines such as spermine [6] and parathyroid hormone [7]. These substances are general bone marrow toxins but are not specific suppressors of erythropoiesis [8]. Because anemia improves after the start of dialysis with cellulose membranes, these inhibitors are thought to be of low molecular weight, but high molecular weight inhibitors cleared only by means of highly porous membranes have also been found [9].

Inflammatory cytokines can also inhibit erythropoiesis. Impaired clearance of cytokines, accumulation of advanced glycation end-products (AGEs), atherosclerosis per se and other inflammatory diseases and unrecognized persistent infections have been all implicated. In addition, the dialysis procedure per se has been linked to increased inflammation. Indeed, the prevalence of elevated levels of C-reactive protein (CRP) is higher after the start of dialysis [10]. Even if available data are not univocal, interleukin (IL)-6 has been found to antagonize the EPO effect on bone marrow proliferation [11]. Its levels were directly related to ESA dose in hemodialysis patients [12] and were found significantly higher in patients treated with the less compatible membranes [13]. Conversely, its reduction by means of treatment with pentoxifylline may improve anemia [14]. IL-1, tumor necrosis factor-α and interferon-γ are also important for EPO resistance [15, 16]. Interestingly, tumor necrosis factor-α was a significant individual predictor of rHuEPO requirements in 34 hemodialysis patients [12].

## Anemia and Dialysis Dose

Adequate dialysis is of paramount importance in correcting anemia by removing small, and possibly medium/large molecules, that may inhibit erythropoiesis. In the early 1980s when ESA therapy was not available yet, Radtke et al. [6] found that starting hemodialysis was associated with an increase in hematocrit levels, which went together with an opposite trend of endogenous serum EPO levels (from 509 to 182 mU/ml). Starting from this observation, it was hypothesized that hemodialysis was able to eliminate some bone marrow inhibitors. After more than 15 years, Ifudu et al. [17] found a direct relationship between hematocrit and dialysis dose in a larger population of hemodialysis patients: after adjustment for other factors, an 11% increase in urea reduction rate (URR) doubled the odds that a patient would have a hematocrit >30%. 20 consecutive patients with baseline URR <65% were selected to receive an increase in dialysis dose and were compared with other 20 consecutive patients with the same characteristics in whom the dialysis schedule was not modified [17]. After 6 weeks, in parallel with an increase of mean URR, hematocrit significantly rose only in the patients receiving increased dialysis dose. Given that this result was also achieved using a highly permeable and biocompatible membrane (high-flux polysulfone), it is possible that biocompatibility or permeability, or both, had an additive effect. The same authors [18] confirmed their initial findings in a retrospective study of 309 hemodialysis patients. Unfortunately, no information was given about dialysis membranes and modality.

Large cohort studies also found a clear relationship between the degree of anemia and dialysis dose [19, 20]. However, none of these studies have been able to discriminate the role of different dialysis modalities in addition to that of adequacy. In order to separate the direct effect of dialysis adequacy per se from that of dialysis modality and membrane biocompatibility, Movilli et al. [21] investigated retrospectively the relationship between ESA and dialysis doses in 68 patients on conventional hemodialysis. Hematocrit did not correlate with Kt/V, but ESA dose and Kt/V were inversely correlated. At multivariate regression analysis with ESA as dependent variable, Kt/V was the only significant variable independently contributing to ESA dose. Some years later, the same authors expanded their observation in a larger sample of 83 patients receiving conventional hemodialysis [22]. Interestingly, regression linear analysis showed a breakpoint for Kt/V at the level of 1.33; the correlation between ESA dose and Kt/V was significant only in the patients with Kt/V below this value. Recently,

Gaweda et al. [23] tested the effect of a number of variables on erythropoietic response in 209 hemodialysis patients treated with epoetin-α. Among these, Kt/V was confirmed not having a linear effect on ESA response with a maximum effect for Kt/V >1.4 (a value similar to that identified by Movilli et al. [22]).

Altogether, these findings suggest that dialysis dose per se has a significant effect on anemia only in patients receiving inadequate treatments. In those receiving adequate dialysis, more permeable membranes and/or convective treatments are more likely of being effective in improving anemia, probably because they remove also medium and large molecules that inhibit erythropoiesis or reduce chronic inflammation.

### Convective Treatments

The main feature of convective treatments is the use of high-flux membranes, characterized (when compared to low-flux membranes) by higher permeability for middle molecular weight solutes (particularly in the range of 1–12 kDa), and lower 'bioincompatibility'. Bioincompatibility can be defined as the sum of specific interactions between blood and the 'foreign' artificial materials of the hemodialysis circuit, which can be ascribed to an 'inflammatory response'.

Starting from the hypothesis that only more permeable membranes can remove medium/large molecular weight inhibitors, Kobayashi et al. [24] firstly reported a significant increase in hematocrit in 2 out of 8 HD patients treated with a large-pore membrane (BK-F polymethylmethacrylate). Similar findings were obtained by other small, uncontrolled studies [25, 26]. Conversely, the secondary analysis of a multicenter trial of 380 patients comparing biocompatible and traditional membranes, convective and diffuse treatment modalities [27] did not find any difference in hematocrit levels in the four groups receiving cuprophane hemodialysis, low-flux polysulfone hemodialysis, high-flux polysulfone hemodialysis, high-flux polysulfone hemodiafiltration (HDF) [28]. However, a significant increase in hematocrit levels was observed in patients on high-flux compared with those on low-flux treatments; a higher dialysis dose in the HDF group may partially explain this observation.

Interestingly, some years later, Ayli et al. [29] were able to demonstrate some beneficial effect of high-flux compared to low-flux hemodialysis with the same membrane on anemia in 48 patients who were hyporesponsive to ESA. These results were obtained without significant changes of dialysis adequacy.

Locatelli et al. [30] performed a multicenter, controlled, randomized trial involving 84 patients aimed at testing whether hemodialysis with high-flux membrane (BK-F polymethylmethacrylate) improves anemia in comparison with conventional hemodialysis with low-flux cellulose membrane. An increase in hemoglobin levels was observed in the population as a whole, but this trend was not significantly different between the two groups. In the experimental group, the tendency of hemoglobin levels to increase was present at each month during the follow-up, possibly indicating an insufficient length of the observation period. The effect of dialysis membrane may have been diluted by the fact that selected patients were receiving adequate dialysis, had no signs of inflammation or malnutrition and were not ESA hyporesponsive.

Data coming from Japanese phase II DOPPS also do not suggest a significant improvement of anemia by dialysis modality, compatibility or increased flux [31].

## Vitamin E-Coated Membranes

Vitamin E is a natural antioxidant that has been shown to increase erythropoiesis dose-dependently in a mouse model [32]. This effect is likely mediated by reduced oxidative stress and possibly by a reduction of IL-6 levels. Accordingly, preliminary data suggest that the use of vitamin E-coated membranes can increase hemoglobin levels and decrease ESA doses in hemodialysis patients [33, 34]. These multilayer membranes are coated with liposoluble vitamin E on the blood surface allowing direct free radical scavenging at the membrane site. Cruz et al. [33] tested the effect of a low-flux membrane containing vitamin E in an uncontrolled study of 172 hemodialysis patients previously treated with high-flux dialyzers. During the 12 months of treatment with the vitamin E membrane, hemoglobin levels had progressively risen (from 10.9 ± 1.2 to 11.7 ± 1.2 g/dl). This went together with a decrease of rHuEPO dose (from 7,762 ± 5,865 to 6,390 ± 5,679 IU/week). Recently, Andrulli et al. [34] tested the hypothesis whether combining the antioxidant properties of vitamin E with those of a high-flux, 'biocompatible' membrane (synthetic polysulfone) may improve anemia management in a controlled, open-label, randomized study. 20 patients on stable ESA therapy and receiving bicarbonate hemodialysis for at least 6 months were randomized to dialysis using a polysulfone dialyzer with or without vitamin E. During the 8-month follow-up, the ESA resistance index (calculated by dividing the weekly ESA dose by the product between hemoglobin and dry body weight) decreased more in the vitamin E group (–37%) than in the group only using the high-flux membrane (–20%). This difference was not statistically significant, probably because of the small sample of this pilot study. In the secondary analysis, including parathyroid hormone and vitamin E levels in the model, the difference between groups in ESA resistance index became significant ($p = 0.042$).

## Online Treatments

Online treatments theoretically may have a stronger effect on anemia compared to conventional treatments or standard HDF techniques by means of

**Table 1.** Anemia and online HDF

| |
|---|
| Water quality and distribution system |
| Dialysate |
| Dialysis dose and frequency |
| Membranes and convective treatments |
| Online treatments |

two mechanisms: higher clearances of medium, and large solutes and reduced microbiological and pyrogenic contamination of the dialysate which can also be important in causing or aggravating anemia in hemodialysis patients by means of a enhanced production of cytokines (table 1). Transmembrane passage of bacterial-derived products from the dialysate to blood, known as backtransport, has been documented in several studies occurring either from backfiltration and/or backdiffusion of dialysate contaminants [35, 36]. Progress in improving dialysate purity has been made possible by inserting an ultrafilter in the dialysate flow path and by using sterile bicarbonate. It has been shown that dialysate prepared by ultrafiltration with filters may be virtually free of bacteria and endotoxins and can be used as substitution fluid.

Maduell et al. [37] were among the first observing the possible favorable effects of online treatments on anemia. 37 patients were switched from conventional HDF (mean fluid replacement of 4 l/session), in which the extent of convection is roughly comparable with that of high-flux HD, to online HDF (mean fluid replacement of 22.5 l/session) and were followed for 1 year. During this period, hemoglobin levels significantly increased (from 10.66 ± 1.1 to 11.4 ± 1.5 g/dl), while rHuEPO doses were decreased (from 3,861 ± 2,446 to 3,232 ± 2,492 IU/week). However, patients also experienced an improvement in dialysis dose (15% increase in Kt/V), possibly contributing to anemia improvement. Some years later, Lin et al. [38] shifted a larger number of patients (n = 92) from conventional hemodialysis to online HDF and found a significant decrease of the median rHuEPO/hematocrit ratio (from 504.6 ± 310.1 to 307.6 ± 334.4). However, the study is limited again by the fact that switching to online HDF went together with a significant increase of Kt/V values (from 1.28 ± 0.99 to 1.63 ± 0.26). Differing from the previous two studies [37, 38], Bonforte et al. [39] studied 32 patients treated by online HDF for at least 9 months in whom Kt/V was kept constant. Anyway, they found a significant increase in hemoglobin levels and a consequent reduction in rHuEPO needs (not statistically significant).

More recently, Vaslaki et al. [40] performed a cross-over study involving 70 hemodialysis patients receiving either HDF or conventional hemodialysis for 6 months. Overall, a higher hematocrit at a lower rHuEPO dose was found during the HDF period. However, data were less distinct when looking at study groups.

**Table 2.** Observational studies on the effect of convective treatments on anaemia correction

| | Design | Treatments | Sample size | Haemoglobin haematocrit | Epo dose |
|---|---|---|---|---|---|
| Kawano et al. 1994 [26] | prospective | LF-HD to HF-HD | 10 | NA | ↓ |
| Villaverde et al. 1999 [25] | prospective | cellulose-HD to polysulphone-HD | 31 | = | ↓ |
| Maduell et al. 1999 [37] | prospective | conventional HDF to online HDF | 37 | ↑ | ↓ |
| Lin et al. 2002 [38] | prospective | conventional HD to online HDF | 92 | ↑ | ↓ |
| Bonforte et al. 2002 [39] | prospective | cuprophan HD to online HDF | 32 | ↑[1] | ↓[2] |
| Yokoyama et al. 2008 [31] | historical, prospective | HF-HD vs. LF-HD and cellulose vs. biocompatible | 1,207 | = | = |

LF-HD = Low-flux haemodialysis; HF-HD = high-flux haemodialysis; HDF = haemodiafiltration; NA = not available.
[1] Only in patients not receiving Epo therapy.
[2] Only in patients receiving Epo therapy.

These observations were not be confirmed by other studies. Ward et al. [41] prospectively compared two convective techniques (online HDF and high-flux HD) in 44 patients, who were followed for 1 year. Although the control of anemia was not a primary outcome, hemoglobin remained unchanged over the course of the study. The average weekly dose of rHuEPO slightly increased, but this variation was independent of the dialysis technique.

Wizeman et al. [42] also failed to confirm the possible effect of online HDF on the correction of anemia. They performed a controlled study of 44 patients who were randomized to undergo either low-flux HD or online HDF for 24 months. To eliminate confounding factors, low molecular efficacy (Kt/V = 1.8), treatment duration (4.5 h) and membrane (polysulfone) were matched. Moreover, the same ultrapure dialysate was used in both groups. At the end of follow-up, hematocrit levels and rHuEPO dose did not differ between the two groups.

Tables 2 and 3 summarize the findings of observational and randomized studies evaluating the role of convective treatments and membranes on Hb levels and ESA doses.

Confirming the importance of dialysate sterility on anemia correction, Sitter et al. [43] found a significant and sustained reduction of rHuEPO dose in patients

**Table 3.** Randomized studies on the effect of convective treatments on anaemia correction

| | Analysis | Treatments (patients) | Sample size | Haemoglobin haematocrit | Epo dose |
|---|---|---|---|---|---|
| Locatelli et al. 1996 [27] | secondary | Cuprophan-HD (132)<br>LF-Ps HD (147)<br>HF-Ps HD (51)<br>HDF Ps (50) | 380 | ↑ (HF-HD vs. LF-HD) | NA |
| Locatelli et al. 2000 [30] | primary | HF-PMMA HD (42)<br>cellulose-HD (42) | 84 | = | = |
| Ward et al. 2000 [41] | primary | online HDF vs. HF-HD | 44 | = | ↑ |
| Wizemann et al. 2000 [42] | primary | LF-HD (21)<br>online HDF (23) | 44 | = | = |
| Ayli et al. 2004 [29] | primary | HF-HD vs. LF-HD | 48 | ↑ | ↓ |
| Vaslaki et al. 2006 [40] | primary (cross-over) | online HDF vs. HD | 70 | ↑ | ↓ |
| Andrulli et al. 2010 [34] | primary analysis<br>secondary analysis | HF-HD + vitamin E-coated membranes (10)<br>HF-HD (10) | 20 | =<br>= | =<br>↓ |

LF-HD = Low-flux haemodialysis; HF-HD = high-flux haemodialysis; HDF = haemodiafiltration; NA = not available; Ps = polysulphone; BK-F polymethylmethacrylate.

switched from conventional bicarbonate HD with potentially microbiologically contaminated dialysate to a similar treatment modality using online produced ultrapure dialysate. The switch also resulted in a lower bacterial contamination with a significant decrease in CRP and IL-6 levels. In a multivariate analysis, IL-6 levels were shown to be strongly predictive of rHuEPO dose in both groups (treatment with conventional or ultrapure dialysate). Testing the same hypothesis, Molina et al. [44] performed a prospective study of 107 patients receiving conventional hemodialysis in whom ultrapure dialysate was obtained by adding two filters (one of hydrophilic nylon and another of polysulfone) to the water treatment process. Similar to Sitter et al. [43], after 1 year with this treatment modality, patients obtained a significant decrease of darbepoetin alfa doses (–34%) despite stable hemoglobin levels. CRP and the endotoxin count were also significantly reduced.

## Conclusions

The possibility that convective treatments, particularly online HDF, may achieve a better control of anemia and reduce ESA doses is intriguing. However, available results are conflicting, mainly because of differences in treatment modalities or membranes, lack of control groups, and small numbers of enrolled patients. Furthermore, online HDF achieved higher dialysis dose than control treatments in many cases, further complicating the interpretation of these observations. The results of prospective, randomized trials aimed at better testing this hypothesis are awaited. Available findings clearly suggest that dialysate quality could also be of importance. Online-produced ultrapure dialysate is a quality target to be reached in the next years, in order to reduce bacterial contamination, pyrogenic production and the consequent chronic inflammatory response.

## References


1 Parfrey PS, Lauve M, Latremouille-Viau D, Lefebvre P: Erythropoietin therapy and left ventricular mass index in CKD and ESRD patients: a meta-analysis. Clin J Am Soc Nephrol 2009;4:755–762.

2 K/DOQI Clinical Practice Guideline and Clinical Practice Recommendations for Anemia in Chronic Kidney Disease, 2007: Update of hemoglobin target. Am J Kidney Dis, Suppl, September 2007.

3 Szczech LA, Barnhart HX, Inrig JK, et al: Secondary analysis of the CHOIR trial epoetin-α dose and achieved hemoglobin outcomes. Kidney Int 2008;74:791–798.

4 Pfeffer MA, Burdmann EA, Chen CY, et al: A trial of darbepoetin alfa in type 2 diabetes and chronic kidney disease. N Engl J Med 2009;361:2019–2032.

5 Singh AK: ESAs in dialysis patients: are you a hedgehog or a fox? J Am Soc Nephrol 2010;21:543–546.

6 Radtke HW, Rege AB, Lamarche B, Bartos D, Bartos F, Cambell RA, Fisher JW: Identification of spermine as an inhibitor of erythropoiesis in patients with chronic renal failure. J Clin Invest 1981;67:1623–1629.

7 Massry SG: Is parathyroid hormone an uremic toxin? Nephron 1977;19:125–130.

8 Caro J, Erslev AJ: Uremic inhibitors of erythropoiesis. Semin Nephrol 1985;5:128–132.

9 Kobayashi H, Ono T, Yamamoto N, Hashimoto T, Fukuda T, Yamada S, Kai C, Kataoka H, Kobayashi T, Sonoda T: Removal of high molecular weight substances with large pore size membrane (BK-F). Kidney Dial 1993;34:154–157.

10 Stenvinkel P, Heimburger O, Paultre F, et al: Strong association between malnutrition, inflammation and atherosclerosis in chronic renal failure. Kidney Int 1999;55:1899–1911.

11 Jongen-Lavrencic M, Peeters HRM, Rozemuller H, et al: IL-6 induced anaemia in rats: possible pathogenetic implications for anaemia observed in chronic inflammations. Clin Exp Immunol 1996;103:328–334.

12 Goicoechea M, Martin J, de Sequera P, Quiroga JA, Ortiz A, Carreno V, Caramelo C: Role of cytokines in the response to erythropoietin in haemodialysis patients. Kidney Int 1998;54:1337–1343.

13 Kletzmayr J, Mayer G, Legenstein E, Heinz-Peer G, Leitha T, Horl WH, Kovarik J: Anemia and carnitine supplementation in hemodialyzed patients. Kidney Int 1999;69(suppl):93–106.

14 Ferrari P, Mallon D, Trinder D, Olynyk JK: Pentoxifylline improves haemoglobin and interleukin-6 levels in chronic kidney disease. Nephrology (Carlton) 2010;15:344–349.

15 Shooley JC, Kullgren B, Allison AC: Inhibition by interleukin-1 of the action of erythropoietin on erythroid precursors and its possible role in the pathogenesis of hypoplastic anaemias. Br J Haematol 1987;67:11–17.
16 Cooper AC, Mikhail A, Lethbridge MW, Kemeny DM, Macdougall IC: Increased expression of erythropoiesis inhibiting cytokines (IFN-γ, TNF-α, IL-10, and IL-13) by T cells in patients exhibiting a poor response to erythropoietin therapy. J Am Soc Nephrol 2003;14:1776–1784.
17 Ifudu O, Feldman J, Friedman EA: The intensity of haemodialysis and the response to erythropoietin in patients with end-stage renal disease. N Engl J Med 1996;334:420–425.
18 Ifudu O, Uribarri J, Rajwani I, Vlacich V, Reydel K, Delosreyes G, Friedman EA: Adequacy of dialysis and differences in haematocrit among dialysis facilities. Am J Kidney Dis 2000;36:1166–1174.
19 Madore F, Lowrie EG, Brugnara C, Lew NL, Lazarus JM, Bridges K, Owen WF: Anemia in haemodialysis patients: variables affecting this outcome predictor. J Am Soc Nephrol 1997;8:1921–1929.
20 Coladonato JA, Frankenfield DL, Reddan DN, Klassen PS, Szczech LA, Johnson CA, Owen WF Jr: Trends in anemia management among US haemodialysis patients. J Am Soc Nephrol 2002;13:1288–1295.
21 Movilli E, Cancarini GC, Zani R, Camerini C, Sandrini M, Maiorca R: Adequacy of dialysis reduces the doses of recombinant erythropoietin independently form the use of biocompatible membranes in haemodialysis patients. Nephrol Dial Transplant 2000;16:111–114.
22 Movilli E, Cancarini GC, Vizzardi V, Camerini C, Brunori G, Cassamali S, Maiorca R: Epoetin requirement does not depend on dialysis dose when Kt/N >1.33 in patients on regular dialysis treatment with cellulosic membranes and adequate iron stores. J Nephrol 2003;16:546–551.
23 Gaweda AE, Goldsmith LJ, Brier ME, Aronoff GR: Iron, inflammation, dialysis adequacy, nutritional status, and hyperparathyroidism modify erythropoietic response. Clin J Am Soc Nephrol 2010;5:576–581.
24 Kobayashi H, Ono T, Yamamoto N, Hashimoto T, Fukuda T, Yamada S, Kai C, Kataoka H, Kobayashi T, Sonoda T: Removal of high molecular weight substances with large pore size membrane (BK-F). Kidney Dial 1993;34(suppl):154–157.
25 Villaverde M, Pérez-Garcia R, Verde E, et al: La polisulfona de alta permeabilidad mejora la respuesta de la anemia a la eritropoyetina en hemodiálisis. Nefrologia 1999;19:161–167.
26 Kawano Y, Takaue Y, Kuroda Y, Minkuchi J, Kawashima S: Effect on alleviation of renal anemia by haemodialysis using the high-flux dialyzer (BK-F). Kidney Dial 1994;34:200–203.
27 Locatelli F, Mastrangelo F, Redaelli B, Ronco C, Marcelli D, La Greca G, Orlandini G: Effects of different membranes and dialysis technologies on patient treatment tolerance and nutritional parameters. The Italian Cooperative Dialysis Study Group. Kidney Int 1996;50:1293–1302.
28 Locatelli F, Del Vecchio L, Andrulli S: Dialysis: its role in optimizing recombinant erythropoietin treatment. Nephrol Dial Transplant 2001;16(suppl 7):29–35.
29 Ayli D, Ayli M, Azak A, Yüksel C, Kosmaz GP, Atilgan G, Dede F, Abayli E, Camlibel M: The effect of high-flux hemodialysis on renal anemia. J Nephrol 2004;17:701–76.
30 Locatelli F, Andrulli S, Pecchini F, Pedrini L, Agliata S, Lucchi L, Farina M, La Milia V, Grassi C, Borghi M, Redaelli B, Conte F, Ratto G, Cabiddu G, Grossi C, Modenese R: Effect of high-flux dialysis on the anemia of haemodialysis patients. Nephrol Dial Transplant 2000;15:1399–1409.
31 Yokoyama H, Kawaguchi T, Wada T, Takahashi Y, Higashi T, Yamazaki S, Fukuhara S, Akiba T, Akizawa T, Asano Y, Kurokawa K, Saito A, J-DOPPS Research Group: Biocompatibility and permeability of dialyzer membranes do not affect anemia, erythropoietin dosage or mortality in Japanese patients on chronic non-reuse hemodialysis: a prospective cohort study from the J-DOPPS II study. Nephron Clin Pract 2008;109:c100–108.

32 Gogu SR, Lertora JJ, George WJ, Hyslop NE, Agrawal KC: Protection of zidovudine-induced toxicity against murine erythroid progenitor cells by vitamin E. Exp Hematol 1991;19:649–652.

33 Cruz DN, De Cal M, Garzotto F, Brendolan A, Nalesso D, Corradi V, Ronco C: Effect of vitamin E-coated dialysis membranes on anemia in patients with chronic kidney disease: an Italian multicenter study. Int J Artif Organs 2008;31:545–552.

34 Andrulli S, Di Filippo S, Manzoni C, Stefanelli L, Floridi A, Galli F, Locatelli F: Effect of synthetic vitamin E-bonded membrane on responsiveness to erythropoiesis-stimulating agents in hemodialysis patients: a pilot study. Nephron Clin Pract 2010;115:c82–c89.

35 Waniewski J, Lucjanek P, Werynski A: Impact of ultrafiltration on back-diffusion in hemodialyzers. Artif Org 1994;18:933–936.

36 Pereira BJ, Sundaram S, Barrett TW, et al: Transfer of cytokine-inducing bacterial products across hemodialyzer membranes in the presence of plasma or whole blood. Clin Nephrol 1996;46:394–401.

37 Maduell F, del Pozo C, Garcia H, Sanchez L, Hdez-Jaras J, Albero MD, Calvo C, Torregrossa I, Navarro V: Change from conventional haemodiafiltration to on-line haemodiafiltration. Nephrol Dial Transplant 1999;14:1202–1207.

38 Lin CL, Huang CC, Yu CC, Wu CH, Chang CT, Hsu HH, Hsu PY, Yang CW: Improved iron utilization and reduced erythropoietin resistance by on-line hemodiafiltration. Blood Purif 2002;20:349–356.

39 Bonforte G, Grillo P, Zerbi S, Surian M: Improvement of anemia in haemodialysis patients treated by hemodiafiltration with high-volume online-prepared substitution fluid. Blood Purif 2002;20:357–363.

40 Vaslaki L, Major L, Berta K, Karatson A, Misz M, Pethoe F, Ladanyi E, Fodor B, Stein G, Pischetsrieder M, Zima T, Wojke R, Gauly A, Passlick-Deetjen J: On-line haemodiafiltration versus haemodialysis: stable haematocrit with less erythropoietin and improvement of other relevant blood parameters. Blood Purif 2006;24:163–173.

41 Ward RA, Schmidt B, Hullin J, Hillebrand GF, Samtleben W: A comparison of on-line hemodiafiltration and high-flux haemodialysis: a prospective clinical study. J Am Soc Nephrol 2000;11:2344–2350.

42 Wizemann V, Lotz C, Techert F, Uthoff S: On-line haemodiafiltration versus low-flux haemodialysis. A prospective randomised study. Nephrol Dial Transplant 2000;15(suppl 1):43–48.

43 Sitter T, Bergner A, Schiffl H: Dialysate related cytokine induction and response to recombinant human erythropoietin in haemodialysis patients. Nephrol Dial Transplant 2000;15:1207–1211.

44 Molina M, Navarro MJ, Palacios ME, de Gracia MC, García Hernández MA, Ríos Moreno F, Pérez Silva FM: Importance of ultrapure dialysis liquid in response to the treatment of renal anaemia with darbepoetin in patients receiving haemodialysis. Nefrologia 2007;27:196–201.



Prof. Francesco Locatelli
Department of Nephrology, Dialysis and Renal Transplant, A. Manzoni Hospital
Via dell'Eremo 9, I–23900 Lecco (Italy)
Tel. +39 0 341489862, Fax +39 0 341489860, E-Mail f.locatelli@ospedale.lecco.it

Kawanishi H, Yamashita AC (eds): Hemodiafiltration – A New Era.
Contrib Nephrol. Basel, Karger, 2011, vol 168, pp 173–178

# Clinical Evaluation Indices for Hemodialysis/Hemodiafiltration in Japan

Toshio Shinoda[a] · Yutaka Koda[b]

[a]Kawakita General Hospital, Tokyo, and [b]Koda Medical Clinic, Niigata, Japan

**Abstract**

Japanese hemodialysis (HD) patients have two remarkable characteristics, that is they have a longer period of chronic HD and better clinical outcome than American and European HD patients. This might be partly explained by the very low prevalence of renal transplantation in Japan. As a result, younger HD patients without serious comorbid conditions, whose prognosis should be good, have not been transplanted but have been treated by chronic HD therapy for a long period. Other potential explanations might be higher prevalence of biocompatible high-flux membrane dialyzers and lower prevalence of arteriovenous graft in Japan than Western countries. Although online hemodiafiltration has potential advantage over high-flux HD, the impact of this therapy has not been evident because of its low prevalence in chronic dialysis therapy in Japan.



Japanese hemodialysis (HD) patients seem to have a better clinical outcome than American and European HD patients. Characteristics of the treatment modality such as low prevalence of renal transplantation, high prevalence of high-flux HD and low prevalence of arteriovenous graft might involve the better clinical outcome. There have been several reports that support the hypothesis [1–4]. In this article we describe the historical review of dialysis therapy and possible impacts of peculiar treatment modality of patients with end-stage renal disease (ESRD), high-flux membrane HD and online Hemodiafiltration (HDF) on clinical indices of dialysis patients in Japan.

**Table 1.** Comparison of crude mortality in HD patients between Japan and five European countries and the USA in the DOPPS study [adapted from 3]

| | Total number of deaths | Total patient-years | Mortality rate per 100 patient-years | p value |
|---|---|---|---|---|
| Japan | 959 | 14,607 | 6.6 | <0.0001 |
| Europe and USA | 12,559 | 61,424 | 20.4 | |

## Historical Review of Chronic HD Therapy in Japan

According to the annual records of the Japanese Society for Dialysis Therapy (JSDT), chronic HD therapy has been applied to patients with ESRD since 1968, when the patient number was only 215. Chronic HD therapy was refunded by the Japanese health insurance system in 1972. The number of chronic dialysis patients increased to 3,631 in 1972, and then rapidly increased thereafter.

Following the development of hemofiltration therapy [5], hemofiltration and hemodiafiltration (HDF) became clinically available in the late 1970s, and high-flux membranes for these treatments were developed one after another. HD with high-flux membrane hemodialyzers was fist applied in the early 1980s, and the Japan High Performance Membrane Society was developed in 1986. Following the report of interleukin hypothesis [6], purification of dialysate and biocompatibility of dialysis membrane were investigated thoroughly. Online HDF with a large volume substitution was developed in order to mainly remove massive large molecules such as $\beta_2$-microglobulin. The Japanese Society of Hemodiafiltration evolved for the investigation and popularization of the treatment in 1995.

## Influence of the Low Prevalence of Renal Transplantation on Chronic HD Therapy in Japan

The above-mentioned characteristics of Japanese HD patients, a longer period of chronic HD [1] and better clinical outcome [2, 3] than American and European HD patients, might be partly explained by the difference in the treatment modality of ESRD patients between Japan and the other countries. The majority of ESRD patients have been treated by chronic HD therapy, because of low prevalence of renal transplantation in Japan. Of a total of 275,119 Japanese dialysis patients, 265,757 (96.6%) were on HD and the remaining 9,362 patients (3.4%) were on peritoneal dialysis at the end of 2007 [1]. Of a total of 264,356

Japanese HD patients, 49.4% were on dialysis for <5 years, 25.0% for 5–9 years, 12.2% for 10–14 years, 6.2% for 15–19 years, 3.6% for 20–24 years, and 3.5% for ≥25 years [1]. The longest time on dialysis therapy was 39 years and 8 months [1]. The annual number of renal transplantations in Japan was only 1,224 (187 cadaveric, 1,037 living donor) in 2007 [4]. Younger HD patients without serious comorbid conditions, whose prognosis was good, were not transplanted but treated by chronic HD therapy for a long period. As a result, the time on HD might be longer and the clinical outcome might be good.

## Impacts of High-Flux Membrane Dialyzers on Clinical Indices of HD Patients

According to the first report of the comparison of survival in HD patients between the USA and Japan, the expected remaining lifetime of HD patients was estimated to be 44.5% of the general population in Japan, but only 15.3% in the USA [2]. A Japanese DOPPS study [3] also demonstrated that the crude mortality of HD patients was 6.6 per 100 patient-years in Japan and 20.4 per 100 patient-years in the USA and 5 European countries (table 1). Other potential explanations for the difference might be a higher prevalence of biocompatible high-flux membrane dialyzers and a lower prevalence of arteriovenous graft in Japan than the other countries. An arteriovenous graft and a high blood flow rate might worsen patient survival because of their potential cardiac load.

According to the annual survey by the JSDT, the ratio of synthetic polymer dialyzers, which are almost synonymous of high-flux dialyzers, was 56.5% in 2002 and 81.0% in 2008 in Japan. On the other hand, the mean ratio of high-flux membrane HD was 25.2 in five European countries (France, Germany, Italy, Spain and UK) in 1998–2001, according to the report by Canaud et al. [7].

Concerning impacts of high-flux membrane hemodialyzers on mortality of HD patients, several studies have been reported. One prospective study demonstrated an improvement of mortality of HD patients treated with high-flux membrane hemodialyzers as compared with those treated with low-flux membrane hemodialyzers [8]. A Japanese retrospective cohort study [9] with a long observation period (5.8 ± 6.4 (SD) years, range 0.1–27.9 years) also demonstrated risk reductions not only in the development of carpal tunnel syndrome (relative risk (RR) 0.503, $p < 0.05$) but also in all-cause mortality (RR 0.613 $p < 0.05$), by the switch from conventional to high-flux membrane in 819 HD patients (fig. 1).

On the other hand, a recent randomized control trial, the HEMO study [10], and a recent observational study, a European DOPPS study [8], did not demonstrate an improvement of HD patients' mortality by the use of high-flux membrane dialyzers. In these studies, observation periods were mean 4.48 years (max. 5 years) and about 3 years, respectively. The subanalysis of the HEMO study [11] however demonstrated risk reductions in all-cause mortality and

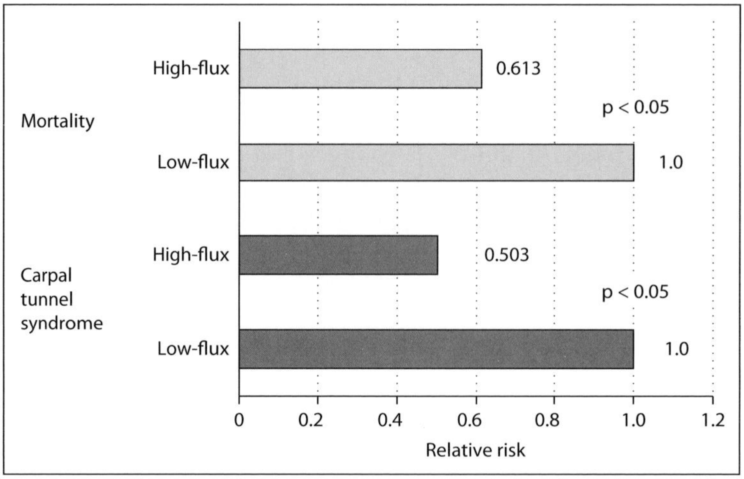


**Fig. 1.** Risk reductions in the development of carpal tunnel syndrome (■) and the all-cause mortality (■) in HD patients by the use of high-flux membrane dialyzers (adapted from Koda et al. [9] and revised).

**Table 2.** Studies on mortality and high-flux membrane in HD patients

| Study | Patients n | Time on dialysis at the start years | Observation period years |
|---|---|---|---|
| Koda et al. [9] | 819 | not shown | 5.8 ± 6.4 SD (range 0.1–27.9) |
| HEMO study [10] | 1,846 | 3.7±4.4 SD | mean 4.48 (max. 5.0) |
| Canaud et al. [7] | 2,165 | mean 4.7 (low-flux HD) mean 5.5 (high-flux HD) | about 3 |

cardiac death in the high-flux membrane group when the analysis was made in HD patients who had been treated for ≥3.7 years before randomization.

Taken together, the beneficial effect of high-flux membrane dialyzers on mortality in HD patients might become evident either by a long-term observation or in patients on HD for a long time (table 2). It is speculated that favorable effects of biocompatible high-flux dialyzers or adverse effects of bioincompatible low-flux dialyzers might become evident after a long-term treatment in HD patients. A randomized controlled study for a long-term observation should be needed in order to confirm the beneficial impacts of high-flux membrane dialyzers on clinical indices of HD patients.

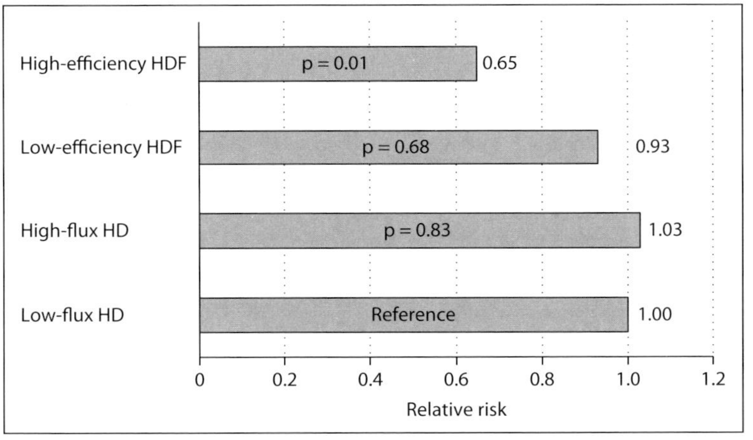


**Fig. 2.** Relative risk of mortality by dialysis type (adapted from Canaud et al. [7]). Adjusted for age, sex, time on dialysis, 14 summary comorbid conditions, weight, catheter use, hemoglobin, albumin, normalized protein catabolic rate, cholesterol, triglycerides, Kt/V, erythropoietin, MCS, and PCS.

## Impacts of HDF on the Clinical Indices of HD Patients

Improvement of clinical indices of HD patients by HDF has been reported less often than with high-flux membrane dialyzers not only in Japan but also the USA and European countries, although many favorable clinical effects by HDF were reported. For example, hemodynamic stability by HDF was demonstrated as compared with HD with bicarbonate-buffered dialysate [12]. Risk reductions of dialysis-related amyloidosis by offline HDF (RR 0.117) and online HDF (RR 0.013) as well as high-flux membrane HD (RR 0.489) were demonstrated in a Japanese observational cohort study [13].

An improvement of patient survival by high-efficiency HDF, or online HDF with a large volume substitution, but not by high-flux HD, was recently demonstrated in the above-mentioned European DOPPS study (fig. 2) [7]. It seems unlikely that an observational study demonstrates an impact of online HDF on survival of HD patients in Japan, because the prevalence of the therapy at the end of 2007 was only 2.5% in 30,510 patients who had begun dialysis in 2007 [1]. The annual survey by the JSDT did not demonstrate an overall prevalence of online HDF among chronic dialysis therapies in Japan.

Online HDF might have potential impacts on clinical indices of chronic dialysis patients such as patient survival, development of dialysis-related amyloidosis, a nutritional status, development of arteriosclerosis, and so on. Potential benefits are more effective removal of large molecules [14] and protein-bound solutes [15], and reduced bioactivation by use of both high-flux synthetic membrane and ultrapure dialysis fluid [16] in addition to the above-mentioned superior hemodynamic stability. A randomized controlled study should be needed in order to confirm also the beneficial impacts of online HDF on clinical indices of HD patients.

## References


1 Nakai S, Masakane I, Shigematsu T, et al: An overview of regular dialysis treatment in Japan (as of 31 December 2007). Ther Aper Dial 2009;13:457–504.

2 Held PJ, Akiba T, Atearns NS, et al: Survival of middle-aged dialysis patients in Japan and the USA, 1988–89; in Friedman EA, et al (eds): Developments in Nephrology, vol 35: Death on Hemodialysis. Dordrecht, Kluwer Academic, 1994, pp 13–23.

3 Akiba T, Akisawa T, Fukuhara S, et al: Results of the international DOPPS hemodialysis study in Japan. J Jpn Soc Dial Ther 2004;37:1865–1873.

4 The Japanese Society for Clinical Renal Transplantation and the Japanese Society for Transplantation: Annual progress report from the Japanese Renal Transplantation Registry, the number of renal transplantations in 2007. Jpn J Transplant 2008;43:206–210.

5 Quellhorst E, Doht B, Schuenemann B: Hemofiltration: treatment of renal failure by ultrafiltration and substitution. J Dial 1977;1:529–543.

6 Schaldon S, Deschodt G, Branger B, et al: Hemodialysis hypotension: the interleukin hypothesis restated. Proc Eur Dial Transplant Assoc 1985;22:229–243.

7 Canaud B, Bragg-Gresham JL, Marshall MR, et al: Mortality risk for receiving hemodiafiltration versus hemodialysis: European results from the DOPPS. Kidney Int 2006;69:2087–2093.

8 Hakim RM, Held PJ, Stannard DC, et al: Effect of dialytic membrane on mortality of chronic hemodialysis patients. Kidney Int 1996;50:566–570.

9 Koda Y, Nishi S, Miyazaki S, et al: Switch from conventional to high-flux membrane reduces the risk of carpal tunnel syndrome and mortality of hemodialysis patients. Kidney Int 1997;52:1096–1101.

10 Eknoyan G, Beck GJ, Cheung AK, et al: Effect of dialysis dose and membrane flux in maintenance hemodialysis. N Engl J Med 2002;347:2010–2019.

11 Cheung AK, Levin NW, Greene T, et al: Effect of high-flux hemodialysis on clinical outcomes: results of the HEMO study. J Am Soc Nephrol 2003;14:3251–3263.

12 Movilli E, Camerini C, Zein H, et al: A prospective comparison of bicarbonate dialysis, hemodiafiltration, and acetate-free biofiltration in the elderly. Am J Kidney Dis 1996;27:541–547.

13 Nakai S, Iseki K, Tabei K, et al: Outcome of hemodiafiltration based on Japanese Dialysis Patient Registry. Am J Kidney Dis 2001;38(suppl 1):212–216.

14 Maduell F, Navarro V, Cruz MC, et al: Osteocalcin and myoglobulin removal in online hemodiafiltration versus low- and high-flux hemodialysis. Am J Kidney Dis 2002;40:582–589.

15 Bammens B, Evenepoel P, Verbeke K, Vanrenterghem Y: Removal of protein-bound solute *p*-cresol by convective transport: a randomized crossover study. Am J Kidney Dis 2004;44:278–285.

16 Guth HJ, Gruska S, Kraatz G: Online production of ultrapure substitution fluid reduces TNF-α- and IL-6 release in patients on hemodiafiltration therapy. Int J Artif Organs 2003;26:181–187.



Toshio Shinoda, MD, PhD, Director
Kawakita General Hospital
1-7-3 Asagaya-Kita, Tokyo 166-8588 (Japan)
Tel. +81 3 3339 2121, Fax +81 3 3339 2986, E-Mail tshinoda@kawakita.or.jp

Kawanishi H, Yamashita AC (eds): Hemodiafiltration – A New Era.
Contrib Nephrol. Basel, Karger, 2011, vol 168, pp 179–187

# Effect of Large-Size Dialysis Membrane and Hemofiltration/Hemodiafiltration Methods on Long-Term Dialysis Patients

Kenji Tsuchida[a] · Jun Minakuchi[b]

Departments of [a]Urology and [b]Clinical Nephrology (Artificial Kidney and Kidney Transplantation), Kawashima Hospital, Tokushima City, Japan

**Abstract**

Over 2,000 substances have been reported as uremic substances that are accumulated or produced due to renal failure that causes various clinical symptoms and complications. These substances include many medium to large molecular weight (MW) substances such as $\beta_2$-microglobulin ($\beta_2$-MG). In hemofiltration/hemodiafiltration (HD/HDF) therapy using high-performance membrane targeting less albumin loss and removal of $\beta_2$-MG with a MW of 11,800, many cases showed insufficient improvement in the clinical outcome contrary to the decrease in serum $\beta_2$-MG concentration. Focusing on these facts, HD/HDF therapy, which associates albumin loss, was implemented targeting the substances in the regions whose MWs are larger than $\beta_2$-MG. HD/HDF therapy with protein-permeable membrane, compared to the therapy without protein-permeable membrane, achieved higher success in the removal of larger MW substances including $\beta_2$-MG, cytokine, homocysteine and complement factor D, and higher clinical outcomes were reported, such as prevention of development of amyloidosis, anemia, osteoarthritis and pruritus, and improvement in life prognosis and biocompatibility in Japan. Therefore, in the current circumstances, it is essential to administer a treatment that can get as close to the glomerular basement membrane as possible, use dialysis membrane to effectively remove a wide range of substances, and aim to remove all of the substances accumulated in the body of patients with kidney dysfunction. 

Blood purification therapy, including dialysis therapy, is a treatment method to route blood out of the body by extracorporeal circulation technology in order to remove disease agents accumulated in the blood and correct the deficit of necessary substances to maintain the concentration level at an acceptable physiological level based on various physical, chemical, or biological principles.

It is presumed that the number of substances that accumulate in the body of patients with kidney dysfunction reaches thousands including the products of metabolism of internal organs. The molecular weight (MW) of the substances vary widely from the low to moderate MW region of urea, creatinine, or uric acid, to low MW protein represented by $\beta_2$-microglobulin ($\beta_2$-MG), or even high MW cut-off that covers from globulin to lipid. Pathogenic mechanisms of some of these substances have been proven, such as $\beta_2$-MG in dialysis-related amyloidosis, however, pathogenic significances in most of the accumulated substances remain to be defined. Safety regarding these substances whose pathogenic significances are not yet clarified also remains to be confirmed. Therefore, in the current circumstances, it is essential to administer a treatment that can get as close to the glomerular basement membrane as possible, use dialysis membrane to effectively remove a wide range of substances, and aim to remove all of the substances accumulated in the body of patients with kidney dysfunction.

## Development of Protein-Permeable Dialysis Membrane

In the 1960s, the early years of dialysis therapy, only low MW uremic substances such as potassium, urea, creatinine, uric acid, and guanidine compounds were removed, which was successful for a limited prolongation of patients' lives.

In 1971, Babb et al. [1] proposed the middle molecules hypothesis, which explains that uremic substances including neurotoxin that causes peripheral nerve disorders exist in the region of middle molecules ranging from 500 to 5,000 MW. In accordance with the middle molecule hypothesis, the square meter-hour hypothesis was formulated, which assumed that it is membrane area and hours of dialysis, not blood or dialysis fluid flow rates, that determine the efficiency in the removal of middle molecules, if using the same dialysis membrane. Following these hypothesis, long-time dialysis using large-size dialysis membrane and the hemofiltration/hemodiafiltration (HF/HDF) methods were more actively implemented based on the ideas that filtration is more effective than dialysis for the removal of middle molecules.

However, as these methods did not produce significant clinical effects, Saito et al. [2] attempted a treatment method to remove substances that are larger than the middle molecules based on the notion that 'glomerular filtration is filtering not only low to middle molecules but also low molecular protein to albumin region', and reported the treatment effects in 1981. Saito et al.'s report stated that symptoms of pruritus, irritable sensation and anemia that had not been improved by HDF using the conventional membrane that did not penetrate protein were improved through HDF using duo-flux membrane that penetrates protein, however, push/pull HDF did not become widespread at this point due in part to the failure to identify the causative substance.

Later, in 1985, Gejyo et al. [3] found that the major constituent protein of dialysis amyloidosis is $\beta_2$-MG. Since then, $\beta_2$-MG has been considered the target in blood purification therapy and the focus is placed on the development of dialysis membrane with high efficiency of $\beta_2$-MG removal. The sieving coefficient for $\beta_2$-MG was <0.5 at that time as opposed to >0.9 of recent years.

However, it was pointed out that the occurrence of pruritus, irritation, anemia and other symptoms associated with amyloidosis is largely influenced by low MW protein, which is larger than $\beta_2$-MG [4, 5]. Based on such facts, the development of hemodialysis (HD)/HDF membrane was promoted aiming to improve the removal ability by enlarging the radius of membrane pore and increasing open pore ratio. In addition, the biocompatibility was also enhanced through the improvement and development of membrane material. Regarding the treatment method, large-amount fluid replacement therapies, such as online HDF or push/pull HDF, were developed aiming to improve the efficiency of the removal of low MW proteins.

## Removal of Uremic Substances and Loss of Albumin in Low MW Protein Region

As mentioned, many cases showed insufficient improvement in the clinical outcome contrary to the decrease in serum $\beta_2$-MG concentration in HD/HDF using high-performance membrane with less albumin leakage targeting $\beta_2$-MG, which suggests that the occurrence of clinical symptoms is affected by substances in larger MW region. One of the proteins in that MW region is $\alpha_1$-microglobulin ($\alpha_1$-MG). It was reported that the observation of the connections between albumin leakage and $\beta_2$-MG and between albumin leakage and $\beta_2$-MG/$\alpha_1$-MG in HD/HDF using polysulfone membrane that causes protein leakage showed no correlation between albumin leakage and $\beta_2$-MG removal rate but a significant correlation with $\alpha_1$-MG removal rate [6] (fig. 1).

As it is shown in the above results, separation of albumin and substances in $\alpha_1$-MG region is limited and needs improvement. The development of high-performance membrane with improved separation characteristics is one idea but is realistically difficult. Hence, a possible solution is the pre-dilution HDF method, through which minimal albumin loss is achieved by a decreased albumin concentration on the membrane surface due to hemodilution. In this method, substitution fluid is added to the blood before the blood enters the hemodiafilter prior to large-scale ultrafiltration in order to remove the solute along with excess water and substitution fluid. Hemodilution helps keep the protein concentration on the filtration membrane surface minimum to cause less clotting of HDF membrane with protein, which prevents the decrease in performance to remove medium/large MW substances. On the other hand, in pre-dilution HDF, it is

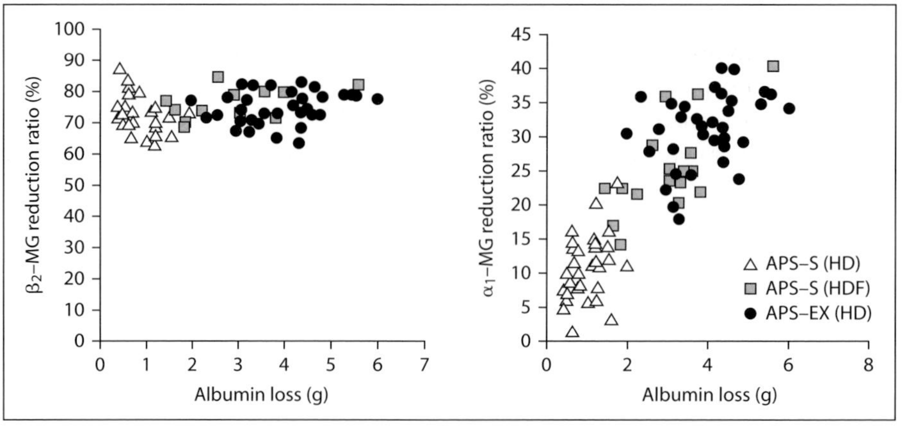


**Fig. 1.** Between albumin leakage and $\beta_2$-MG and between albumin leakage and $\beta_2$-MG/$\alpha_1$-MG in HD/HDF using polysulfone membrane.

also expected to lessen the albumin loss as the concentration level on the membrane surface is lower due to hemodilution. Therefore, higher success might be achieved with pre-dilution HDF than post-dilution HDF in the separation of albumin and medium/large MW substances that are to be removed. Another method to maximize the characteristics of pre-dilution HDF is to increase the filtration area. Through this, it becomes possible to achieve larger $\alpha_1$-MG clearance than albumin clearance [7] (fig. 2). Large-volume pre-dilution HDF (HF) using large-size membrane will allow the separation of substances in $\alpha_1$-MG region and albumin and the original purpose of HDF, whose target is to remove large MW substances, shall be achieved. If the filtration performance through development of HDF membrane can be secured, there will be no limit to the volumes of substitution fluid and ultrafiltration in pre-dilution HDF and we can achieve a higher solute removal performance.

## Clinical Efficiency

Over 2,000 substances have been reported as uremic substances that are accumulated or produced due to renal failure that causes various clinical symptoms and complications. These substances include many medium to large MW substances such as $\beta_2$-MG. In HD/HDF therapy using high-performance membrane targeting less albumin loss and removal of $\beta_2$-MG with a MW of 11,800, many cases showed insufficient improvement in the clinical outcome contrary to the decrease in serum $\beta_2$-MG concentration. Focusing on these facts, HD/HDF therapy, which associates albumin loss, was implemented targeting the

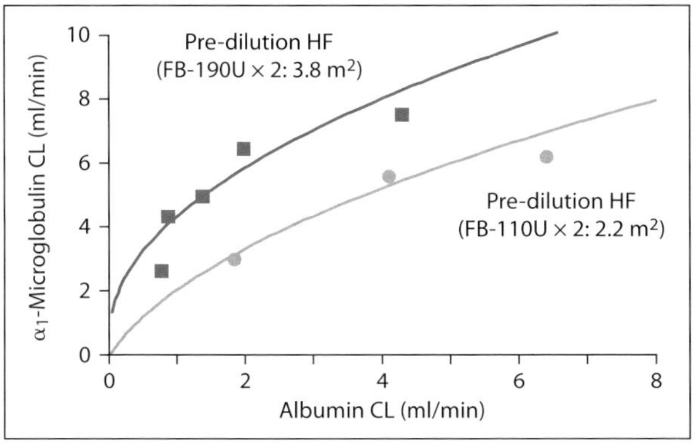


**Fig. 2.** Relationship between $\alpha_1$-MG clearance and albumin clearance in different sizes of dialysis membrane.

substances in the regions whose MWs are larger than $\beta_2$-MG. HD/HDF therapy with protein-permeable membrane, compared to the therapy without protein-permeable membrane, achieved higher success in the removal of larger MW substances including $\beta_2$-MG, cytokine, homocysteine and complement factor D, and higher clinical outcomes were reported, such as prevention of development of amyloidosis, anemia, osteoarthritis and pruritus, and improvement in life prognosis and biocompatibility in Japan.

*Improvement in Anemia, Osteoarthritis, Pruritus and Irritable Sensation*

Since the report by Saito et al. [2] on the improved symptoms of anemia, osteoarthritis, pruritus and irritable sensation through the use of protein-permeable membrane, additional examinations were performed in many facilities and the results were reported. The protein-permeable membranes used at that time were ethylene vinyl alcohol (EVAL)-C, cuprophane, PS, polymethyl-methacrylate and polyacrylonitrile. The improvement effects based on the Japanese reports were 30–44% for anemia in short term (1–3 months), 75–83% for anemia in long term (6–12 months), 40–75% for osteoarthritis (2 weeks to 12 months), and 60–100% for pruritus (1–12 months). These reports on the symptom improvements include patients' subjective perceptions, not based on the objectively evaluated control studies, however the patients should be valued to some extent as they were reported by many different facilities. It these, symptom improvements resulted from increased volume in the removal of larger MW substances, the causative factors for anemia, osteoarthritis, pruritus, and irritable sensation are highly likely medium/large molecular size substances, however we are not yet able to identify the causative factors.

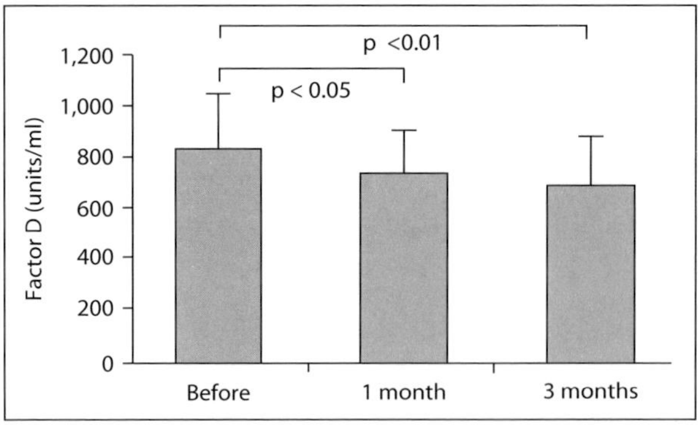


**Fig. 3.** Removal of complement factor D through HDF is implemented using EVAL-CH.

*Attempts Towards the Improvement of Biocompatibility Through the Removal of Complement Factor D*

Complement factor D is a serine protease with a MW of approximately 24 kDa that functions to activate the alternate pathway in the complement system and increase the production of mediator of tissue inflammation within the complement cascade. It is filtered from glomerulus, decomposed into amino acid and reabsorbed in the tubule, which, in the case of renal insufficiency, accumulates in blood at 10–20 times higher concentration level in the serum of maintenance dialysis patients.

The removal of complement factor D through HDF is implemented using EVAL-CH that permeates 6–8 g of protein per session and reported the prevention of the production of anaphylatoxin C3a (fig. 3) [8]. An improvement in the biocompatibility is expected through an active removal of complement factor D that facilitates the biological reaction. In order to hinder biological reaction, it is necessary to develop treatment materials with higher biocompatibility, however the examination suggested that it is also useful to actively remove the substances that facilitate biological reaction.

*Effects on the Life Prognosis and the Occurrence of Snapping Finger and Carpal Tunnel Syndrome*

Five-year follow-ups on 35 cases that underwent push/pull HDF with large volume albumin loss (6–8 g per session) (push/pull HDF group) and 30 cases that underwent HDF without albumin loss (standard HDF group) are conducted. During this clinical examination, the mortality risk was significantly lower in push/pull HDF group (fig. 4). Although there was no difference in the incidence of snapping finger or carpal tunnel syndrome during the examination period, we have obtained the result of possible extension of recurrence interval through push/pull HDF. The dialysis records in the push/pull HDF group were significantly long and the Standard HDF group included high-risk cases whose

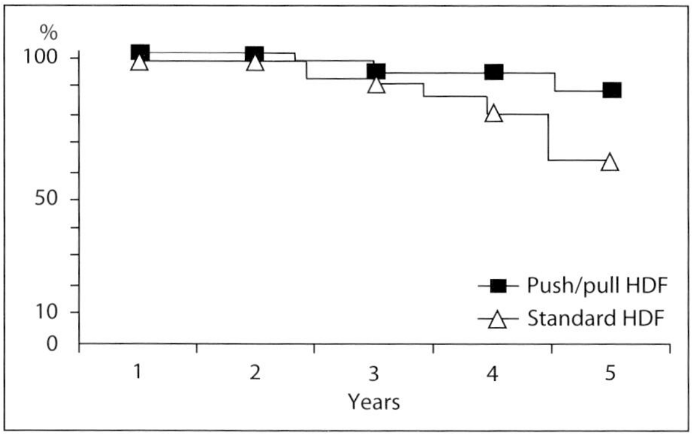


**Fig. 4.** Effect of the protein-permeable dialysis membrane on the frequencies of hospitalization and occurrence of complication events.

amyloidosis symptoms did not improve, thus we consider push/pull HDF to be useful for the prevention of disease prevention.

*Decrease in Hospitalization and Complication*

Three-year studies on the groups that underwent dialysis treatment are conducted using dialysis membrane that allows albumin leakage of 7.69 ± 1.0 g per treatment and otherwise about the frequency of hospitalization and complication events such as cardiovascular complication, cancer, gastrointestinal bleeding, infection or dialysis amyloidosis. The frequencies of hospitalization and occurrence of complication events were 22.0 and 28.0%, respectively, for the albumin-permeable membrane group and 35.4 and 61.5%, respectively, for the non-albumin-permeable membrane group; we have reported that frequencies for both hospitalization and occurrence of complication events were lower in the albumin-permeable membrane group (fig. 5) [9].

*Variation in the Serum Albumin Value in HD/HDF Using Protein-Permeable Membrane*

One concern is that the implementation of HD/HDF using protein-permeable membrane may cause hypoproteinemia. It is reported that when using protein-permeable membrane for a long period of time, serum albumin value decreases in the first 1–3 months and then rises up to or close to the previous value (fig. 6) [9].

## Conclusion

Most of dialysis membranes in recent years have improved $\beta_2$-MG clearance that does not allow albumin leakage to a maximum extent. However, the cases that

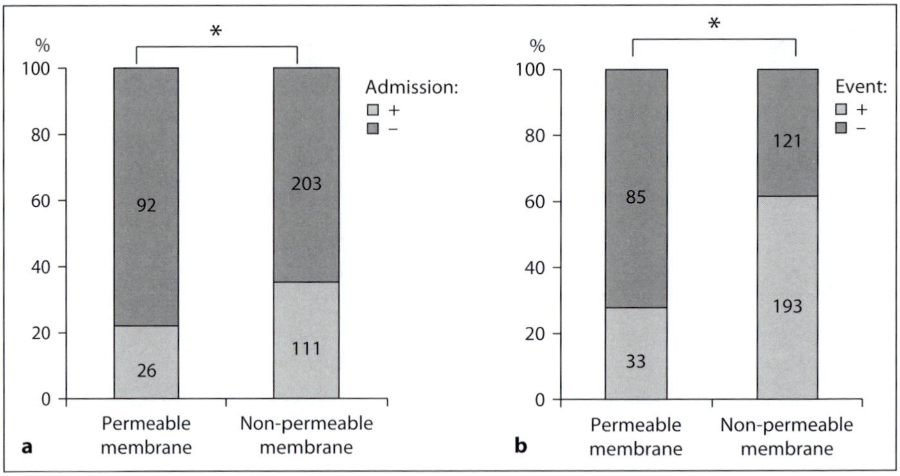


**Fig. 5.** Mortality risk between push/pull HDF group (**a**) and standard HDF group (**b**). $^*p < 0.05$ by $\chi^2$ test.

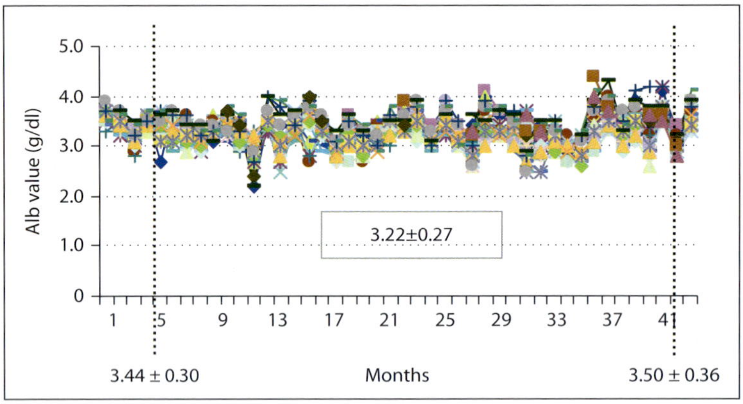


**Fig. 6.** Effect of the protein-permeable dialysis membrane on serum albumin value.

underwent HD/HDF therapy using high-performance membrane with less albumin leakage showed insufficient improvement in the clinical outcome contrary to the decrease in serum $\beta_2$-MG concentration, which suggests that the occurrence of clinical symptoms is affected by substances in a larger MW region.

The primary idea regarding albumin leakage in dialysis therapy is that a certain level of albumin leakage cannot be avoided in order to increase the volume of the removal of low MW substances and low molecular protein that are accumulated in blood. Meanwhile, albumin has various roles in the body such as maintaining colloid osmotic pressure, transportation and absorption of hormone, fatty acid, medical substances and other biologically active substances, pH buffer action and antioxidant action. In normal renal function, approximately 10 g of albumin is filtered in glomerulus per day, decomposed in renal tubule and reabsorbed as amino acid, and resynthesized into albumin in the liver. To the contrary, in dialysis patients, albumin that is bound to biologically active substances and/or an oxidized form of albumin that lost its antioxidant effect cannot be filtered from kidney and accumulate. Therefore, the second idea regarding albumin leakage is to remove biologically active substances that bind to albumin and function as uremic toxin, remove albumin without the antioxidant effect, and facilitate synthesis of new albumin with antioxidant effect. Acceleration of albumin metabolism not only helps the removal of uremic toxic substances, but also the maintenance of albumin functions.

## References


1 Babb AL, Popovich RP, Christopher TG, Scribner BH: The genesis of the square meter-hour hypothesis. Trans Am Soc Artif Intern Organs 1971;17:81–91.

2 Saito A, Suzuki I, Chung TG, Okamoto T, Hotta T: Separation of an inhibitor of erythropoiesis in 'middle molecules' from hemodialysate from patients with chronic renal failure. Clin Chem 1986;32:1938–1941.

3 Gejyo F, Yamada T, Odani S, Nakagawa Y, Arakawa M, Kunitomo T, Kataoka H, Suzuki M, Hirasawa Y, Shirahama T, et al: A new form of amyloid protein associated with chronic hemodialysis was identified as $\beta_2$-microglobulin. Biochem Biophys Res Commun 1985;129:701–706.

4 Splendiani G, Albano V, Tancredi M, Daniele M, Pignatelli F: Our experience with combined hemodialysis-hemoperfusion treatment in chronic uremia. Biomater Artif Cells Artif Organs 1987;15:175–181.

5 Meert N, Eloot S, Waterloos MA, Van Landschoot M, Dhondt A, Glorieux G, Ledebo I, Vanholder R: Effective removal of protein-bound uraemic solutes by different convective strategies: a prospective trial. Nephrol Dial Transplant 2009;24:562–570.

6 Tomo T: Effect of high permeable dialysis membrane on dialysis patients (in Japanese). Kidney Dial 2008;56:13–17.

7 Minakuchi J, Tsuchida K, Nakamura M: Removal of low molecular weight uremic toxin and albumin loss (in Japanese). Kidney Dial 2008;65:18–22.

8 Minakuchi J, Naito H, Saito A, et al: Effect of hemodiafiltration on removal of factor D and biocompatibility (in Japanese). Kidney Dial 1998;45:20–24.

9 Tsuchida K, Nakamura M, Yoshikawa K, Minakuchi J: Efficacy of various high-flux membrane on long-term dialysis patients (in Japanese). Kidney Dial 2008;65:33–38.



Kenji Tsuchida
Department of Urology, Kawashima Hospital
1-39 Kita-Sako Ichiban-cho
Tokushima-City, Tokushima 770-0011 (Japan)
Tel. +81 88 631 0110, Fax +81 88 631 5500, E-Mail ktsuchida@khg.or.jp

Kawanishi H, Yamashita AC (eds): Hemodiafiltration – A New Era.
Contrib Nephrol. Basel, Karger, 2011, vol 168, pp 188–194

# Who Needs Acetate-Free Biofiltration?

Tsutomu Kuno

Ikebukuro Kuno Clinic, Tokyo, Japan

**Abstract**

Acetate-free biofiltration (AFB) is a hemodiafiltration (HDF) technique that is performed with a base-free dialysate and simultaneous infusion of sodium bicarbonate solution. In Japan 3 years ago, a new form of acetate-free dialysate containing 2.0 mEq/l citric acid was approved. Recently, we have had a 76-year-old male subject who switched from AFHD to AFB, mainly because of cardiovascular stability. Several factors may contribute to hemodynamic adaptation during AFB. One theory is that an increase in peripheral vascular tone and vascular refilling rate is caused by the high sodium concentration of the substitution fluid. AFB has all the premises for being a perfectly biocompatible technique capable of satisfying even the demands of critical patients laden with comorbidities. 

## Background

Over the past few years, patients with a critical clinical status on chronic hemodialysis (HD) have increased because of the progressive increase in the mean age of patients and greater comorbidity, particularly with cardiovascular pathologies and diabetes mellitus [1]. Cardiovascular disease is the most frequent cause of morbidity and mortality in patients with chronic kidney disease. Moreover, cardiovascular disease-associated risk is partly explainable by cofactors such as uremia per se, systemic inflammation, and oxidative stress due to the exposure that occurs during dialysis treatment. Bioincompatible factors also enhance the risk for patients on HD.

## Concept of Acetate-Free Biofiltration

It is well known that acetate is directly and indirectly involved in generating several side effects. Among these are hypoxia, vasodilatation and the increased production of inflammatory cytokines, such as IL-1β, IL-6, and TNF-α. It has also been proposed that acetate can induce NO synthase (NOS-2) by triggering the release of proinflammatory mediators from both endothelial and smooth muscle cells [2]. These factors increase the risk of cardiovascular instability. However, almost all dialysis techniques contain some acetate in the dialysis fluid in order to maintain chemical stability. Acetate mainly had a chemical role, allowing for the improvement of the dialysis fluid's electrolytic stability. Consequently, despite the small proportion of acetate in bicarbonate dialysis, the level of plasma acetate may rise [3]. It could be reinforced by repeated dialysis treatment.

Acetate-free biofiltration (AFB) is a hemodiafiltration (HDF) technique that combines both diffusion and convective solute transport, performed with a base-free dialysate and simultaneous infusion in post-dilutional mode of sterile isotonic sodium bicarbonate solution. Hence, with AFB there is no simultaneous mixing of calcium and $HCO_3$. Only $HCO_3$ is infused into blood (as $NaHCO_3$), whereas calcium is supplied only by the electrolyte-containing, buffer-free dialysate. Hence, there is no need for acetate. This idea of an acetate-free dialysis technique, with no buffer at all, was first introduced about 26 years ago by Zucchelli et al. [4].

The absence of acetate is expected to provide much better cardiovascular stability and also improve biocompatibility by avoiding the acetate-induced cytokine activation [5]. In addition, the single base-free dialysate concentrate can reduce the risk of contamination by bacteria or endotoxins. AFB has all the premises for being a perfectly biocompatible technique capable of satisfying even the demands of critical patients laden with comorbidities.

## Indication for AFB

Rapid removal of fluid and solute by HD and intermittent blood purification therapy may result in symptomatic hypotension, which is the most common acute complication. 20–30% of dialysis sessions are complicated by dialysis hypotension and associated symptoms of muscle cramp, nausea, vomiting, and headache [6]. Elderly patients and those with diabetes, as well as those with autonomic insufficiency and structural heart disease, are particularly affected. Reduction in the frequency of this complication could contribute significantly to improve the quality of life of patients on HD. Santoro et al. [7] have analyzed nine clinical studies on AFB, focusing particularly on cardiovascular stability, specifically on the capacity of AFB to prevent dialysis-related hypotension. The overall population is made up of around 200 patients. The probability of intradialysis hypotension in AFB is about 40% of probability of dialysis hypotension in bicarbonate HD. On the other hand, metabolic acidosis commonly complicates chronic kidney disease and has adverse effects on bone,

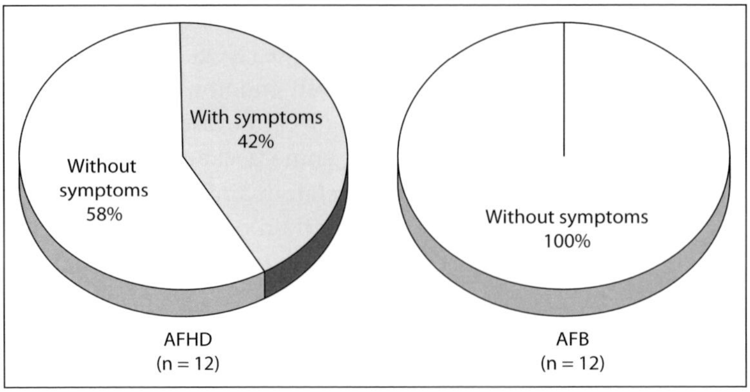


**Fig. 1.** Incidence of clinical symptoms during both AF-HD and AFB sessions.

nutrition, and metabolism. For patients treated with dialysis, the National Kidney Foundation Kidney Disease Outcomes Quality Initiative (K/DOQI) guidelines recommended maintaining serum bicarbonate levels >22 mmol/l to help prevent these complications [8]. Some clinical observations reported that AFB could improve both acid-base control and hemodynamics in patients on HD [9–11].

## AFHD vs. AFB

In Japan 3 years ago, a new form of acetate-free commercial dialysate containing 2.0 mEq/l of citric acid for pH adjustment in the fluid was approved. We have been routinely using acetate-free dialysate in our clinic for 3 years. Therefore, AFB can be compared to new acetate-free hemodialysis (AF-HD). Recently, we have had a male subject who switched from AFHD to AFB.

*Case Report:* A 76-year-old man had been receiving HD since June 2007 for end-stage renal disease due to diabetic nephropathy. After initiation of dialysis the patient's urine volume was decreased according to loss of residual renal function. Thereafter, interdialytic weight gain increased (2.5–3.0 kg). He had acquired symptomatic hypotension due to ultrafiltration despite receiving AFHD. Therefore, we proposed him to change treatment time to 4 h/session from 3 h/session. However, he rejected this proposal. His dialysis procedure was therefore switched to AFB from AFHD using the same polysulfone membrane dialyzer. The dialysis sessions lasted 180 min and were performed 3 times a week. Blood flow rate was kept at 200 ml/min and dialysate flow rate was kept constant at 500 ml/min. In AFB treatment, the substitution fluid (Na 166 mEq/l, $HCO_3$ 166 mEq/l) was infused at a constant rate of 1.8 l/h.

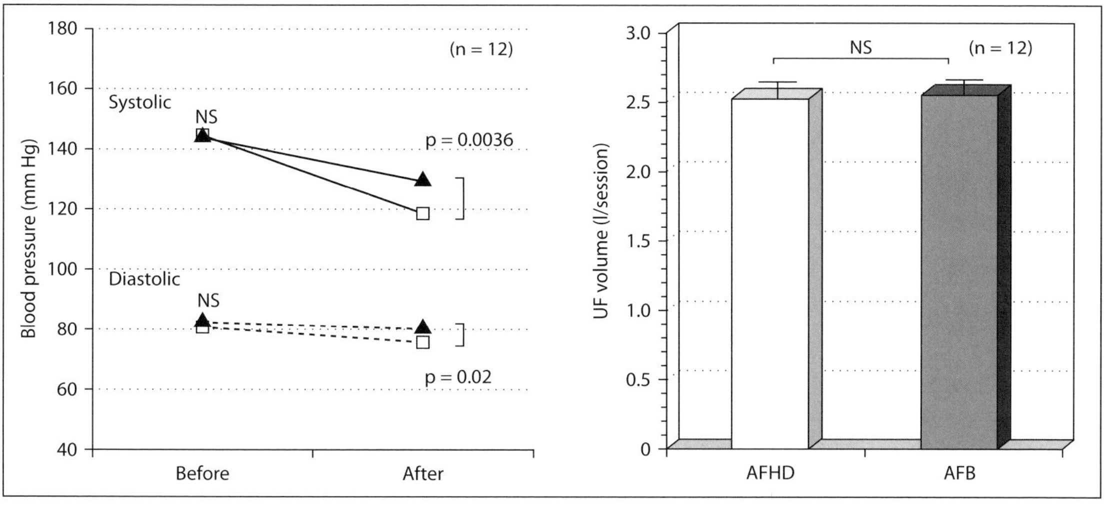


**Fig. 2.** Blood pressure and ultrafiltration volume.

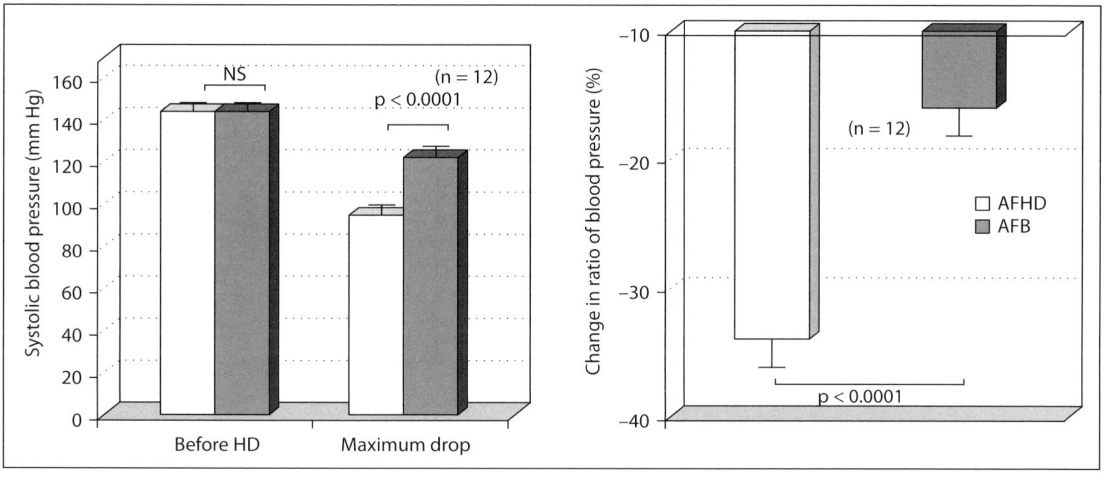


**Fig. 3.** Blood pressure before dialysis and maximum drop during the session, and change in ratio of blood pressure.

In AF-HD, the composition in dialysate was Na 140, K 2.0, Ca 1.5, Mg 1.0, Cl 111.0, $HCO_3$ 35 mEq/l, and glucose 150 mg/dl. Figure 1 shows the incidence of clinical symptoms during both AFHD and AFB sessions. In 42% of AF-HD sessions some clinical symptoms were observed, compared to 0% of AFB sessions. Figure 2 shows the patient's blood pressure and ultrafiltration volume. Although there were no differences of the ultrafiltration volume between AFHD and AFB,

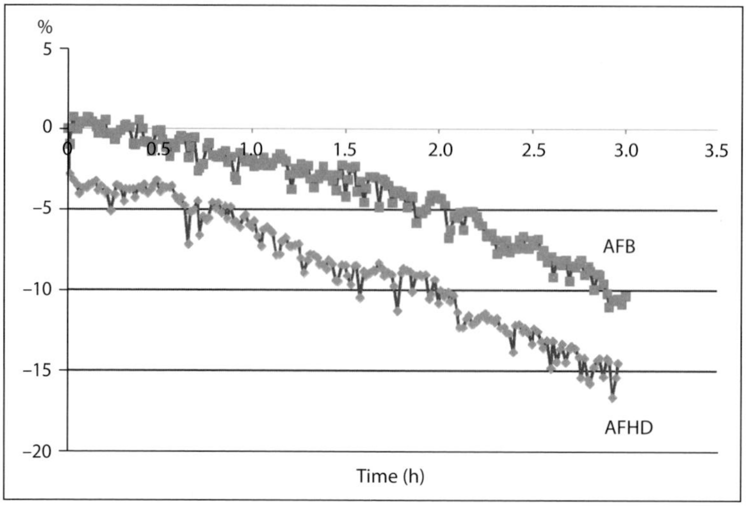


**Fig. 4.** Blood volume (BV) monitoring during the AF-HD and AFB sessions. BV changes were observed by non-invasive continuous hematocrit measurement during AFHD and AFB sessions. Both ultrafiltration rates were nearly the same (2.8 kg/session).

blood pressure after dialysis significantly decreased on AFHD compared to AFB. Also, although there were no differences of blood pressure before dialysis between AFHD and AFB, blood pressure at the maximum drop on AFHD was significantly lower than that of AFB (fig. 3). Figure 4 shows a typical pattern for blood volume changes during both AFBF and AFB session. This observation suggested that AFB might lead to better plasma refilling compared to AFHD. This is a successful case of change from AFHD to AFB. Table 1 indicates the main characteristics for both AFHD and AFB. Dialysis-inducing hypotension can be seen as being linked to both non-autonomic and autonomic causes. One of the causes of cardiovascular instability is intolerance to the acetate present in the dialysate. In this case however, acetate is absent in both AF-HD and AFB (table 1). Several factors may contribute to this hemodynamic adaptation during AFB. One theory is that an increase in peripheral vascular tone and vascular refilling rate is caused by the high sodium concentration of the substitution fluid.

## Conclusion

AFB permits personalized optimal correction of metabolic acidosis in patients on HD. It leads to a beneficial effect on uremic metabolic abnormalities. The absence of both acetate and citric acid loading during AFB might be one of the

**Table 1.** Comparison between AF-HD and AFB

| | AF-HD | AFB |
|---|---|---|
| Modality | HD | HDF |
| Acetate loading | no | no |
| Buffer in dialysate | $NaHCO_3$ (fixed concentration) | buffer-free |
| Substitution fluid | no | 1.4% sodium bicarbonate |
| Citrate | 2.0 mEq/l | no |
| Buffer supply | depends on concentration gradient of bicarbonate between the dialysate and blood | intravenous infusion of sodium bicarbonate (strongly related to QB*/Qsf ratio) |
| Acid-base balance | not personalized | personalized correction of acidosis |

reasons for asymptomatic dialysis treatment in patients on HD. Also, a high sodium concentration of substitution fluid on AFB can lead to a better vascular stability in patients on HD with a critical clinical status.

## References


1 Nakai S, Masakane I, Shigematsu T, et al: An overview of regular dialysis treatment in Japan (as of 31 December 2007). Ther Apher Dial 2009;13:457–504.

2 Grandi E, Govoni M, Furini S, et al: Induction of NO synthase-2 in ventricular cardiomyocytes incubated with a conventional bicarbonate dialysis bath. Nephrol Dial Transplant 2008;23:2192–2197.

3 Kuno T, Kikuchi F, Yanai M, et al: Clinical advantage of acetate-free biofiltration. Contrib Nephrol. Basel, Karger, 1994, vol 108, pp 121–130.

4 Zucchelli P, Santro A, Raggiotto G, et al: Biofiltration in uremia preliminary observation. Blood Purif 1984;2:187–195.

5 Higuchi T, Kuno T, Takahashi S, et al: Chronic effect of long-term acetate-free biofiltration in the production of interleukin-1β and interleukin-1 receptor antagonist by peripheral blood mononuclear cells. Am J Nephrol 1997;17:428–434.

6 Donauer J, Schweiger C, Rumberger B, et al: Reduction of hypotensive side effect during online hemodiafiltration. Nephrol Dial Transplant 2003;18:1616–1622.

7 Santoro A, Guarnieri F, Ferramosca E: Acetate-free biofiltration. Contrib Nephrol. Basel, Karger, 2007, vol 158, pp 138–152.

8 National Kidney Foundation: K/DOQI clinical practice guidelines for nutrition in chronic renal failure. Am J Kidney Dis 2000;35(suppl 2):S38.

9 Galli G, Bianco F, Pannzetta G: Acetate-free biofiltration: an effective treatment for high-risk dialysis patients; in Man NK, Rotella J, Zucchelli P (eds): Blood Purification in Perspective: New Insights and Future Trends. Cleveland, ICAOT Press, 1992, No 320, vol 2.

10 Movilli E, Bossini N, Viola BF, et al: Evidence for independent role of metabolic acidosis on nutritional status in hemodialysis patients. Nephrol Dial Transplant 1998;13:125–131.

11 Chiappini MG, Moscatelli M, Batoli R: Effect of different hemodialysis methods on the nutritional status of HD patients. Ren Fail 1990;12:277–278.

Tsutomu Kuno
Ikebukuro Kuno Clinic, 9F, 2-26-5 Minami-Ikebukuro
Toshima-ku, Tokyo 171-0022 (Japan)
E-Mail tkuno@med.nihon-u.ac.jp

Kawanishi H, Yamashita AC (eds): Hemodiafiltration – A New Era.
Contrib Nephrol. Basel, Karger, 2011, vol 168, pp 195–203

# Improvement of Autonomic Nervous Regulation by Blood Purification Therapy Using Acetate-Free Dialysis Fluid – Clinical Evaluation by Laser Doppler Flowmetry

Takashi Sato[a] · Masahiro Taoka[a] · Takaaki Miyahara[b]

[a]Kaikokai Medical Corporation Meiko Kyoritsu Clinic, Nagoya, and [b]Tokyo Women's Medical University Medical Center East, Tokyo, Japan

**Abstract**

In Japan, acetate-free biofiltration (AFBF) became commercially available in the year 2000, and these products have been reported to be clinically effective for controlling the decrease of blood pressure during dialysis or various types of dialysis intolerance. And more, acetate-free dialysis fluid was made clinically available in 2007, acetate-free hemodialysis (AFHD) is expected to inhibit the malnutrition-inflammation-atherosclerosis syndrome, improve anemia and the nutritional status of patients, stabilize hemodynamics, and reduce inflammation and oxidative stress. In a broad sense, AFBF can be classified as hemodiafiltration (HDF), and its clinical effects seem to be associated with multiple factors, including use of acetate-free dialysis fluid, massive removal of low molecular weight proteins by convection, and the sodium concentration of the replacement fluid. Therefore, the clinical significance of acetate-free dialysis fluid could be demonstrated more clearly by comparing AFHD with conventional hemodialysis (conv. HD) using dialysis fluid containing about 10 mEq/l acetate. Since 2005, we have been investigating the efficacy of various modalities of blood purification therapy by continuously monitoring changes of tissue blood flow in the lower limbs and earlobes (head) using non-invasive continuous monitoring method (NICOMM). In this report, we assess the clinical effectiveness of AFHD on the basis of clinical findings and head stability index (head SI) obtained by NICOMM, particularly with respect to the influence on autonomic regulation. After switching to AFHD from conv. HD, anemia, stored iron utilization, and the frequency of treatments for dialysis hypotension and of muscle cramps were significantly improved. Further, the head SI was also significantly smaller with AFHD than conv. HD. This finding suggests that AFHD improved the maintenance of homeostasis by the autonomic nervous regulation system. In addition, we could not find clinical features of excessive alkalosis during an observation period of about 1 year, even if online HDF using acetate-free dialysis fluid as the substitution fluid. Our conclusion is that the advent of acetate-free dialysis fluid has led to investigations into new clinical effectiveness of AFHD or online HDF/HF using ultrapurified acetate-free dialysis fluid as the substitution fluid. 

Since acetate-free biofiltration – a modified form of hemodiafiltration (HDF) – became available clinically, it has been reported to have various clinical effects by acetate-free blood purification, including stabilization of hemodynamics, improvement of biocompatibility and reduction of chronic inflammation [1–3].

In 2007, acetate-free dialysis fluid was also made clinically available in Japan. This new dialysis fluid allows acetate-free hemodialysis (AFHD) to be performed, which is expected to inhibit the malnutrition-inflammation-atherosclerosis syndrome and improve its prognosis. Specifically, it will improve anemia and the nutritional status of patients, stabilize hemodynamics, and reduce inflammation and oxidative stress [4]. And it is supposed that the clinical significance of acetate-free dialysis fluid could be demonstrated more clearly by comparing AFHD with conventional hemodialysis (conv. HD) using dialysis fluid containing about 10 mEq/l acetate. Since 2005, we have been investigating the efficacy and mechanisms of different modalities of blood purification therapy by continuously monitoring changes of tissue blood flow in the lower limbs and earlobes (corresponding to head tissue blood flow) with a laser Doppler flowmeter (LDF), as well as the mean arterial pressure, and analyzing data by non-invasive continuous monitoring method (NICOMM) [5–7]. This report assesses the usefulness of blood purification therapy with acetate-free dialysis fluid on the basis of the results obtained by NICOMM, particularly with respect to the influence on autonomic nervous regulation.

## Evaluation of Autonomic Function by NICOMM

Our NICOMM system can record data on changes of tissue blood flow in the lower limbs and the earlobe during blood purification therapy by using two LDFs (CDF-2000, Nexis Corp.), as well as data on changes of the mean arterial pressure obtained from an oscillometric sphygmomanometer, and can display the data on trend graphs. This system also allows comparison of the mean values of each parameters and assessment of correlations by statistical processing of the accumulated data with analytical software (fig. 1). In 1959, Lassen [8] reported that cerebral blood flow remained constant when the mean arterial pressure was between 60 and 120 mm Hg, while there was a positive correlation between these parameters when the mean arterial pressure was outside that

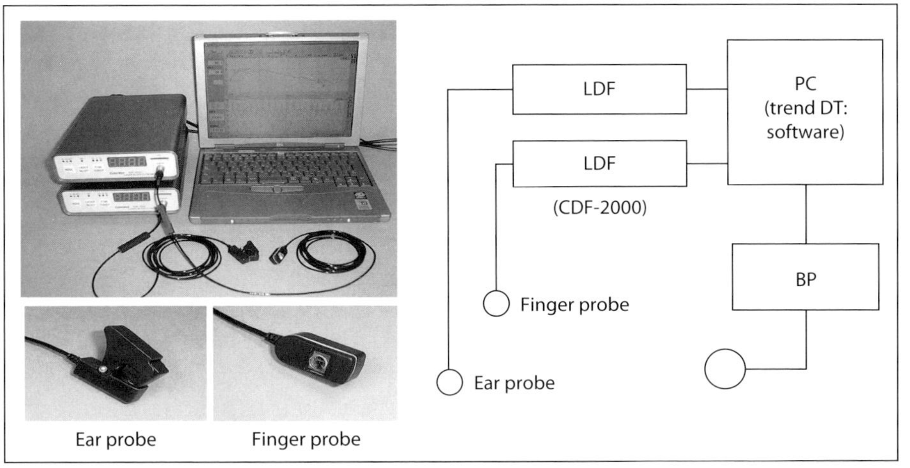


**Fig. 1.** Outline of the NICOMM system. This system continuously collects data on changes of skin tissue blood flow obtained via LDF probes attached to an earlobe and the tip of a toe, as well as data on changes of the mean arterial pressure obtained by an oscillometric sphygmomanometer. Analysis of the data can be done with special software.

range. Further, in 1973, Wiederhielm and Weston [9] experimentally demonstrated that there was a positive correlation between the skin tissue blood flow and the mean arterial pressure, while the tissue blood flow in the brain and kidneys was constant and independent of changes in the mean arterial pressure. In 1992, Izumi and Karita [10] reported that the tissue blood flow in the trunk and skin was controlled by sympathetic nerves, while that in the face and head was controlled by both sympathetic and parasympathetic nerves. These findings strongly suggested that cerebral blood flow is controlled by autonomic nervous regulatory mechanism. Our previous investigation of the possible correlation between tissue blood flow in the earlobe and the mean arterial pressure in healthy subjects using NICOMM has revealed that earlobe tissue blood flow is constant and independent of changes in blood pressure, as was reported by Lassen [8] and Wiederhielm and Weston [9], while there is a positive correlation between earlobe tissue blood flow and the mean arterial pressure during dialysis related hypotension. These findings suggest that changes of earlobe tissue blood flow obtained by laser Doppler studies indirectly reflect head blood flow (HBF). Therefore, regulation of blood flow by the autonomic nervous system can be assessed by continuously monitoring earlobe (head) tissue blood flow and assessing the relationship with mean arterial pressure. And smaller changes of earlobe (head) tissue blood flow seem to indicate adequate homeostatic function of the autonomic nervous regulation system. To evaluate autonomic regulation of blood flow, we therefore focused on the stability index (SI) of earlobe

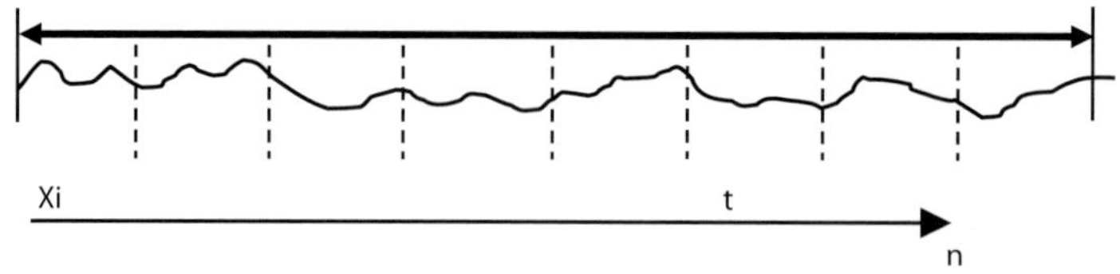


SI = STBF/MTBF
STBF: standard deviation of tissue blood flow
MTBF: mean tissue blood flow
Tissue blood flow (X)
$MTBF = \Sigma xi^{n} \cdot xi/n$
$STBF = \sqrt{\Sigma xi^{n}(Xi - X^{-})^{2}/n}$

**Fig. 2.** The SI represents tissue blood flow homeostasis. A small SI indicates good homeostasis, while a high value shows impaired homeostasis.

(head) tissue blood flow, and investigated the effects of different blood purification modalities by comparing their SI values.

## Stability Index of Tissue Blood Flow in the Head

Skin tissue blood flow in the lower limbs normally changes linearly with fluctuations of blood pressure. A laser Doppler study of skin SI in patients with diabetes mellitus showed that this parameter could be employed for evaluation of autonomic imbalance [11]. However, the skin SI is easily affected by water removal, plasma refilling, blood pressure, and other factors during blood purification therapy, and accordingly it fluctuates greatly. On the other hand, HBF is constantly controlled by a sympathetic and a parasympathytic nervous system during treatment as long as the patient is not in a state of intradialytic hypotension. Therefore, assuming that stability of HBF is important for homeostasis of the body during blood purification therapy, we calculated the HBF SI (head SI), and employed it as a parameter to evaluate autonomic regulation of blood flow. The head SI is the coefficient of variation, which was calculated as the standard deviation of the HBF determined from initiation to completion of blood purification therapy divided by the mean value (fig. 2). A small head SI indicates HBF stability, while a high value indicates loss of homeostasis or impaired regulation by the autonomic nervous system.

Equation for calculating the head SI:
SI = SHBF/MHBF
Mean head tissue blood flow (MHBF)
Standard deviation of head tissue blood flow (SHBF)

Head tissue blood flow (X)
$MHBF = \Sigma xi^n \, xi/n$
$SHBF = \sqrt{\Sigma xi^n (Xi - X-)^2/n}$

## Evaluation of Blood Purification Modalities with the Head SI

*Comparison between Healthy Subjects and Stable Dialysis Patients*
Previous studies have revealed that, in healthy volunteers who are not on extracorporeal circulation, HBF is constant and independent of changes in blood pressure, with no correlation between the percent change of HBF and that of the mean arterial pressure, while tissue blood flow in the lower limbs varies with fluctuations of blood pressure and there is a significant positive correlation between the percent change of tissue blood flow in the lower limbs and that of the mean arterial pressure. In patients on HD with stable blood pressure, tissue blood flow in the head is constant and independent of changes in blood pressure, as it is in healthy volunteers, while tissue blood flow in the lower limbs shows a positive or negative correlation with changes of the mean arterial pressure. These findings suggest that tissue blood flow in the lower limbs is influenced by ultrafiltration, plasma refilling, and other factors during extracorporeal circulation. In contrast, since tissue blood flow in the head was found to be constant, homeostasis of cerebral blood flow, which is vital organ for the body, seems to be maintained by autonomic nervous regulation system [5, 6]. Comparison of the head SI between HD patients with stable blood pressure and healthy volunteers revealed that the SI value was significantly higher in the former group. Moreover, the head SI value was higher in diabetic patients on dialysis than in non-diabetic patients on dialysis (fig. 3). These findings suggest that HD patients have less stable regulation of homeostasis by the autonomic nervous system compared with healthy volunteers and that this difference is more pronounced in diabetic patients on dialysis than in non-diabetic patients. Therefore, HD itself seems to impose stress on regulation of the circulation by the autonomic nervous system.

*Comparison between Conventional Hemodialysis and AFHD*
In 2007, acetate-free dialysis fluid became available clinically in Japan, and has been shown to have various benefits, i.e., improvement of anemia, improvement of the nutritional status, and correction of chronic inflammation [3, 4]. In Japan, dialysis fluid is mainly supplied by a central dialysis fluid delivery system (CDDS) at each dialysis center, and some dialysis doctors hesitate to use acetate-free dialysis fluid for all patients. We investigated the benefits of the acetate-free dialysis fluid supplied by the CDDS by comparing clinical parameters for about 1 year before and after switching to the fluid from conventional dialysis fluid (containing about 11 mEq/l acetate) (table 1). After dialysis, the

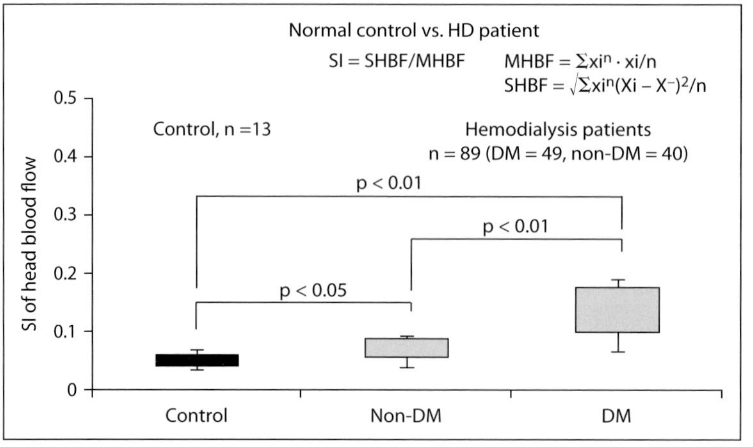


**Fig. 3.** Comparison of SI values. The SI was significantly larger in patients on hemodialysis than in healthy volunteers, and it was larger in diabetic patients on dialysis than in non-diabetic patients.

**Table 1.** Comparison of the composition of conventional dialysis fluid and acetate-free dialysis fluid

| | $Na^+$ mEq/l | $K^+$ mEq/l | $Ca^{2+}$ mEq/l | $Mg^{2+}$ mEq/l | $Cl^-$ mEq/l | $HCO_3^-$ mEq/l | $CH_3COO^-$ mEq/l | Glucose mg/l |
|---|---|---|---|---|---|---|---|---|
| Acetate-free dialysis fluid | 140 | 2.0 | 3.0 | 1.0 | 111 | 35 | (–) | 150 |
| Conventional dialysis fluid | 143 | 2.0 | 2.5 | 1.0 | 112 | 27.5 | 11 | 100 |

$HCO_3^-$ concentration was increased significantly with either type of dialysis fluid. The $HCO_3^-$ concentration was similar before dialysis with either dialysis fluid, but increased significantly after dialysis with AFHD. These findings indicate that acidosis was adequately corrected after dialysis (fig. 4). We also assessed the improvement of anemia. There was no significant difference of the hemoglobin level over a 6-month period before and after switching the dialysis fluid (before: 10.68 mg/dl, after: 10.58 mg/dl, $p = 0.12$, $n = 86$), but the dose of erythropoietin decreased significantly after switching (before: 2,187.83 ± 49.65 U, after: 2,015 ± 37.23 U, $p = 0.0001$, $n = 86$). There were no significant differences of the transferrin saturation or ferritin levels, while the total dose of iron decreased significantly after switching to acetate-free dialysis fluid. These

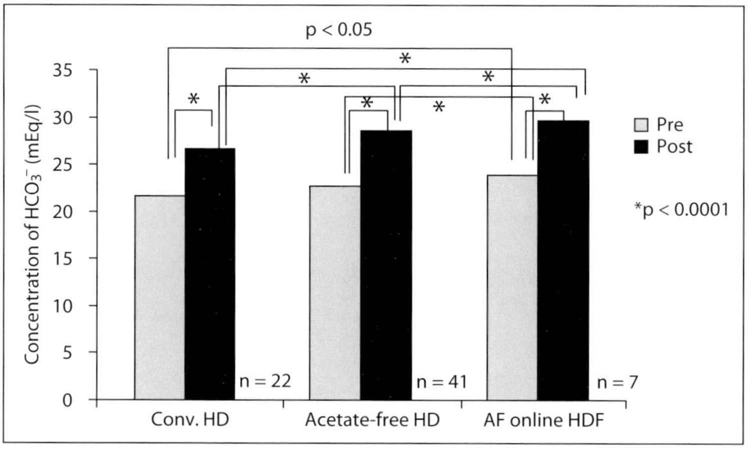


**Fig. 4.** Changes of $HCO_3^-$ pre- and post-dialysis: the $HCO_3^-$ concentration was compared before and after HD using conventional dialysis fluid, HD using acetate-free dialysis fluid, and online HDF using acetate-free dialysis fluid. The pretreatment $HCO_3^-$ concentration was significantly higher for online HDF using acetate-free dialysis fluid than for HD using conventional dialysis fluid. After treatment, the $HCO_3^-$ concentration increased significantly with all of these modalities. It increased significantly more for HD or online HDF using acetate-free dialysis fluid than for HD using conventional dialysis fluid.

findings suggest that anemia is improved by using acetate-free dialysis fluid because of more efficient incorporation of stored iron, but the details should be investigated in future studies. There were no significant differences of any of the other clinical parameters that we assessed before and after switching the dialysis fluid. However, assessment of symptoms revealed that the frequency of fluid replacement or discontinuation of water removal for treatment of dialysis hypotension, as well as the frequency of muscle cramps, were also decreased significantly after switching the dialysis fluid. The head SI was also significantly smaller with acetate-free dialysis fluid than with conventional dialysis fluid (fig. 5). This finding suggests the usefulness of AFHD for maintenance of homeostasis by the autonomic nervous regulation system. The above-mentioned improvement of symptoms seems to have been mainly related to the use of acetate-free dialysis fluid and intensive correction of acidosis, but the possible role of citrate (which is contained in acetate-free dialysis fluid) requires further investigation.

*Future Prospects for Acetate-Free Dialysis Fluid*

AFHD will be expected to improve various symptoms, such as malnutrition, inflammatory condition, unstable circulatory condition and anemia. We have investigated the safety and usefulness of long-term supply of acetate-free dialysis fluid via the CDDS, especially focusing on the SI of tissue blood flow in the head.

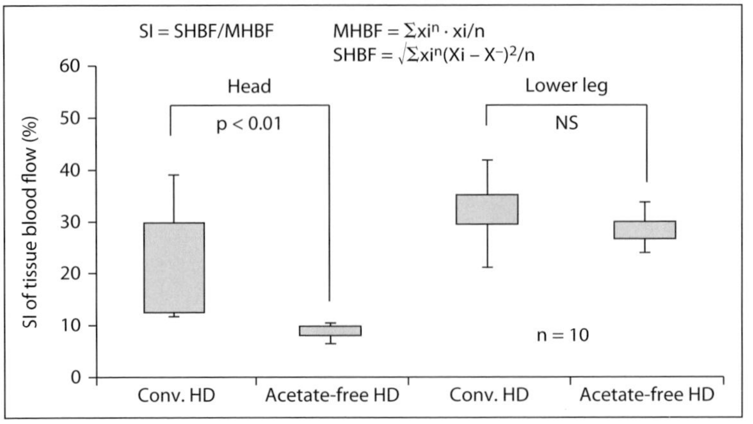


**Fig. 5.** Changes of the SI during acetate-free dialysis. The SI for the earlobe (head) tissue blood flow was significantly smaller when HD was performed using acetate-free dialysis fluid.

In the present study, the head SI was lower in AFHD than with conv. HD. The factors of AFHD consist of intensive correction of acidosis and no containing acetate. Further studies seem to be required to determine the relative contribution of these factors to reduction of the head SI, which corresponds to improved blood flow regulation by the autonomic nervous system. Of the subjects in the present study, 7 patients underwent online HDF using acetate-free dialysis fluid as the substitution fluid. None of these patients had clinical features of excessive alkalosis or significant symptoms during an observation period of about 1 year. At the 15th Annual Meeting of the Japanese Society for Hemodiafiltration, Tomo et al. reported that online HDF using acetate-free dialysis fluid improved various factors (including C-reactive protein, interleukin-6, and pentosidine) that predict the outcome of cardiovascular complications. In the future, use of acetate-free dialysis fluid with different blood purification modalities may lead to reports about various new clinical effects.

## Conclusions

To contribute to prevention and treatment of the complications of long-term dialysis, we have tried high-performance membrane HD, internal filtration-enhanced HD, high-volume HDF/hemofiltration (HF), and other modalities based on ultrapure dialysis fluid. We have attempted to increase the efficiency of removal of solutes and the clinical response by controlling dialysis conditions, including the filtration volume, dialysis session duration, and blood flow rate.

The advent of acetate-free dialysis fluid has led to investigations into new clinical effects of HD or online HDF/HF using purified acetate-free dialysis fluid as the substitution fluid. Although some physicians hesitate to use acetate-free dialysis fluid for all patients, we have experienced no problems with this type of dialysis fluid during a 1-year period. The advent of acetate-free dialysis fluid has provided us with a new method of blood purification. At the same time, further long-term studies seem to be required to increase its efficacy and investigate various issues, including the influence of citrate in the dialysis fluid and regulation of the volume of substitution fluid during online HDF.

## References


1 Noris M, Todeschini M, Cashiragi F, et al: Effect of acetate bicarbonate dialysis, and acetate-free biofiltration on nitric oxide synthesis: implication for dialysis hypotension. Am J Kidney Dis 1998;32:115–124.

2 Movilli E, Camerini C, Zein H, et al: A prospective comparison of bicarbonate dialysis, hemodiafiltration, and acetate-free biofiltration in elderly. Am J Kidney Dis 1996;27:541–547.

3 Higuchi T, Yamamoto C, Kuno T, et al: A comparison of bicarbonate hemodialysis, hemodiafiltration, and acetate-free biofiltration on cytokine production. Ther Apher Dial 2004;8:460–467.

4 Saito A: Clinical efficacy of hemodialysis with acetate-free dialysate. J Jpn Assoc Dial Physicians 2008;23:257–263.

5 Sato T, Miyahara T, Niwayama J, et al: Measurement of tissue blood volume at head and foot with LDF (laser Doppler flowmeter) during dialysis treatment – clinical application of NICOMM (non-invasive continuous monitoring method) for blood purification treatment. Jpn J Clin Dial 2006;22:537–544.

6 Niwayama J, Sato T, Komatsu M, et al: Analysis of hemodialysis during blood purification therapy using a newly developed noninvasive continuous monitoring method. Ther Apher Dial 2006;10:380–386.

7 Ebihara I, Sato T, Hirayama K, et al: Blood flow analysis of the head and lower limbs by the laser Doppler blood flowmeter during LDL apheresis. Ther Apher Dial 2007;11:325–330.

8 Lassen NA: Cerebral blood flow and oxygen consumption in man. Physiol Rev 1959;39:183–238.

9 Wiederhielm C, Weston BV: Microvascular, lymphatic and tissue pressures in the unanesthetized mammal. Am J Physiol 1973;225:992–996.

10 Izumi H, Karita K: Somatosensory stimulation causes autonomic vasodilation in cat lip. J Physiol 1992;450:191–202.

11 Hatanaka Y, Maeda Y, Hata F, et al: Measurement of skin blood flow by periflux laser Doppler flowmeter in diabetic patients, stability of microcirculation and its clinical evaluation. Jpn J Clin Pathol 1986;36:343–347.



Takashi Sato, MD, PhD
Meiko Kyoritsu Clinic, 8-202, Kiba, Minato
Nagoya, Aichi 4550021 (Japan)
Tel. +81 52 698 3077, Fax +81 52 698 3166
E-Mail tsato@touseki.jp

Kawanishi H, Yamashita AC (eds): Hemodiafiltration – A New Era.
Contrib Nephrol. Basel, Karger, 2011, vol 168, pp 204–212

# Preservation of Residual Renal Function with HDF

Toru Hyodo[a,b] · Naoko Koutoku[c]

[a]Department of Urology, Yokohama Dai-ichi Hospital, Yokohama, [b]Department of Urology, Kitasato University School of Medicine, Sagamihara, and [c]Department of Nephrology, Mitajiri Hospital, Houfu, Japan

**Abstract**

Previous studies have shown that the presence of the residual renal function (RRF) is associated with a lower mortality risk in hemodialysis (HD) patients. A factor promoting a decrease in the RRF has been reported to be dehydration. Therefore, we performed HD or online hemodiafiltration (HDF) without water removal, in which intravascular dehydration due to water removal during dialysis are avoided. We also examined the RRF-maintaining effects of online HDF. *Water removal-free dialysis study:* The subjects were 44 HD patients within 3 months after the introduction of dialysis. They were divided into two groups: a group undergoing water removal-free dialysis at least for more than 3 months (group A) and a group undergoing dialysis with water removal (group B). Group A consisted of 28 patients including 5 in whom online HDF was initially introduced. Group B consisted of 16 patients on HD with water removal. In each group, the 24-hour urine volume was examined. The follow-up period was 36 months. In group A, the daily urine volume after 6 months or more was significantly larger. The mean water removal-free dialysis period was 18.1 ± 16.2 months. *Study of the effects of online HDF on the RRF:* The subjects were 49 patients undergoing maintenance dialysis. The 24-hour urine volume was measured. We compared an online HDF group (n = 37) with a HD group (n = 12). We examined the relationship between the duration of dialysis and urine volume. In the HDF group the r value was 0.333 (p = 0.044) and in the HD group it was 0.834 (p = 0.007). There was a significant difference in the correlation coefficient between the two groups (p = 0.024), suggesting that HDF is more useful than HD for maintaining the urine volume for a prolonged period. *Conclusion:* The online HDF and dialysis without water removal are useful to preserve the RRF. 

## Background

Previous studies have shown that a better reserved residual renal function (RRF) is associated with longer survival periods in patients receiving peritoneal dialysis, and with better nutritional states in patients receiving hemodialysis (HD) [1–3]. The presence of the RRF, even at a low level, is associated with a lower mortality risk also in HD patients [4]. A factor promoting a decrease in the RRF has been reported to be hypotension during dialysis in patients receiving HD and also the presence of a dehydration state period during the treatment course in patients receiving peritoneal dialysis [5]. In daily clinical practice, patients with chronic renal failure in the conservative state are given instructions to prevent dehydration outdoors in summer to avoid decreasing the renal function. Based on the above studies, dehydration clearly promotes a decrease in the RRF. Therefore, we performed HD or online hemodiafiltration (HDF) without water removal, in which both overhydration from the time of the introduction of dialysis and intravascular dehydration due to water removal during dialysis are avoided.

A previous study reported that the use of ultrapure dialysis fluid inhibited hypofunction of the residual kidney in patients undergoing HD [6]. According to another study, HD with ultrapure dialysis fluid and a high-flux biocompatible dialysis membrane made it possible to maintain the RRF as favorably as on using peritoneal dialysis [7]. To our knowledge, no study has examined such effects of online HDF. A recent study compared the effects of online HDF between patients in whom the RRF was and those in whom it was not maintained [8]. Based on these findings, we compared the RRF-maintaining effects of HD using ultrapure dialysis fluid and a high-flux biocompatible dialysis membrane with those of online HDF.

## Study 1

*Evaluation of the Condition for the Initiation of Water Removal*
*Purpose.* To determine the degree of water retention as a condition for the initiation of water removal in HD patients with the RRF, the average body weight in the week was evaluated in patients with a negligible RRF.

*Subjects and Methods.* The subjects consisted of 54 patients with a urine volume/day ≤200 ml receiving HD 3 times per week (32 males and 22 females; mean age 61.9 ± 12.8 years; presence of diabetes mellitus in 12 patients; its absence in 42; mean dialysis period 9.2 ± 4.7 years). At intervals of 3 days (Friday–Monday or Saturday-Tuesday), 2 days (Monday–Wednesday or Tuesday–Thursday), and 2 days (Wednesday–Friday or Thursday–Saturday), the mean water retention compared with the dry weight (DW) was expressed in terms of the percentage of the DW using the following equation: 100 × (body weight before dialysis – that after previous dialysis)/DW/2.

*Results.* Mean water retention was 1.95 ± 0.56% at an interval of 3 days, 2.09 ± 0.61% at an interval of 2 days in the middle of the week, and 1.93 ± 0.79% at an interval of 2 days at the end of the week. The mean value at an interval of 2 days in the middle of the week was significantly higher than that at an interval of 3 days. However, the mean value was about 2% at each interval.

## Study 2

*Dialysis without Water Removal*

*Purpose.* Water removal during HD may cause a decrease in the RRF (urine volume). We examined the effect to preserve the RRF by dialysis without water removal.

*Subjects and Methods.* The subjects were 44 patients on maintenance HD at Atsugi Clinic who were referred to the single attending physician within 3 months after the introduction of dialysis. They were divided into two groups: a group undergoing water removal-free dialysis for at least more than 3 months (group A) and a group undergoing dialysis with water removal (group B). We excluded cystic kidney patients, as the primary disease allows the residual renal to function for a longer period compared to other diseases. In the two groups, dialysis fluid containing 0.01 EU/ml (detection limit) or less of endotoxin was used. We employed the dialyzers with high-flux membranes measuring 1.8–2.1 $m^2$ in area. The blood flow volume was established as 200–250 ml/min, and the dialysis fluid flow rate as 400 ml (pre-dilution online HDF: 600 ml containing substitution fluid). Dialysis time was 4–5 h. In addition, if necessary, hypotensive agents such as angiotensin receptor blocker (ARB), calcium antagonists, and angiotensin converting enzyme inhibitor (ACEI) were prescribed in the two groups so that the home systolic/diastolic blood pressures were maintained at <140/80 mm Hg, respectively. When administering contrast medium, dialysis was performed for 4–5 h on the same day. If possible, no analgesic agent was employed.

Group A consisted of 28 HD patients including 5 in whom online HDF was initially introduced (18 males, 10 females; 11 diabetics, 17 non-diabetics; mean age 62.0 ± 14.1 years), and group B consisted of 16 patients on maintenance HD with water removal (13 males, 3 females; 7 diabetics, 9 non-diabetics; mean age 58.7 ± 11.9 years).

There were no significant differences in the presence or absence of diabetes or gender between the two groups (Fisher's direct method). There was also no significant difference in the mean age (Student's t test).

In each group, the 24-hour urine volume on the first Sunday or Monday of the month was examined to evaluate the efficacy of water removal-free dialysis. The follow-up period was 36 months. In group A, the number of patients after 0/3/6, 12/18, 24, and 30/36 months was 28, 27, 20, and 8, respectively. In group B, that after 0/3/6/12, 18, 24, and 30/36 months was 16, 14, 13, and 10, respectively.

Conditions for water removal-free HD were established based on the results of study 1: water removal was only performed when the body weight before the start of dialysis on each dialysis day exceeded 102.0% as a percentage of the

DW, until the body weight reached DW. When water removal was consecutively required 3 times a week, the first day of the week was regarded as the date of discontinuation of water removal-free HD.

*Results.* The changes in the daily urine volume are shown in figure 1. In group A, the urine volume was significantly larger (Student's t test). The mean water removal-free dialysis period was 18.1 ± 16.2 months.

## Study 3

*Examination of the Effects of Online HDF on the RRF*

*Purpose.* We investigated whether online HDF is useful for maintaining the RRF.

*Subjects and Methods.* The subjects were 49 patients undergoing maintenance dialysis in Mitajiri Hospital (mean age 66.8 ± 10.8 years, 29 males, 20 females). The 24-hour urine volume was measured the day before dialysis at the beginning of the week. Dialysis fluid containing 0.01 EU/ml (detection limit) or less of endotoxin was used. We employed a dialyzer with high-flux polysulfone membranes measuring 1.8–2.1 $m^2$ in area. The dialysis time was 4–6 h. The blood flow volume was established as 250–300 ml/min, and the dialysis fluid flow rate as 500 ml (HDF group: containing substitution fluid). The inferior vena cava (IVC) diameter was periodically measured using echography before and after dialysis, and the DW was determined based on the cardiothoracic ratio and IVC. Water removal was carried out if necessary (patients with overhydration/pulmonary edema) while measuring the IVC during dialysis to prevent excessive dehydration when there was a fall in the blood pressure during dialysis. Briefly, in this study, water removal-free dialysis was performed if possible. However, water removal was conducted when physicians considered it necessary.

We compared a group in which online HDF (pre-dilution: 72 l) was started 1 month after the introduction of dialysis (HDF group, n = 37) with a group in which HD was continued after the introduction of dialysis (HD group, n = 12). The mean ages in the HDF and HD groups were 65.3 ± 10.4 and 71.3 ± 10.9 years, respectively (p = 0.11, Student's t test). The mean duration of dialysis was 59.3 ± 35.9 and 42.6 ± 30.7 months, respectively (p = 0.13, Student's t test). The proportions of patients receiving insulin were 29.3 and 25%, respectively, showing no significant difference. In the HDF group, the proportion of patients with ischemic heart disease who had undergone percutaneous transluminal coronary angioplasty or coronary artery bypass grafting was 21.6%, higher than that in the HD group (8.3%).

*Results.* We examined the relationship between the duration of dialysis (x) and urine volume (y). In the HDF group, the r value was 0.333 (p = 0.044) (y = –231.1 In (x)+1,294). In the HD group, it was 0.834 (p = 0.007) (y = –632 In (x)+2,776.3) (fig. 2). There was a significant difference in the correlation

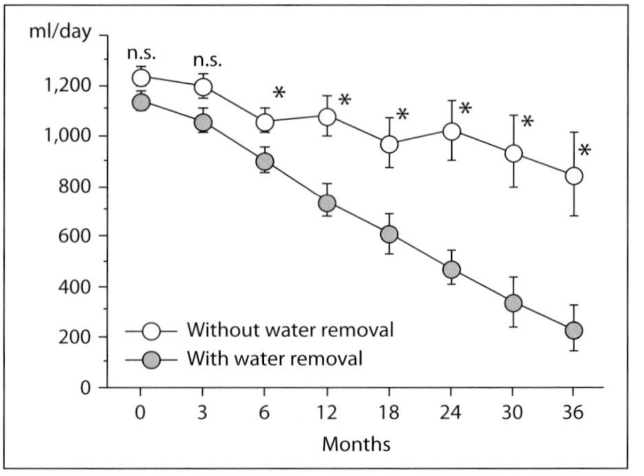


**Fig. 1.** There were no significant differences in the daily urine volume at the start of dialysis and after 3 months between two groups with and without water removal. However, the daily urine volume after 6 months or more of dialysis was significantly larger in patients on water removal-free dialysis; the RRF was significantly maintained. *$p < 0.05$.

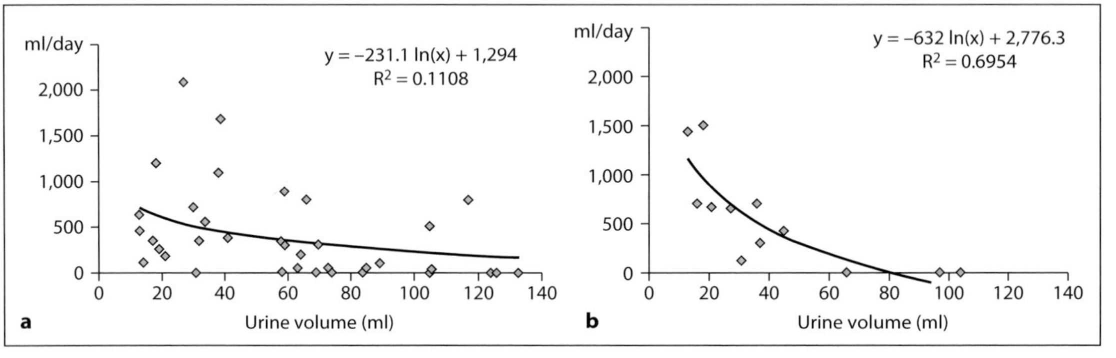


**Fig. 2. a** With respect to the relationship between the duration of dialysis and daily urine volume, there was only a weak correlation in the HDF group. **b** The HD group showed a strong correlation. There was a significant difference in the correlation coefficient between the HDF and HD groups ($p = 0.024$), indicating that the urine volume was maintained for a longer period in the HDF group.

**Fig. 3. a** Percent changes in the circulating plasma volume determined on a Crit-Line monitor during dialysis in a patient undergoing online HDF without water removal. There were only slight changes. The pre- and post-dialysis body weights were 54.7 and 54.9 kg, respectively. **b** Percent changes in the circulating plasma volume determined on a Crit-Line monitor during dialysis in a patient undergoing HD without water removal. There were only slight changes, although they were more marked than in the patient undergoing online HDF. The pre- and post-dialysis body weights were 49.5 and 50.1 kg, respectively. **c** Percent changes in the circulating plasma volume determined on a Crit-Line monitor during dialysis in a patient undergoing HD with water removal. The circulating plasma flow rate decreased to 25% of the baseline at maximum. The pre- and post-dialysis body weights were 49.1 and 46.7 kg, respectively.

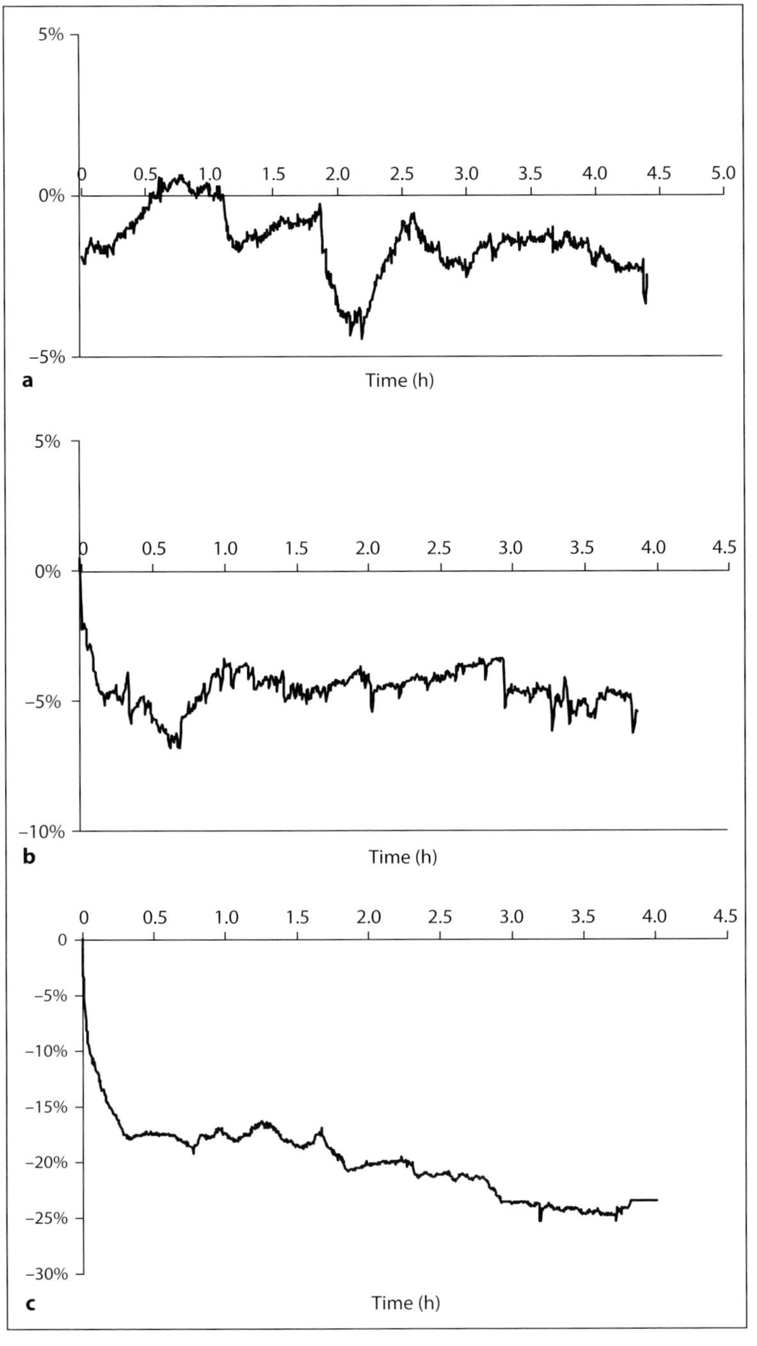
5%
0%
−5%
0
0.5
1.0
1.5
2.0
2.5
3.0
3.5
4.0
4.5
5.0
a
Time (h)
5%
0%
−5%
−10%
b
Time (h)
0
−5%
−10%
−15%
−20%
−25%
−30%
c
Time (h)

3

coefficient between the two groups ($p = 0.024$), suggesting that HDF is more useful than HD for maintaining the urine volume for a prolonged period.

## Discussion

The reported factors promoting a decrease in the RRF in dialysis patients include: hypotension during HD, dehydration during peritoneal dialysis, and high diastolic blood pressures and high urinary protein values in both HD and peritoneal dialysis [5]. The reported measures to preserve the RRF are the avoidance of: the use of drugs (anti-inflammatory analgesics/antibiotics) and contrast agents that decrease the renal function, promotion of salt and water excretion by diuretics, use of ACEI/ARB as antihypertensive drugs [9].

In the general dialysis with water removal, in addition to changes in the plasma osmotic pressure, acute changes in the body fluid volume due to water removal occur. Even when selecting water removal-free dialysis, the circulating blood volume may decrease, depending on changes in the plasma osmotic pressure. However, the rate of decrease is smaller than in the presence of water removal; this procedure is advantageous with respect to the renal hemodynamics, and may be useful to maintain the RRF (fig. 3). As shown in figure 3 (results of observation with a Crit-Line monitor, Hema Metrics, Inc., USA), dialysis with water removal markedly decreased the circulating plasma volume.

There is room for discussion regarding the validity of the initiation of water removal in the presence of 2% water retention compared with the DW in HD or HDF without water removal. This condition was used because the actual average body weight of the patients with a urine volume/day ≤200 ml was the DW + about 2% DW. Since safe, long-term dialysis is performed in many patients even with a low urine volume, this condition may be safe. Indeed, no patient receiving dialysis without water removal developed overhydration such as pulmonary edema under this condition. The cardiothoracic ratio was also maintained within the safety range (data not shown). As the number of patients was small, further investigation is needed. However, the urine volume was significantly maintained in patients on water removal-free dialysis (fig. 1). The absence of water removal is concluded as effective.

For study 3, we compared HD with online HDF, considering that HDF may favorably influence the kidney function in comparison with HD under the same condition, that is, in the absence of water removal, since HDF facilitates the convection-related removal of uremic toxin in the middle-molecular-weight area. In the two procedures, we used pure dialysis fluid and a high-flux dialysis membrane, whose biocompatibility is considered to be favorable. The results suggested that online HDF is more useful for maintaining the RRF, as expected. A recent study indicated that kidney clearance of $\beta_2$-microglobulin (and possibly other middle-molecular-weight solutes) seems to be much more important than convective clearance by HDF in patients with a glomerular filtration rate exceeding 4.2 ml/min/1.72 $m^2$, emphasizing the importance of the RRF [8]. In addition, patients undergoing online HDF show a favorable prognosis [10]. Online HDF provides superior solute removal to high-flux HD over a wide molecular weight range [11–13]. The presence of the RRF, even at a low level, is associated with a lower mortality risk also in HD patients [4]. Based on these results and the present study, online HDF with preservation of the RRF may improve the prognosis of patients undergoing dialysis. In the future, the usefulness of RRF-based dialysis should be investigated in a larger number of patients with respect to the survival rate and incidence of complications.

## Acknowledgments

We thank Masami Kurihara and Sumiko Yamamoto at Atsugi Clinic and Takashi Sahara at the Dialysis Center of Mitajiri Hospital for the support of the studies.

## References

1 Canada-USA (CANUSA) Peritoneal Dialysis Study Group: Adequacy of dialysis and nutrition in continuous peritoneal dialysis: association with clinical outcomes. J Am Soc Nephrol 1996;7:198–207.

2 Bargman JM, Thorpe KE, Churchill DN, for the CANUSA Peritoneal Dialysis Study Group: Relative contribution of residual renal function and peritoneal clearance to adequacy of dialysis: a reanalysis of the CANUSA Study. J Am Soc Nephrol 2001;12:2158–2162.

3 Suda T, Hiroshige K, Ohta T, Watanabe Y, Iwamoto M, Kanegae K, Ohtani A, Nakashima Y: The contribution of residual renal function to overall nutritional status in chronic hemodialysis patients. Nephrol Dial Transplant 2000;15:396–401.

4 Shemin D, Bostom AG, Laliberty P, Dworkin LD: Residual renal function and mortality risk in hemodialysis patients. Am J Kidney Dis 2001;38:85–90.

5 Jansen MAM, Hart AAM, Korevaar JC, Dekker FW, Boeschoten EW, Krediet RT, for the NECOSAD Study Group: Predictors of the rate of decline of residual renal function in incident dialysis patients. Kidney Int 2002;62:1046–1053.

6 Schiffl H, Lang SM, Fischer R: Ultrapure dialysis fluid slows loss of residual renal function in new dialysis patients. Nephrol Dial Transplant 2002;17:1814–1818.

7 McKane W, Chandna SM, Tattersall JE, Greenwood RN: Identical decline of residual renal function in high-flux biocompatible hemodialysis and CAPD. Kidney Int 2002;61:256–265.

8 Penne BL, van der Weed NC, Blankestijn PJ, van den Dorpel MA, Grooteman MPC, Nube MJ, ter Wee PM, Levesque R, Bots ML, on behalf of the CONTRAST Investigators: Role of residual kidney function and convective volume on change in $\beta_2$-microglobulin levels in hemodiafiltration. Clin J Am Soc Nephrol 2010;5:80–86.

9 Bargman JM, Golper TA: The importance of residual renal function for patients on dialysis. Nephrol Dial Transplant 2005;20:671–673.
10 Canaud B, Bragg-Gresham JL, Marshall MR, Desmeules S, Gillespie BW, Depner T, Klassen P, Port FK: Mortality risk for patients receiving hemodiafiltration versus hemodialysis: European results from the DOPPS. Kidney Int 2006;69:2087–2093.
11 Ward RA, Schmidt B, Hullin J, Hillerbrand GF, Samtleben W: A comparison of on-line hemodiafiltration and high-flux hemodialysis: a prospective clinical study. J Am Soc Nephrol 2000;11:2344–2350.
12 Lin CL, Yang CW, Chiang CC, Chang CT, Huang CC: Long-term on-line hemodiafiltration reduces predialysis $\beta_2$-microglobulin levels in chronic hemodialysis patients. Blood Purif 2001;19:301–307.
13 Schiffl H: Prospective randomized cross-over long-term comparison of online hemodiafiltration and ultrapure high-flux hemodialysis. Eur J Med Res 2007;12:26–33.

Toru Hyodo
Department of Urology, Yokohama Dai-ichi Hospital
2-5-5 Takashima, Nishi-Ku, Yokohama City
Kanagawa 220-0011 (Japan)
E-Mail thyodomd@yahoo.co.jp

# Author Index

# Subject Index